Families Carin

Committee on Family Caregiving for Older Adults

Board on Health Care Services

Health and Medicine Division

Richard Schulz and Jill Eden, *Editors*

A Report of
The National Academies of
SCIENCES · ENGINEERING · MEDICINE

THE NATIONAL ACADEMIES PRESS
Washington, DC
www.nap.edu

THE NATIONAL ACADEMIES PRESS 500 Fifth Street, NW Washington, DC 20001

This activity was supported by Grant No. 14-02-39 from Archstone Foundation, Grant No. 18203 from California Health Care Foundation, Grant No. 20130622 from The Commonwealth Fund, Grant No. 940 from Health Foundation of Western and Central New York, Grant No. 2014-0094 from The John A. Hartford Foundation, Grant No. 2013-247 from The Retirement Research Foundation, Contract No. VA101-14-C-0014 from the U.S. Department of Veterans Affairs, and grants from Alliance for Aging Research, Alzheimer's Association, an anonymous donor, The Fan Fox and Leslie R. Samuels Foundation, May and Stanley Smith Charitable Trust, The Rosalinde and Arthur Gilbert Foundation, Santa Barbara Foundation, and Tufts Health Plan Foundation. Any opinions, findings, conclusions, or recommendations expressed in this publication do not necessarily reflect the views of any organization or agency that provided support for the project.

International Standard Book Number-13: 978-0-309-44806-2
International Standard Book Number-10: 0-309-44806-9
Digital Object Identifier: 10.17226/23606
Library of Congress Control Number: 2016956939

Additional copies of this publication are available for sale from the National Academies Press, 500 Fifth Street, NW, Keck 360, Washington, DC 20001; (800) 624-6242 or (202) 334-3313; http://www.nap.edu.

Printed in the United States of America

Suggested citation: National Academies of Sciences, Engineering, and Medicine. 2016. *Families caring for an aging America*. Washington, DC: The National Academies Press. doi: 10.17226/23606.

The National Academies of

SCIENCES · ENGINEERING · MEDICINE

The National Academies of
SCIENCES · ENGINEERING · MEDICINE

Reports document the evidence-based consensus of an authoring committee of experts. Reports typically include findings, conclusions, and recommendations based on information gathered by the committee and committee deliberations. Reports are peer reviewed and are approved by the National Academies of Sciences, Engineering, and Medicine.

Proceedings chronicle the presentations and discussions at a workshop, symposium, or other convening event. The statements and opinions contained in proceedings are those of the participants and have not been endorsed by other participants, the planning committee, or the National Academies of Sciences, Engineering, and Medicine.

For information about other products and activities of the Academies, please visit nationalacademies.org/whatwedo.

COMMITTEE ON FAMILY CAREGIVING FOR OLDER ADULTS

RICHARD SCHULZ (*Chair*), Director, University Center for Social and Urban Research, University of Pittsburgh
MARIA P. ARANDA, Associate Professor, University of Southern California School of Social Work
SUSAN BEANE, Vice President and Medical Director, Healthfirst, Inc.
SARA J. CZAJA, Leonard M. Miller Professor and Scientific Director, Center on Aging, University of Miami Miller School of Medicine
BRIAN M. DUKE, System Director, Senior Services, Main Line Health
JUDY FEDER, Professor, McCourt School of Public Policy, Georgetown University
LYNN FRISS FEINBERG, Senior Strategic Policy Advisor, AARP Public Policy Institute
LAURA N. GITLIN, Director and Professor, Center for Innovative Care in Aging, Johns Hopkins University School of Medicine
LISA P. GWYTHER, Director, Duke Family Support Program; Associate Professor, Department of Psychiatry and Behavioral Sciences, Duke University
ROGER HERDMAN, Retired
LADSON HINTON, Geriatric Psychiatrist and Professor, Department of Psychiatry and Behavioral Sciences, University of California, Davis
PETER KEMPER, Professor Emeritus, Health Policy and Administration; Demography, Pennsylvania State University
LINDA O. NICHOLS, Co-Director, Caregiver Center, Memphis Veterans Affairs Medical Center; Professor, Preventive and Internal Medicine, University of Tennessee Health Science Center
CAROL RODAT, New York Policy Director, PHI (Paraprofessional Healthcare Institute), Inc.
CHARLES P. SABATINO, Director, Commission on Law and Aging, American Bar Association
KAREN SCHUMACHER, Professor, College of Nursing, University of Nebraska Medical Center
ALAN STEVENS, Director, Center for Applied Health Research Program on Aging and Care, Baylor Scott & White Health
DONNA WAGNER, Dean, College of Health and Social Services, New Mexico State University
JENNIFER L. WOLFF, Associate Professor, Department of Health Policy and Management, Bloomberg School of Public Health, Johns Hopkins University

Study Staff

JILL EDEN, Study Director
KATYE MAGEE, Senior Program Assistant
AMY BATCHELOR, Research Associate (*through May 2015*)
KATHRYN ELLETT, U.S. Department of Health and Human Services Detail (*April through July 2015*)
GUS ZIMMERMAN, Research Associate (*starting July 2015*)
SHARYL NASS, Director, Board on Health Care Services

Consultant

VICKI FREEDMAN, University of Michigan

Reviewers

This report has been reviewed in draft form by individuals chosen for their diverse perspectives and technical expertise. The purpose of this independent review is to provide candid and critical comments that will assist the institution in making its published report as sound as possible and to ensure that the report meets institutional standards for objectivity, evidence, and responsiveness to the study charge. The review comments and draft manuscript remain confidential to protect the integrity of the deliberative process. We wish to thank the following individuals for their review of this report:

ELISABETH BELMONT, MaineHealth
CHRISTOPHER M. CALLAHAN, Indiana University Center for Aging Research and Regenstrief Institute, Inc.
ANDREW CHERLIN, Johns Hopkins University
EILEEN CRIMMINS, University of Southern California
PEGGYE DILWORTH-ANDERSON, University of North Carolina at Chapel Hill
DAVID GRABOWSKI, Harvard Medical School
PAMELA HYMEL, Walt Disney Parks and Resorts
JUDY D. KASPER, Johns Hopkins Bloomberg School of Public Health
ARTHUR KLEINMAN, Harvard Medical School
CAROL LEVINE, United Hospital Fund
MARGARET NEAL, Portland State University
CHARLES E. PHELPS, University of Rochester

ALAN ROSENFELD, Steward Health Care (*Retired*)
ROBYN I. STONE, LeadingAge Center for Applied Research
COURTNEY HAROLD VAN HOUTVEN, Durham Veterans Affairs Medical Center and Duke University Medical Center
KENNETH W. WACHTER, University of California, Berkeley
GAIL R. WILENSKY, Project HOPE
DONNA L. YEE, ACC Senior Services
HEATHER M. YOUNG, University of California, Davis

Although the reviewers listed above have provided many constructive comments and suggestions, they were not asked to endorse the conclusions or recommendations nor did they see the final draft of the report before its release. The review of this report was overseen by **DAVID B. REUBEN,** University of California, Los Angeles, and **STEPHEN E. FEINBERG,** Carnegie Mellon University. They were responsible for making certain that an independent examination of this report was carried out in accordance with institutional procedures and that all review comments were carefully considered. Responsibility for the final content of this report rests entirely with the authoring committee and the institution.

Acknowledgments

The committee and staff are indebted to a number of individuals and organizations for their contributions to this report. The following individuals provided testimony to the committee:

DONNA BENTON, Director, Older Adults Pacific Clinic
MARIE A. BERNARD, Deputy Director, National Institute on Aging, National Institutes of Health
CLIFF BURT, Caregiver Specialist, Georgia Division of Aging Services
CYNTHIA CALVERT, Founder and Principal, WORKFORCE 21C; Senior Counsel, WorkLife Law
MARIE-THERESE CONNOLLY, Director, Life Long Justice; Senior Scholar, Woodrow Wilson International Center for Scholars
EILEEN CRIMMINS, AARP Professor of Gerontology, Davis School of Gerontology, University of Southern California
TOM DELBANCO, Co-Director, OpenNotes; Richard and Florence Koplow-James Tullis Professor of General Medicine and Primary Care, Harvard Medical School
KAREN FREDRIKSEN-GOLDSEN, Professor and Director, Hartford Center of Excellence, University of Washington School of Social Work
WINSTON GREENE, Family Caregiver
KATHY KELLY, Executive Director, National Center on Caregiving, Family Caregiver Alliance
KATHY KENYON, Family Caregiver

NINA KOHN, Professor of Law, Syracuse University College of Law
CAROL LEVINE, Director, Families and Health Care Project, United Hospital Fund
SUSAN C. REINHARD, Senior Vice President and Director, AARP Public Policy Institute; Chief Strategist, Center to Champion Nursing in America
ZALDY S. TAN, Medical Director, Alzheimer's and Dementia Care Program; Associate Professor, David Geffen School of Medicine, University of California, Los Angeles
LAURA TREJO, General Manager, Los Angeles Department of Aging
MARIKO YAMADA, Former State Assembly Member for California's 4th Assembly District
DONNA L. YEE, Chief Executive Officer, Asian Community Center
HEATHER YOUNG, Associate Vice Chancellor for Nursing, Betty Irene Moore School of Nursing, University of California, Davis

We also extend special thanks to the following individuals who were essential sources of information, generously giving their time and knowledge to further the committee's efforts:

EILEEN APPELBAUM, Senior Economist, Center for Economic and Policy Research
SCOTT BEACH, Center for Social and Urban Research, University of Pittsburgh
ELLEN BLACKWELL, Senior Advisor, Centers for Medicare & Medicaid Services
TERRY FULMER, Former Dean, Bouvé College of Health Sciences, Northeastern University
BARBARA J. GAGE, Expert, Center for Health Policy, Brookings Institution
MARISSA GORDON, Senior Health Information Privacy Specialist, U.S. Department of Health and Human Services (HHS)
CHRISTINA HEIDE, Acting Deputy Director, Health Information Privacy, Office for Civil Rights, HHS
SUSAN JENKINS, Administration for Community Living, HHS
MEG KABAT, National Director, Caregiver Support Program, U.S. Department of Veterans Affairs
HELEN LAMONT, Office of the Assistant Secretary for Planning and Evaluation, HHS
SHARI LING, Deputy Chief Medical Officer, Center for Clinical Standards and Quality, Centers for Medicare & Medicaid Services

GREG LINK, Aging Services Program Specialist, Administration for Community Living, HHS
ELIZABETH McGLYNN, Director, Center for Effectiveness and Safety Research, Kaiser Permanente
COLES MERCIER, Health Insurance Specialist, Centers for Medicare & Medicaid Services
D. E. B. POTTER, Senior Survey Statistician, Agency for Healthcare Research and Quality, HHS
RUTHIE ROSENFELD, Family Caregiver
JANET SCHLARB, Center for Social and Urban Research, University of Pittsburgh
RACHEL SEEGER, Senior Advisor, Public Affairs and Outreach, Office for Civil Rights, HHS
JOAN WEISS, Senior Advisor, Health Resources and Services Administration

Funding for this study was provided by the Alliance for Aging Research, Alzheimer's Association, an anonymous donor, Archstone Foundation, California Health Care Foundation, The Commonwealth Fund, The Fan Fox and Leslie R. Samuels Foundation, Health Foundation of Western and Central New York, The John A. Hartford Foundation, May and Stanley Smith Charitable Trust, The Retirement Research Foundation, The Rosalinde and Arthur Gilbert Foundation, Santa Barbara Foundation, Tufts Health Plan Foundation, and the U.S. Department of Veterans Affairs. The committee appreciates the opportunity and support extended by the sponsors for the development of this report.

Many within the Health and Medicine Division of the National Academies of Sciences, Engineering, and Medicine were helpful to the study staff. We would like to thank Patrick Burke, Chelsea Frakes, Greta Gorman, Nicole Joy, Tracy Lustig, Bettina Ritter, and Lauren Shern.

Contents

APPENDIXES

Boxes, Figures, and Tables

BOXES

FIGURES

TABLES

Summary[1]

Family caregiving affects millions of Americans every day, in all walks of life. At least 17.7 million individuals in the United States are family caregivers of someone age 65 and older who needs help because of a limitation in their physical, mental, or cognitive functioning. As a society, we have always depended on family caregivers to provide the lion's share of long-term services and supports (LTSS) for our elders. Yet the need to recognize and support caregivers is among the most significant overlooked challenges facing the aging U.S. population, their families, and society.

For decades, demographers, gerontologists, health researchers, health care professionals, economists, and other experts have called attention to the nation's rapidly aging population. However, little action has been taken to prepare the health care and LTSS systems for this unprecedented demographic shift. By 2030, 72.8 million—more than one in five U.S. residents—will be age 65 or older. The greatest growth will be in the numbers of the "oldest old," the population that is most in need of help because they are the most likely to have physical, cognitive, and other functional limitations.

The increasing diversity of older Americans may further increase the demand for caregivers because data indicate that older African-American and Hispanic adults have been more likely than white adults to have functional impairments. In less than 15 years, nearly 3 in 10 older Americans will identify as a member of a minority group. Differences in culture, along with differences in income, education, neighborhood environments, lifetime access to health care, and occupational hazards will have a significant

[1] This summary does not include references. Citations appear in subsequent chapters.

impact on the need for care, the availability and willingness of family caregivers to provide it, and the most effective and appropriate ways to provide caregiver support. Developing programs and services that are accessible, affordable, and tailored to the needs of diverse communities of caregivers presents significant challenges.

While the need for caregiving is rapidly increasing, the pool of potential family caregivers is shrinking. Families have fewer children, older adults are more likely to have never married or to be divorced, and adult children often live far from their parents or may be caring for more than one older adult or their own children. In the past, families could rely on women to provide what is often referred to as eldercare, especially daughters, daughters-in-law, and wives who were not in the workforce. Today, the typical caregiver is still female. But that caregiver is almost as likely as a male caregiver to be employed, to need employment income, and to have limited schedule flexibility to juggle caregiving, work, and other responsibilities.

OBJECTIVE OF THE STUDY

In 2014, 13 private foundations, the Alliance for Aging Research, Alzheimer's Association, Archstone Foundation, California Health Care Foundation, The Commonwealth Fund, The Fan Fox and Leslie R. Samuels Foundation, Health Foundation of Western and Central New York, The John A. Hartford Foundation, May and Stanley Smith Charitable Trust, The Retirement Research Foundation, The Rosalinde and Arthur Gilbert Foundation, Santa Barbara Foundation, and Tufts Health Plan Foundation, as well as the U.S. Department of Veterans Affairs (VA), and an anonymous donor came together to ask the National Academies of Sciences, Engineering, and Medicine to develop a report with recommendations for family caregiving of older adults.

Box S-1 presents the charge to the committee. This study has three principal objectives:

1. to assess the prevalence and nature of family caregiving of older adults as well as the impact of caregiving on individuals' health, employment, and overall well-being
2. to examine available evidence on the effectiveness of programs, supports, and other interventions designed to support family caregivers
3. to assess and recommend policies to address the needs of family caregivers and to minimize the barriers that they encounter in trying to meet the needs of older adults

BOX S-1
Charge to the Committee on Family Caregiving for Older Adults

An ad hoc Institute of Medicine committee will develop a report with recommendations for public- and private-sector policies to support the capacity of family caregivers to perform critical caregiving tasks, to minimize the barriers that family caregivers encounter in trying to meet the needs of older adults, and to improve the health care and long-term services and supports provided to care recipients.

The committee will focus on family caregivers of older adults, typically age 65 and older. The report will analyze the prevalence of family caregiving and the demographic, societal, and technological trends that influence it. It will also examine caregivers' roles and responsibilities, both current and expected in the future, and the impact of the caregiver role on individual health, employment, and well-being. Caregivers' unmet needs and the gap between the projected demand for caregivers and the population available to serve as caregivers will be assessed and differences associated with race/ethnicity, culture, rural residence, and geography will be examined.

The report will also review the evidence of the effectiveness of potential supports for family caregivers and care recipients across a range of settings, including, for example, in medical homes and other primary care settings, home- and community-based settings, acute care hospitals, and residential facilities. These might include, for example, models of team-based care that include the family caregiver as member; approaches to training providers regarding the caregiver role; and models for training caregivers for their various roles.

The committee's charge raises questions about the boundaries among the responsibilities of individuals, families, and government. By its very nature, family caregiving of older adults is both a personal and private issue as well as a public and societal concern. From the individual perspective, one's involvement in caregiving for his or her elders is, in part, a matter of personal, spousal, or filial responsibility. Yet, for generations, the American public has also assumed collective responsibility in helping to protect the well-being of the nation's older adults through government programs such as Social Security, Medicare, Medicaid, the Area Agencies on Aging, and others. The committee recognizes that the role of the individual versus that of society overall is often a matter of public debate.

WHO IS A FAMILY CAREGIVER?

The committee agreed that the term "family caregiver" should be used to reflect the diverse nature of older adults' family and helping relationships. Some caregivers do not have a family kinship or legally defined relationship with the care recipient, but are instead partners, neighbors, or friends. Many older adults receive care from more than one family caregiver, and some caregivers may help more than one older adult. The circumstances of individual caregivers and the caregiver context are extremely variable. Family caregivers may live with, nearby, or far away from the person receiving care. Regardless, the family caregiver's involvement is determined primarily by a personal relationship rather than by financial remuneration. The care they provide may be episodic, daily, occasional, or of short or long duration.

Although this study focuses on caregivers of adults ages 65 and older, the committee recognizes that many other people need caregiving. This report's conclusions and recommendations are likely to apply to family caregivers regardless of the care recipient's age.

WHAT CAREGIVERS DO

Families traditionally have provided emotional support and assisted their older members with household tasks and personal care. Today, family caregivers still assume these roles but they also provide health and medical care at home, navigate complicated and fragmented health care and LTSS systems, and serve as surrogate decision makers. Medicare and other payer's financial incentives encourage shorter hospital stays with the implicit expectation that family members can support the older adult at home and manage the transition from hospital to home and back again. Providers expect family caregivers—with little or no training—to handle technical procedures and equipment for older adults at home, such as feeding and drainage tubes, catheters, and tracheostomies, and to manage and monitor their condition. Family caregivers describe learning by trial and error and fearing that they will make a life-threatening mistake.

In order to fulfill the numerous roles that they play, family caregivers must interact with a wide range of providers in a variety of systems. They communicate with physicians, physician assistants, nurses, nurse practitioners, social workers, psychologists, pharmacists, physical and occupational therapists, certified nursing assistants, home health and personal care aides, and others. They provide information about older adults' health histories, social supports, medications, past diagnoses, and previous treatments and surgeries (especially if the older adult is forgetful or has dementia). They also work with and arrange the services of community-based organizations.

Despite the integral role that family caregivers play in the care of older adults with disabilities and complex health needs, they are often marginalized or ignored in the delivery of health care and LTSS, and are often ignored in public policy as well. Paradoxically, family caregivers may be excluded from treatment decisions and care planning while the providers who exclude them assume their availability to perform the wide range of tasks prescribed by the older adults' care plan. Numerous systemic barriers impede effective engagement with family caregivers, including emphasis on the bioethical concept of individual autonomy, misinterpretation of the privacy requirements of the Health Insurance Portability and Accountability Act, payment rules that discourage providers from spending time communicating with caregivers, and a health insurance model oriented to individual coverage.

THE PERSONAL IMPACT OF CAREGIVING

Substantial evidence indicates that family caregivers of older adults are at risk compared to non-caregivers; they have higher rates of depressive symptoms, anxiety, stress, and emotional difficulties. Evidence also suggests that caregivers have lower self-ratings of physical health, elevated levels of stress hormones, higher rates of chronic disease, and impaired health behaviors. Numerous factors predispose caregivers to adverse outcomes, including sociodemographic factors; intensity or type of caregiving; perceptions of the care recipient's physical, psychological, and existential suffering; lack of choice in taking on the caregiving role; the caregiver's health and physical functioning; the social and professional supports they receive; and the care recipient's home physical environment. Caregivers transitioning from a low- to high-intensity role also report greater adverse effects compared to others.

Research also shows that family caregivers of significantly impaired older adults are at the greatest risk of economic harm, in part because of the many hours of care and supervision and the costs of hiring help. Caregiver surveys find that several other factors are associated with financial harm including co-residence with or residing a long distance from the older adult; limited or no availability of other family members to share responsibilities and costs; and, if employed, limited or no access to paid leave or a flexible workplace. Caregivers who cut back on paid work hours or leave the workforce to meet caregiving responsibilities lose income, receive reduced Social Security and other retirement benefits (because of fewer hours in paid employment), and may incur significant out-of-pocket expenses for the older adult's care.

Despite the array of negative consequences, caregivers also report positive outcomes. Numerous surveys suggest that, for some people, caregiving instills confidence, provides lessons on dealing with difficult situations, brings them closer to the care recipient, and assures them that the care recipient is well cared for.

EFFECTIVE CAREGIVER INTERVENTIONS

A robust body of research demonstrates that interventions aimed at supporting caregivers can significantly improve the quality of care delivered as well as improve the well-being and quality of life for both caregivers and care recipients. Interventions that have been tested through well-designed randomized clinical trials have involved a broad range of therapeutic techniques, have been applied in a variety of settings, and have been evaluated for a broad set of impacts on caregivers and care recipients. Well-designed randomized controlled trials (RCTs) have shown that education and skills training can improve caregiver confidence in managing daily care challenges; caregiver skill building and environmental modifications can improve quality of life for family caregivers and care recipients. They also demonstrate that these interventions may yield cost savings. When caregivers receive personal counseling and participate in care management programs, for example, nursing home admissions for older adults with dementia can decline. Integrating caregivers into the hospital discharge process has been shown to decrease re-hospitalizations and shorten lengths of stay. These approaches hold promise for meeting the needs of an increasingly diverse population of older adults and family caregivers.

A VISION FOR THE FUTURE

This study confirms how essential family caregivers are to the health and well-being of older Americans. It also raises profound concerns about our dependence on family caregivers and the potentially serious health and economic risks that caregiving can entail. It is time to publicly acknowledge caregiving families. In today's world, family caregivers cannot be expected to provide complex care and support on their own. Family caregivers need greater recognition, information, and support to fulfill their roles and responsibilities and to maintain their own health, financial security, and well-being.

Effectively engaging and supporting caregivers of older Americans cannot happen overnight. New caregiver programs and policy reforms will carry new costs and require financing. As noted above, some portion of new investments may be offset by savings—from reductions in use of nursing home, home health, emergency room, and inpatient hospital care. These savings are not likely to fully support all of this report's recommendations. Rigorous evaluation and transparency as to costs as well as benefits will be essential.

The committee also recognizes that the context for this report is a time of economic constraints, concerns about future financing of Medicare and Social Security, a wide range of competing demands for public dollars, and deep divisions among Americans about the role and size of government. Nevertheless, the rapid aging of the U.S. population and its impact on families and health care expenditures should not be ignored. If the needs of our older adults' caregivers are not addressed, we, as a society, risk compromising the well-being of our elders and their families. Failure to take on these challenges also means a lost opportunity to discover the potential societal benefits of effectively engaging and supporting family caregivers in the care of older adults—both economic and otherwise. The public's investment in family caregiving for older adults should be carefully considered and public dollars shepherded responsibly. As federal and state agencies move to develop new programs and supports to address the needs of family caregivers, it will be important to prioritize the needs of the most vulnerable caregivers and tailor eligibility appropriately.

RECOMMENDATIONS

Family caregiving is a critical issue of public policy. The committee calls for a transformation in the policies and practices affecting the role of families in the support and care of older adults. Today's emphasis on person-centered care needs to evolve into a focus on person- and family-centered care. The committee urges that support of family caregivers be recognized as an integral part of the nation's collective responsibility for caring for older Americans.

RECOMMENDATION 1: The committee calls upon the Administration that takes office in January 2017 to take steps to address the health, economic, and social issues facing family caregivers of older Americans. Specifically, the committee recommends that:

The Secretary of the U.S. Department of Health and Human Services, in collaboration with the Secretaries of the U.S. Departments of Labor and Veterans Affairs, other federal agencies, and private-sector organizations with expertise in family caregiving, develop and execute a National Family Caregiver Strategy that, administratively or through new federal legislation, explicitly and systematically addresses and supports the essential role of family caregivers to older adults. This strategy should include specific measures to adapt the nation's health care and long-term services and supports (LTSS) systems and workplaces to effectively and respectfully engage family caregivers and to support their health, values, and social and economic well-being, and to address the needs of our increasingly culturally and ethnically diverse caregiver population.

The Secretaries should publicly announce and begin to implement the strategy by

1. executing steps allowable under current statutory authority;
2. proposing specific legislative action, where appropriate, to address additional steps;
3. convening and establishing partnerships with appropriate government (federal, state, and local) and private-sector leaders to implement the strategy throughout education, service delivery, research, and practice; and
4. addressing fully and explicitly the needs of our increasingly culturally and ethnically diverse caregiver population.

The Secretaries should issue biannual reports on progress and actions of the National Family Caregiver Strategy.

This strategy should include the following steps:

RECOMMENDATION 1-a: Develop, test, and implement effective mechanisms within Medicare, Medicaid, and the U.S. Department of Veterans Affairs to ensure that family caregivers are routinely identified and that their needs are assessed and supported in the delivery of health care and long-term services and supports.

Most health and LTSS providers do not assess the health, skills, employment, and willingness of family caregivers. Family caregivers are typically provided little, if any, information and training to carry out the complicated medical procedures, personal care, and care coordination tasks they are expected to provide. Indeed, the lack of systematic assessment of family participation in health and LTSS not only affects the experience of caregivers and care recipients, it also precludes knowledge of how their involvement influences the quality of clinical care and social services, limits the spread of evidence-based interventions that strengthen the well-being of family caregivers and their ability to promote and provide quality care, and undermines credible accounting of the value family caregivers bring to the health care delivery system and to society.

Given the growing national commitment to accountability and efficiency in care delivery, the committee concludes that the time is ripe to elevate family-centered care alongside person-centered care to the forefront of delivery system reform—rationalizing the roles of family caregivers and better supporting their involvement in the delivery process. Achieving that goal will require systematic attention to the identification, assessment, and support of caregivers throughout the care delivery process by

- identifying caregivers in both the care recipient's and the caregiver's medical record;
- screening family caregivers to identify those who are at risk themselves, or whose circumstances place older adults they assist in harm's way;
- assessing at-risk caregivers' strengths, limits, needs, and risks across the full range of expected tasks—medical care, personal care, and coordination—and that, at a minimum, asks family caregivers about their own health and well-being, level of stress, and types of training and supports they might need to continue their role; and
- assuring that identification, screening, and appropriate caregiver assessment occurs at each point in care delivery for the care recipient—including delivery of publicly funded LTSS, annual wellness exams, physician visits, admission and discharge for hospitals and emergency rooms, and chronic care coordination and care transition programs.

RECOMMENDATION 1-b: Direct the Centers for Medicare & Medicaid Services to develop, test, and implement provider payment reforms that motivate providers to engage family caregivers in delivery processes, across all modes of payment and models of care.

As the predominant payers of care for older adults, Medicare, Medicaid, and the VA are essential to motivating appropriate provider practice. A number of recent initiatives have been taken to advance recognition of caregivers in Medicare and Medicaid coverage, payment, and delivery policies. In Medicare, hospitals are now expected to engage and support family caregivers in the discharge planning process as a part of the hospital's conditions of participation. New chronic care management and transitional care services codes allow providers to be paid for non-face-to-face communication with individuals and their caregivers about a beneficiary's care. Innovative delivery mechanisms implicitly encourage providers (through shared savings for quality care at lower costs) to actively engage caregivers as a resource in the care delivery process. In Medicaid, many states formally or informally assess family caregivers as part of the process for developing LTSS care plans. In the VA, the Caregivers and Veterans Omnibus Health Services Act of 2010 established a mechanism for reimbursement/workload credit for services provided to caregivers (mainly of younger veterans).

For the most part, however, these advances create the potential for, rather than a commitment to, payment practices that support provider engagement with caregivers. That commitment requires

- the development and application of payment mechanisms to promote providers' interaction with family caregivers when care recipients are not present;
- the development and application of performance standards that hold providers accountable for caregiver engagement, training, and support in accessing the full range of health care and LTSS they require, by explicitly including caregiver outcomes in quality measures;
- the inclusion of family caregivers in CMS payment and service delivery demonstrations; and
- adherence to the National Standards for Culturally and Linguistically Appropriate Services in Health and Health Care to provide quality care that is effective, equitable, understandable, respectful, and responsive to older adults' and caregivers' cultural health beliefs and practices, preferred languages, health literacy, and other communication needs.

RECOMMENDATION 1-c: Strengthen the training and capacity of health care and social service providers to recognize and to engage family caregivers and to provide them evidence-based supports and referrals to services in the community.

To ultimately ensure high-quality person- and family-centered care by the health and LTSS workforce, providers should see family caregivers not just as a resource in the treatment or support of an older person, but also as both a partner in that enterprise and as someone who may need information, training, care, and support. Achieving and acting on that perspective requires that all types of providers be able to

- recognize a family caregiver's presence;
- assess whether and how the caregiver can best participate in overall care;
- engage and share information with the caregiver;
- recognize the caregiver's own health care and support needs; and
- help caregivers to obtain needed support by referring caregivers to appropriate services.

Given the growing diversity of the older adult population as well as their caregivers, cultural competence in exercising these skills is essential to their effectiveness.

A range of professionals and direct care workers are likely to serve older people with family caregivers—physicians, nurses, physician assistants, social workers, psychologists, pharmacists, occupational therapists, physical and other rehabilitation therapists, certified nursing assistants, and home care aides. Professional organizations in social work and nursing have led the way in taking steps to build a workforce with the competencies necessary for person- and family-centered care. However, work to date falls far short of a systematic and comprehensive effort that should include

- identification of specific competencies, by provider type, to demonstrate effective practice, including competencies related to working with diverse family caregivers;
- development of educational curricula and training to instill those competencies;
- incorporation of those competencies into requirements for licensure, certification, and accreditation;
- articulation of standards of practice; and
- evaluation of practice using standardized quality-of-care metrics.

The federal government, in collaboration with professional societies, education programs, licensure and certification bodies, accrediting bodies, and other organizations, should move this effort forward. Specifically, action requires

- federal support for the development and enforcement of competencies for identifying, assessing, and supporting family caregivers by health care and human service professionals and regulatory and accrediting organizations;
- the U.S. Department of Health and Human Services (HHS) Office for Civil Rights to clarify caregivers' access to information by providing administrative guidance to health care and social service providers regarding the permitted uses and disclosures of protected health information to family caregivers and encourage providers to train their workforce regarding that clarification;
- convening professional societies, training programs, accrediting bodies, and other organizations to develop educational curricula and to support their systematic evaluation and implementation; and
- convening and collaborating with state agencies and professional organizations to incorporate competencies into standards for licensure and certification.

RECOMMENDATION 1-d: Increase funding for programs that provide explicit supportive services for family caregivers such as the National Family Caregiver Support Program and other relevant U.S. Department of Health and Human Services programs

to facilitate the development, dissemination, and implementation of evidenced-based caregiver intervention programs.

A robust body of research demonstrates that interventions aimed at supporting caregivers can significantly improve quality of care as well as the well-being and quality of life for both caregivers and care recipients. Interventions that have been tested through well-designed RCTs have involved (separately or in combination) a broad range of therapeutic techniques, been applied in a variety of settings, and been evaluated for a broad set of impacts on caregivers and care recipients. Despite demonstrated effectiveness, however, promising interventions have not been disseminated and adopted in everyday settings. As a result, few caregivers have access to services that may lessen their health risks or improve their ability to help older adults effectively.

RECOMMENDATION 1-e: Explore, evaluate, and, as warranted, adopt federal policies that provide economic support for working caregivers.

Caregiving and employment are increasingly intertwined. Already about half of the nation's caregivers for older adults are employed. As noted above, working caregivers—especially those who care for people with dementia or with substantial personal care needs—are at risk of significant economic costs: loss of income; out-of-pocket cost for the care recipient; and lower lifetime earnings, savings, and retirement benefits. Low-wage and part-time workers are particularly vulnerable. Job discrimination may also affect caregivers' job security.

The Family and Medical Leave Act (FMLA) of 1993 was an important step toward providing working caregivers some help in balancing job and family responsibilities. However, FMLA covers only certain family relationships, excluding daughters- and sons-in-laws, grandchildren, nieces and nephews, siblings, and other friends and relatives who are caring for older adults; and it does not apply to employers with fewer than 50 employees. Perhaps even more important—eligible caregivers may be unable to afford the unpaid leave FMLA protects—and many American workers—especially low-wage workers—lack access to paid time off of any kind.

Four states—California, New Jersey, New York, and Rhode Island—have enacted paid family leave statutes, and five states—California, Connecticut, Massachusetts, Oregon, and Vermont—have paid sick leave laws that require employers to allow workers a reasonable number of earned sick days to care for an ill family member (including some older adults). The states finance paid family leave through an insurance model that relies on minimal payroll taxes paid by employees. Although some employers report additional costs, initial evidence suggests that many have adapted to family leave requirements. These programs have the potential both to facilitate family caregiving and alleviate some of its economic hardships.

Other policy measures have the potential to help safeguard caregivers' immediate and long-term economic security. An array of worthy proposals merits serious consideration. These include, for example, refundable tax credits to increase caregiver incomes; Social Security caregiving credits to reduce the impact of foregone wages on retirement benefits; including family caregiver status as a protected class under federal employment discrimination laws; and providing employers with guidance and training on best practices to better support workers with caregiving responsibilities. Exploring the feasibility of these options will require economic impact assessments that include not only the caregiver but also employers and federal and state agencies. Evaluating feasibility will also require that analyses take into account unintended consequences, such as the impact on caregivers' labor force participation.

As reliance on working caregivers grows, federal policy action across some or all of these lines is essential to promote economic security for all the nation's caregivers of older Americans. Federal, state, and local governments should accelerate efforts to expand and evaluate paid family and medical leave and paid sick leave policies.

RECOMMENDATION 1-f: Expand the data collection infrastructures within the U.S. Departments of Health and Human Services, Labor, and Veterans Affairs to facilitate monitoring, tracking, and reporting on the experience of family caregivers.

The nation lacks a basic data infrastructure and knowledge base to inform policy and monitor progress in supporting caregivers. Current data collection does not capture essential details on caregivers' characteristics or the outcomes of their caregiving activities. A robust surveillance system is needed. Routine, longitudinal, population surveys should assess family caregivers and be sufficiently powered to allow analyses of important subgroups of caregivers. Key variables include age, race and ethnicity, sexual orientation, rural or urban location, employment status, geographic proximity to care recipients, and care recipient condition. Concerted federal leadership and the engagement of experts (statisticians, care providers, researchers, and policy makers) and professionals in public and private organizations will be essential.

RECOMMENDATION 1-g: Launch a multi-agency research program sufficiently robust to evaluate caregiver interventions in real-world health care and community settings, across diverse

conditions and populations, and with respect to a broad array of outcomes.

Despite the valuable lessons learned from research on caregiver interventions, there are significant barriers to moving existing evidence-based interventions from the test phase into implementation in diverse clinical practice settings. Progress in caregiver support requires a new approach to research among federal agencies and private foundations to support large-scale multi-site research studies evaluating efficacy and cost-effectiveness of a range of caregiver interventions. The research agenda should be guided by a consensus conference among key stakeholders.

RECOMMENDATION 2: State governments that have yet to address the health, economic, and social challenges of caregiving for older adults should learn from the experience of states with caregiver supports, and implement similar programs.

As noted above, several states have led the nation in addressing working caregivers' access to family or sick leave. Twenty-nine states have also enacted the Caregiver Advise, Record, Enable (CARE) Act, requiring hospitals to ask people whether they wish to designate a family caregiver, and, if so, record the name of the caregiver when individuals are admitted; notify the family caregiver if the individual is to be discharged to another facility or back home; and provide effective explanation of and instruction on the medical/nursing tasks (e.g., medication management, injections, wound care) that the family caregiver will need to perform at home.

In addition to efforts by the federal government to build on this experience in developing and implementing the recommended Caregiver Strategy, states can also independently advance caregiver and care recipient well-being by learning from other states and adopting best practices.

RECOMMENDATION 3: The Secretaries of the U.S. Departments of Health and Human Services, Labor, and Veterans Affairs should work with leaders in health care and long-term services and supports delivery, technology, and philanthropy to establish a public–private, multi-stakeholder innovation fund for research and innovation to accelerate the pace of change in addressing the needs of caregiving families.

Addressing caregiver issues will require not only changes in the public sector but also the support and guidance of the private sector. Employers of all types have a vested interest in supporting caregivers. Insurance, health care, and technology companies, for example, can bring to bear both financial resources and expertise to address current and emerging challenges for caregivers. Multiple national and local private foundations, as well as non-profit organizations, have already begun to invest in the implementation of a caregiver agenda. The public sector cannot achieve all necessary progress on its own; a public–private innovation fund could leverage private funding to complement public resources and fill gaps in public funding.

The fund, for example, could sponsor the development of market-driven approaches for lessening the strain of caregiving on families—targeting innovative services and products that are scalable and sustainable. Potential products include assistive technologies, remote monitoring and sensing systems, telehealth applications, and other tools to assist family caregivers and to enable older adults to continue living in their home and communities. These systems could also be linked to health care and social service providers to aid in care coordination efforts.

> RECOMMENDATION 4: **In all the above actions, explicitly and consistently address families' diversity in assessing caregiver needs and in developing, testing, and implementing caregiver supports.**

The future of caregiving for older Americans will be shaped not only by the growing older adult population needing care but also by the increasing ethnic and racial diversity of older people and their families. The National Family Caregiver Strategy should address the needs and values of diverse family caregivers. The strategy, including all of the above recommendations, should include specific goals for advancing support for diverse caregivers and the biannual report should specifically address progress of the strategy in meeting these goals. Specific steps that can be taken include the following:

- Making cultural competence a core aspect of provider competencies in working with family caregivers.
- Addressing critical gaps in our knowledge about the effectiveness of interventions for diverse populations are through both research and implementation efforts.
- Conduct monitoring in a way that allows for meaningful data on the health and well-being of diverse family caregivers as well as on the quality and outcomes of care.

1

Introduction

ABSTRACT: This introductory chapter describes the background for the study, the scope of the inquiry, and the committee's methods and vision for the future. It also reviews current federal programs that provide direct support to family caregivers. The committee's charge was to develop recommendations to support the nation's family caregivers so that they can effectively advocate and care for older adults without harm to themselves. The report examines what is known about the characteristics of caregivers and the older adults they care for, the evolving role of caregivers and the impact of caregiving on their health and well-being, the economic impact of caregiving especially on those caregivers who are employed, the evidence on the effectiveness of existing caregiver programs and interventions, and the challenges that caregivers face in health care and long-term care systems.

Millions of Americans are providing care and support to an older parent, spouse, friend, or neighbor who needs help because of a limitation in their physical, mental, or cognitive functioning. For decades, demographers, gerontologists, health researchers and providers, economists, and other experts have raised concerns about the rapid aging of our population and its implications for the health care system, Social Security, and local, state, and federal resources (Brody, 1966; IOM, 1991, 2008, 2012; MedPAC, 2015; NRC, 1988, 1994, 2003, 2012). Billions of public dollars are being invested in much needed research and development to find ways to improve

Box 1-1
Sponsors of the Study

Alliance for Aging Research
Alzheimer's Association
Anonymous
Archstone Foundation
California Health Care Foundation
The Commonwealth Fund
The Fan Fox and Leslie R. Samuels Foundation
Health Foundation of Western and Central New York
The John A. Hartford Foundation
May and Stanley Smith Charitable Trust
The Retirement Research Foundation
The Rosalinde and Arthur Gilbert Foundation
Santa Barbara Foundation
Tufts Health Plan Foundation
U.S. Department of Veterans Affairs

the value and quality of the U.S. health care system (CMS, 2016a,b). Far less attention has been given to family caregivers who provide the lion's share of long-term services and supports (LTSS)[1] to our older adult population. Many are unaware that, today, family caregivers are also expected to provide complex health care services once only delivered by licensed health care personnel in a hospital or other institutional setting.

In 2014, 13 private foundations, the U.S. Department of Veterans Affairs (VA), and an anonymous donor came together to ask the National Academies of Sciences, Engineering, and Medicine to develop a report with recommendations for family caregiving of older adults (see Box 1-1). The committee's charge is presented in Box 1-2. This study has three principal objectives: (1) to assess the prevalence and nature of family caregiving of older adults as well as the impact of caregiving on caregivers' health, employment, and overall well-being; (2) to examine available evidence on the effectiveness of programs, supports, and other services designed

[1] Long-term services and supports (LTSS), sometimes referred to as long-term care, include the array of paid and unpaid personal care, health care, and social services generally provided over a sustained period of time. Services can include personal care (such as bathing or dressing), help with medication management, paying bills, transportation, meal preparation, and health maintenance tasks. Services can be provided in a variety of settings such as nursing homes, residential care facilities, and individual homes.

BOX 1-2
Charge to the Committee on Family Caregiving for Older Adults

An ad hoc Institute of Medicine committee will develop a report with recommendations for public- and private-sector policies to support the capacity of family caregivers to perform critical caregiving tasks, to minimize the barriers that family caregivers encounter in trying to meet the needs of older adults, and to improve the health care and long-term services and supports provided to care recipients.

The committee will focus on family caregivers of older adults, typically age 65 and older. The report will analyze the prevalence of family caregiving and the demographic, societal, and technological trends that influence it. It will also examine caregivers' roles and responsibilities, both current and expected in the future, and the impact of the caregiver role on individual health, employment, and well-being. Caregivers' unmet needs and the gap between the projected demand for caregivers and the population available to serve as caregivers will be assessed and differences associated with race/ethnicity, culture, rural residence, and geography will be examined.

The report will also review the evidence of the effectiveness of potential supports for family caregivers and care recipients across a range of settings, including, for example, in medical homes and other primary care settings, home- and community-based settings, acute care hospitals, and residential facilities. These might include, for example, models of team-based care that include the family caregiver as member; approaches to training providers regarding the caregiver role; and models for training caregivers for their various roles.

to support family caregivers; and (3) to assess and recommend policies to address the needs of family caregivers and to minimize the barriers that they encounter in trying to meet the needs of older adults.

The Committee on Family Caregiving for Older Adults was appointed in October 2014 to conduct the study and prepare this report. The committee included 21 individuals with research or clinical experience related to family caregiving of older adults in home- and community-based settings; physicians' offices; clinics; hospitals; VA facilities; and senior residential, assisted living, and skilled nursing facilities.[2] The committee members had specific expertise in gerontology, geriatric psychiatry, social work, home- and community-based services, psychology, anthropology, diversity and health disparity issues, nursing and medicine, health services research, health policy, economics and finance, employee benefits and workplace

[2] Due to personal circumstances, three members of the committee withdrew from the study before its completion.

programs, elder law, and the design and effectiveness of interventions to improve outcomes for caregivers and older adults. The committee also included a retired physician and health policy expert in his 80s. Brief biographies of committee members and the study staff are provided in Appendix B.

CONTEXT FOR THIS REPORT

The committee's charge raises questions about the boundaries among the responsibilities of individuals, families, and government. By its very nature, family caregiving of older adults is both a personal and private issue as well as a public and societal concern. From the individual perspective, one's involvement in caregiving for his or her elders is, in part, a matter of personal, spousal, or filial responsibility. Yet, for generations, the American public has also assumed collective responsibility in helping to protect the well-being of the nation's older adults through government programs such as Social Security, Medicare, Medicaid, the Area Agencies on Aging (AAAs), and others. The committee recognizes that the role of the individual versus that of society overall is often a matter of public debate.

Who Is a Family Caregiver?

The committee agreed that the term "family caregiver" should be used to reflect the diverse nature of older adults' family and helping relationships. Some family caregivers do not have a family kinship or legally defined relationship with the care recipient, but are instead partners, neighbors, or friends. Many older adults receive care from more than one family caregiver, and some caregivers may help more than one older adult.

The circumstances of individual caregivers and the caregiver context are extremely variable. Family caregivers may live with, nearby, or far away from the person receiving care. Regardless, the family caregiver's involvement is determined primarily by a personal relationship rather than by financial remuneration. The care they provide may be episodic, daily, occasional, or of short or long duration. The caregiver may help with simple household tasks; self-care activities such as getting in and out of bed, bathing, dressing, eating, or toileting; or provide complex medical care tasks, such as managing medications and giving injections. The older adult may have dementia and, thus, require a caregiver's constant supervision. Or, the caregiver may be responsible for all of these activities.

In developing policy regarding family caregiving of older adults, it is important to recognize that not all older adults need a family caregiver and not all family caregivers need support or services. As Chapter 2 will describe, the committee focused on the overall population of caregivers of older adults who receive help because of a physical, mental, cognitive, and/or functional limitation. The committee also focused on the "high-need" subgroup of caregivers who help an older adult who either has dementia or who needs help with at least two self-care activities (i.e., bathing, dressing, eating, toileting, or getting in and out of bed) or both.

This report uses the terms "family caregiver" and "caregiver" interchangeably to refer to these two groups. It does not use the terms "informal" or "unpaid" although they are often used in the economics and medical literature to differentiate family caregivers from "formal" caregivers—paid direct care workers (such as home care aides) or health and social service professionals. "Informal" does not capture the complexity of what family caregivers do or their connection to the older adults they are helping.

The term "care recipient" is used to refer to the older adults for whom they care. The committee focused on older adults, defined as the 65 and older age group, because of the sponsors' specific interests, the dramatic aging of the older U.S. population, and the available data that often draw from datasets describing older Medicare beneficiaries.

Providing care to an older family member is a normative developmental experience that presents universal challenges and opportunities. Some caregiving demands and responses to these demands in late life cut across all families regardless of socioeconomic class, gender, race, ethnicity, national origin, language, sexual orientation, gender identity, rural versus urban residence, etc. For example, normative stressors experienced by older adults such as increased physical dependence and bereavement signal a need for physical and emotional support among all older adults. Diversity may influence the breadth and nature of exposure to stress events and demands, responses to stressors, access to resources and supports, and values and beliefs about help-seeking. Throughout the report, the committee addresses issues of diversity in the caregiving context, and where scientific evidence is specifically available, results are discussed.

Many Faces of Caregiving

The nation's population is becoming one in which no racial or ethnic group is a majority.

This report takes a broad view of diversity that goes beyond multicultural caregiving to include socioeconomic status, rural residence, sexual orientation, gender, and other factors that are relevant to caregiving policies, services, and programs. Among lesbian, gay, bisexual, and transgender (LGBT) and ethnic minority caregivers, for example, caregiving tasks and decision making are more likely to be shared by multiple family members or with members of the extended family or non-kin (Apesoa-Varano et al., 2015). Services and programs will be more effective in engaging and supporting family caregivers if they incorporate a family's values, taking care to avoid terms that are likely to be misunderstood or convey stigma. Words matter. Commonly used terms such as "caregiver," "caregiver burden," or "dementia" do not readily translate into other languages and may have negative connotations. For example, among Latinos, the term "caregiver burden" may be misinterpreted as suggesting that caring for one's loved one is an inconvenience rather than a filial, marital, or intimate partner obligation. In fact, the term actually denotes freight or cargo associated with transporting goods. Regardless of language or cultural background, many family caregivers in the United States do not relate to the term "caregiver" or describe the help they provide as "caregiving"; instead, they view their interactions as part of their familial roles and expectations justified by longstanding spousal or kin relations.

Background on Federal Involvement in Family Caregiving

Historically, the Medicare and Medicaid programs—like other third-party payers—have focused on beneficiaries with only limited, if any, attention to their caregivers. Thus, their impact on family caregivers is indirect (Doty and Spillman, 2015). Regardless, the benefits of Medicare and Medicaid for caregivers are significant when they enable older adults to obtain needed health care and LTSS.

For the most part, Medicare and Medicaid do not fund caregiver services and supports. Medicaid-funded, home- and community-based services (HCBS) are an important exception. Under 1915(i) Medicaid waivers, states have the option to cover respite care, and caregiver education and training. State Medicaid programs may also offer self-directed service programs (e.g., Cash and Counseling) that allow eligible older adults to use their Medicaid home care benefits to pay a family caregiver for LTSS under certain circumstances. Use of the programs has been limited however.

The Centers for Medicare & Medicaid Services (CMS) is beginning to address other areas that may help support caregivers. The agency, for example, is piloting new models of care delivery designed to integrate health care and LTSS for high-need, low-income older adults. However, best practices for involving family caregivers and their specific needs have yet to be defined (CMS, 2016c; Grabowski et al., 2015). CMS is also testing potential performance-based incentives using quality measures to improve quality and value (CMS, 2016c). The agency has issued a draft plan for developing clinician quality measures that will, for the first time, include a focus on family caregivers (CMS, 2015; NQF, 2016). Presumably, this will lead to inclusion of family caregivers in older adults' home care plans as well. However, the role of family caregivers of older adults has not yet received substantive attention in these initiatives.

Federal Programs That Provide Direct Support to Family Caregivers of Older Adults

While CMS has focused on the beneficiary, direct services for caregivers have been developed by other U.S. Department of Health and Human Services (HHS) agencies including the Administration for Community Living (ACL) and the Health Resources and Services Administration (HRSA), as well as the VA and the U.S. Department of Labor (DOL). Federal programs that focus directly on caregivers of older adults are described below and in Tables 1-1 and 1-2.

Administration for Community Living

National Family Caregiver Support Program (NFCSP) In 2000, Congress explicitly recognized the importance of family caregivers by creating NFCSP under the Older Americans Act—the first and only federal program to specifically address the needs of family caregivers of older individuals and also grandparents (and other relatives) raising grandchildren. With its establishment 16 years ago, family caregivers are now recognized as consumers of information and supportive services in their own right (Feinberg and Newman, 2006). Before NFCSP, only seven states had funded programs with the family caregiver as the explicit client and recipient of services (Feinberg, 2004). With its creation, programs could be created in every state, and existing programs could be expanded.

NFCSP is run by the Administration on Aging, a unit of ACL, an agency of HHS[3] and the primary federal agency charged with supporting family caregivers. NFCSP requires State Units on Aging (SUAs) to work in partnership with AAAs and local service providers to provide five required services (see Box 1-3): information; assistance in gaining access to services; individual counseling, education, and support groups; respite; and supplemental services, on a limited basis. Most of the other ACL caregiver support programs, described in Table 1-1, are administered at the state level. States often expand the programs by broadening eligibility criteria or raising the caps on benefits (e.g., for respite care services), and, in many states, caregiving task forces, coalitions, and other organizations supplement the federal programs (Ramchand et al., 2014).[4] These organizations

[3] In 2012, the Secretary of the U.S. Department of Health and Human Services (HHS) merged its agencies—the Administration on Aging, the Administration on Intellectual and Developmental Disabilities, and the HHS Office on Disability—under the umbrella of a new Administration for Community Living (http://www.acl.gov).

[4] For details on state caregiving programs, see *The State of the States in Family Caregiving: A 50-State Study* at: https://www.caregiver.org/caregiving-across-states-50-state-profiles-2014 (accessed August 22, 2016).

TABLE 1-1 Administration for Community Living Programs That Support Caregivers of Older Adults

Program	Description	Funding (FY 2015)	Older Adult Target Population	Use by Caregivers of Older Adults
National Family Caregiver Support Program (NFCSP)	• Requires state units on aging to partner with the AAAs and local providers to provide five services: information; assistance in gaining access to services; individual counseling, education, caregiver (CG) training, and support groups; respite services; and some supplemental services	$145.5 million	• CGs of older adults (age 60+); • CGs of individuals of any age with ADRD	• >1.3 million CG units (i.e., counseling, respite, information, access assistance) • 115,585 CGs received counseling, training, or support groups • >64,000 CGs received respite
National Eldercare Locator	• Assists CGs in identifying community resources	$2 million	• Older adults and their CGs	• 754,430 individuals
National Alzheimer's Call Center	• Provides information, referrals, and counseling via a grantee (currently Alzheimer's Association)	$0.9 million	• People with ADRD; their CGs and family members	• 319,216 calls
Aging and Disability Resource Centers	• Grants to states to provide information to CGs and improve access to LTSS	$6.1 million	• CGs of older adults and persons with disabilities	• 86,871 CGs age 60+
Native American Caregiver Support Initiative	• Grants to tribal organization to provide CGs with respite, training, information and outreach, counseling, and support groups	$6 million	• American Indian, Alaskan Native, and Native Hawaiian CGs of older adults with a chronic disability or illness	• 92,259 CGs

Alzheimer's Disease Supportive Services Program	• Grants to states for home- and community-based service systems for persons with dementia and their CGs, including information, counseling and assistance, screening, service coordination, and referral and access to evidence-based LTSS	$4.8 million	• CGs of individuals with ADRD	• 14,656 CGs
Alzheimer's Disease Initiative Specialized Support Services	• Grants to states, tribal entities, and localities to improve LTSS and CG training and consultations on behavioral symptom management	$10.5 million	• CGs of individuals with ADRD or I/DD	• Not available (new program)
Lifespan Respite Care Program	• Grants to states to provide respite care	$2.3 million	• All CGs	

NOTES: NFCSP also serves caregivers (age 55+) of children and younger adults with disabilities. Unless noted otherwise, data are for the most recent 12-month period available. AAA = Area Agency on Aging; ADRD = Alzheimer's disease and related dementias; I/DD = intellectual/developmental disabilities; LTSS = long-term services and supports.
SOURCES: ACL, 2016a,b; Alzheimer's Association, 2015; Barretto et al., 2014; Colello, 2007; Doty and Spillman, 2015; Draper, 2010; Gould et al., 2014; Napili and Colello, 2013; National Association of Area Agencies on Aging, 2014.

TABLE 1-2 U.S. Department of Veterans Affairs Programs and Services for Caregivers

Program	Description	Target Population	Utilization
U.S. Department of Veterans Affairs (VA) Caregiver Support Program	• Provides training and education, support, and coordination for caregivers (CGs) • Total FY 2015 budget of $478 million for all caregiving programs including, but not limited to, those below	• CGs of veterans	See below
• Caregiver education and training	• Building better caregivers		• 4,742 CGs received training (27 percent were CGs of older veterans) (2012 to 2015) • 8,505 CGs completed the course (15 percent were CGs of older veterans)
	• Self-management/self-care courses (solving problems, managing stress, identifying resources)		
• Caregiver Support Line	• Toll-free phone line staffed by licensed social workers • Provides information, referral, and support • Designed to serve as a single entry point for veterans' CGs' access to resources and referrals	• CGs of veterans	• 57,118 calls; more than 228,000 calls (2011 to 2015) • 7,859 referrals to Caregiver Support Coordinators • More than 3,200 telephone education group participants

	• Facilitates national monthly telephone education calls		• CGs of veterans
• Caregiver Support Coordinators (CSCs)	• Designated social workers, nurses, and psychologists who provide support, referral to local resources, and care coordination • Coordinators act as intermediaries between CGs and VA staff • Every VAMC is required to have one full-time CSC	• CGs of veterans at VA medical centers (VAMCs)	• Not available
• Peer Support for Caregivers	• Trained volunteer peer mentors are assigned to CGs to provide guidance to resources and decrease feelings of isolation	• CGs of veterans	• More than 300 CGs trained (2012 to 2015)
• Resources for Enhancing Alzheimer's Caregiver Health (REACH)	• Skills-building intervention designed to provide support, education, and skills building to individual CGs	• CGs of veterans with Alzheimer's disease or related dementias, spinal cord injury or disorder, PTSD, ALS, MS	• 1,208 VA clinical staff (social workers, counselors, psychologists, and nurses) received REACH training (2011 to 2015)

TABLE 1-2 Continued

Program	Description	Target Population	Utilization
	• CGs receive 4+ one-on-one sessions focusing on problem solving, stress and coping techniques, and strategies for managing everyday problems		
• Telephone support groups for caregivers	• Skills-building intervention designed to provide support, education, and training for CGs via telephone-based support groups • Topics include techniques for problem solving, behavioral management, stress reduction, and coping	• CGs of veterans with Alzheimer's disease or related dementias, spinal cord injury or disorder, PTSD, ALS, and MS	• 150 VA clinical staff (social workers, counselors, psychologists, nurses) received training (2012 to 2015)
VA Geriatrics and Extended Care			
• Adult Day Health Care (ADHC)	• Day programs for social interaction, support, and recreation; may be provided by the VA or a community provider closer to veteran's residence	• Older veterans who need assistance with activities of daily living, isolated, or whose CGs need respite	• VA provided and/or purchased ADHC for 16,604 unique veterans
• Homemaker and Home Health Aide Program	• Provides homemaker or home health aides to come to the home	• Veterans who need skilled services, case management, and help with self-care	• 101,843 veterans

• Respite Care	• Respite services provided at veterans' homes, nursing homes, or adult day care programs • 30-day maximum per year	• Veterans with functional impairments	• 20 percent of CGs of older veterans (65+) report using VA respite services in the previous year
• Home Hospice Care	• Hospice services, including grief counseling for CGs	• Older veterans who have a terminal condition	• 8,278 veterans received hospice services paid for by the VA, but provided by community providers

NOTES: Services may be provided in a VA facility or under contract by a community provider. Hospice services are limited to veterans who have less than 6 months to live and are not seeking curative treatment. Unless noted otherwise, utilization data are for the most recent 12-month period available (fiscal year). ALS = amyotrophic lateral sclerosis; I/DD = intellectual/developmental disabilities; MS = multiple sclerosis; PTSD = post-traumatic stress disorder.
SOURCES: Dupke et al., 2016; VA, 2015a,b, 2016a,b,c; Wright et al., 2015.

BOX 1-3
State Units on Aging and Area Agencies on Aging

State Units on Aging (SUAs): These state and territorial agencies administer, manage, design, and advocate for programs and services that support older adults, people with disabilities, and their caregivers. SUAs work with Area Agencies on Aging and other service providers to ensure that populations receive the federal, state, and local benefits for which they are eligible.

Area Agencies on Aging (AAAs): Established in 1973 under the Older Americans Act (OAA), these local agencies help plan, develop, coordinate, and deliver long-term services and supports to adults age 60 and older and their caregivers in a given local planning and service area. The OAA requires that AAAs offer five core service areas: elder rights, caregiver supports, nutrition, health and wellness activities, and supportive services. AAAs may offer additional services past these core areas and may also service additional populations including disabled individuals of all ages and veterans.

SOURCES: National Association of Area Agencies on Aging, 2016; National Association of States United for Aging and Disabilities, 2016.

may work with state agencies through contracts or grants to implement the state caregiving programs.

Caregivers are eligible for NFCSP services if they are caring for someone age 60 or older. Caregivers age 60 and older are eligible regardless of the care recipients' age. The annual appropriation for the program has remained at around $150 million despite the marked growth in the older adult population (Doty and Spillman, 2015). Funds are allotted to the states based on the number of state residents age 70 and older, and states are required to match at least 25 percent of the federal contribution. Most states and territories use an intrastate funding formula to disseminate funds to local AAAs (Link, 2015/2016).

In fiscal year 2015, with a total budget of $145.6 million, NFCSP served more than 900,000 individual caregivers of older adults.[5] Of these, 115,585 received counseling or training, and more than 64,000 caregivers received respite care; the remainder was provided information about available services and supports or assistance with accessing services (see Table 1-1). The extent of public awareness of the availability of these

[5] Personal communication, G. Link, Aging Services Program Specialist, Administration for Community Living (e-mail March 3, 2016).

services is not known. The number of family caregivers who might benefit from NFCSP services is likely to far exceed the current capacity of the program.

ACL is currently conducting the first national evaluation of NFCSP's implementation at the state and local levels; its impact on family caregivers and care recipients; and its integration with and impact on long-term-care policies and home- and community-based service systems (Barretto et al., 2014; Link, 2015/2016).[6] The implementation evaluation found that NFCSP is the only specific source of caregiver support provided by AAAs in three-quarters of the service areas (Lewin Group and ACL, 2016). In addition, it substantially increased the number of caregivers served in the 15 states that had created caregiver programs before the advent of NFCSP. The ACL evaluation of caregiver outcomes is underway and is expected to be completed in 2017.

Other ACL Programs That Support Caregivers of Older Adults

As Table 1-1 indicates, ACL also administers seven smaller state-based caregiver programs with budgets ranging from just below $1 million, for the National Alzheimer's Call Center, to more than $10 million for the recently created Alzheimer's Disease Initiative Specialized Support Services for caregivers of individuals with Alzheimer's disease and related disorders or intellectual and developmental disorders.

Established in 2006, the Lifespan Respite Program supports efforts at the state and local levels to help family caregivers by improving the quality of and access to respite, the temporary relief of caregiving duties. As of 2015, the program has provided agencies in 33 states and the District of Columbia with grants of up to $200,000 to initiate or improve access to respite services and training of respite care providers. Although the program is relatively small, respite is one of the most important caregiver supports (see Chapter 5 for more details).

In 2016, ACL announced a research collaborative, the Family Support Research and Training Center (FSRTC), to synthesize and generate knowledge about the needs of families caring for children and adults with disabilities (FSRTC, 2016). Although FSRTC does not serve family caregivers directly, the initiative is noteworthy because of its emphasis on engaging family caregivers in the research process. Current plans are for families to be involved in developing the center's research priorities. The research center is based at the University of Illinois, Chicago. Participating organizations include the National Council on Aging, The Lurie Institute for

[6] The evaluation was delayed for years because of budget constraints (Doty and Spillman, 2015).

Disability Policy at Brandeis University, The National Resource Center for Participant-Directed Services at Boston College, and the Research Training Center (RTC) on Community Living at the University of Minnesota.

U.S. Department of Veterans Affairs (VA)

Caregiver Support Program The VA provides a wide range of services to caregivers of veterans, both young and old (see Table 1-2). The mission of the Caregiver Support Program is to promote the health and well-being of veterans' caregivers through education, resources, support, and services (Kabat, 2015). The total budget for the VA Caregiver Support Program was $478 million in FY 2015. The share of the funding that reached caregivers of older veterans is not known, but is likely to be substantial. Several VA caregiver programs specifically target caregivers of older veterans with Alzheimer's disease or related dementias, spinal cord injury or disease, post-traumatic stress disorder (PTSD), amyotrophic lateral sclerosis (ALS), and multiple sclerosis (MS).

Geriatrics and extended care The VA has provided home-based primary care and other targeted services for older veterans for decades (O'Shaughnessy, 2013). These services include clinical services as well as an array of important caregiver supports, including adult day health care, homemaker/home health aide services, respite care, and hospice care (see Table 1-2). One in five (or 20 percent of) caregivers of veterans older than age 65 reported using VA respite services in FY 2015.

U.S. Department of Labor (DOL)

The Family and Medical Leave Act (FMLA) was enacted in 1993 to require employers to provide unpaid, job-protected leave to workers in certain settings to attend to their own health needs, to bond with a new child, or to care for a parent, spouse, or child with a serious health condition.

FMLA only applies to governmental agencies and private employers with more than 50 employees. DOL is charged with monitoring and ensuring that employers comply with the Act. By 2013, most private employers were in compliance (Lipson, 2015).

Health Resources and Services Administration (HRSA)

Geriatric Workforce Enhancement Program (GWEP)[7] This program focuses on improving competencies in geriatrics among not only health professionals, but also family caregivers and direct care workers. Although GWEP awards most of its funding to training primary care and direct service personnel, its awardees are also tasked with educating and training older adults and caregivers. Since the start of the program in July 2015 through March 2016, GWEP awardees have trained approximately 13,384 paid and family caregivers on a variety of topics. The top five training topics are

1. basics of Alzheimer's disease and related dementias;
2. evidence-based programs for family caregivers;
3. promoting self-care by the caregivers;
4. community resources to support caregivers; and
5. managing dementia.[8]

Over the course of the 3-year grants, HRSA expects that 52,352 paid and family caregivers will participate in a training program.

Federal Tax Benefits

The Internal Revenue Code currently provides a limited tax deduction for the medical and LTSS expenses of a dependent, non-spouse who resides with the taxpayer and whom the taxpayer provides more than 50 percent of their support. The deductible medical and LTSS costs are those that exceed 10 percent of the taxpayer's adjusted gross income or 7.5 percent[9] if the taxpayer is age 65 or older (IRS, 2014). The taxpayer qualifies by his or her level of financial support and not by meeting any criteria for being a caregiver, so the deduction does not apply to all caregivers, such as spousal or long-distance caregivers (IRS, 2014). Another tax benefit available at the option of employers is the federal Dependent Care Assistance Plan, which allows individuals to exclude up to $5,000 of expenses incurred in caregiving from their taxable income (IRS, 2016). However, only persons whose employers have set up a dependent care assistance benefit for their

[7] In 2015, HRSA merged several programs—Comprehensive Geriatric Education Program; Geriatrics Education Centers; Geriatric Training for Physicians, Dentists, and Behavioral/ Mental Health Professionals; and Geriatric Academic Career Awards—into this one competitive program (HHS, 2016).

[8] Personal communication, Joan Weiss, Senior Advisor, Division of Medicine and Dentistry, HRSA (e-mail March 28, 2016).

[9] In 2017, deductible costs for taxpayers age 65 or older will be subject to the same threshold as younger persons (i.e., those medical and LTSS costs that exceed 10 percent of adjustable gross income) (IRS, 2015).

employees may take advantage of the deduction, and only 39 percent of civilian workers had access to such an account in 2013 (BLS, 2015).

A VISION FOR THE FUTURE

The committee agreed early on to adopt and build on the basic principles described in the Institute of Medicine report *Crossing the Quality Chasm: A New Health System for the 21st Century* (IOM, 2001). A focus on the individual experience of care requires attention to six dimensions of health care quality: safety, effectiveness, patient-centeredness, timeliness, efficiency, and equity (IOM, 2001). However, these principles alone do not explicitly address the critical role of family members and close friends in meeting the health care and LTSS needs of the older adult population or the challenges that family caregivers face.

The committee's assessment confirms how essential family caregivers are to both health care and LTSS for older Americans. But there are other important reasons to call for a system-wide reorientation that takes into account both the individual and the family. As noted earlier, there is a growing gap between the numbers of older people in need of support and the numbers of potential family caregivers. In just 10 years (2026), the leading edge of the baby boomers will enter their 80s, placing new demands on both the health care and LTSS systems. Despite this reality, there is a significant disconnect between providers' continued reliance on family caregivers, their exclusion of family caregivers from care planning, and their lack of attention to providing meaningful caregiver supportive services. Ignoring family caregivers' presence leaves them unprepared for the tasks they may be expected to perform, carrying significant economic and personal costs, and with their own health needs unassessed and unaddressed. It may also diminish the quality of care for the care recipient.

The committee concludes that family caregiving has become a critical issue of public policy, linked to important social, health, and economic goals and essential to the growing needs of a population whose demographics foretell a new reality. The committee also concludes that the time has come for public acknowledgment of caregiving families—to make caregiving an integral part of the nation's collective responsibility for caring for its older adults. Family caregivers are the mainstay of support for older people with a chronic, disabling, or serious health condition. But in today's world, family caregivers cannot be expected to provide an array of complex care and support on their own. Family caregivers need greater recognition, information, and support to both help them care for older relatives or friends, and to maintain their own health, financial security, and well-being. If their needs are not recognized and addressed, family caregivers risk burnout from the prolonged distress and physical demands of caregiving, and the nation will bear the costs.

To that end, the committee calls for a transformation in the policies and practices affecting the role of families in the support and care of older adults. The emphasis on person-centered care needs to evolve into a focus on person- and family-centered care. The markers of a transformed system will result in a society in which family caregivers:

- Have their own health and well-being considered:
  - Health, well-being, and experiences of family caregivers are assessed and addressed.
- Have rights and protections:
  - Where family caregivers of older people have rights and protections in health care, LTSS, and in the workplace.
  - Where family caregivers have the right to up-to-date health information and support they need, when they need it.
- Have their preferences, needs, and strengths recognized and supported:
  - Where the uniqueness and diversity of families are properly recognized, and their caregiving preferences, needs, and strengths provide the foundation for care planning and services.
  - Where providers serving older people and their caregivers have the technical and communication skills and competencies to provide high-quality (best practice), culturally appropriate, person- and family-centered services.
- Are supported as caregiving changes and evolves:
  - Where federal and state governments monitor progress toward this vision and adapt policy in response to changing demographic, social, technological, and economic circumstances.

METHODS OF THE STUDY

The committee deliberated over six in-person meetings and numerous teleconferences between November 2014 and March 2016. Two in-person meetings included public workshops featuring invited speakers on relevant related topics. The first workshop focused on caregiver experiences, their interactions with the health care and LTSS systems, and relevant legal issues. The second workshop examined the implications of demographic trends on family caregiving, meeting the needs of diverse caregiver populations broadly defined to include race and ethnicity as well as rural and lesbian, gay, bisexual, and transgender (LGBT) caregiving, and a husband's experiences in caring for his wife with dementia. Appendix C contains the workshop agendas. The webcasts of these events are available on the Academies' website.[10]

Several committee workgroups were formed to review and assess the quality of the available evidence and to draft summary materials for the full committee's review. The workgroups conducted in-depth reviews of the epidemiology of caregiving; the tasks that caregivers undertake and how caregiving affects their mental and physical health; the economic impact of caregiving (overall and in the workplace); the effectiveness of programs for supporting caregivers; and caregivers' interactions with the health care and LTSS systems.

The data workgroup oversaw a commissioned analysis of the National Health and Aging Trends Study (NHATS) and its companion survey, the National Study of Caregiving (NSOC). NHATS is a longitudinal survey, funded by the National Institute on Aging, that is specifically designed to document how functioning in life changes with age (Freedman et al., 2011). It draws from a nationally representative sample of Medicare beneficiaries, age 65 and older, who live independently or in a senior community, assisted living facility, nursing home, or other organized setting (Freedman et al., 2013; Kasper and Freedman, 2014; Kasper et al., 2014). NSOC is a survey of the caregivers named by the NHATS respondents (except those living in nursing homes). The purpose of the commissioned study was to estimate the average number of years someone currently age 20 will spend during his or her lifetime as a caregiver of an older adult. The full analysis appears in Appendix D.

The committee also used the NHATS and NSOC public use files to develop tables and figures describing the characteristics of older adults who need help with living because of a health or functional limitation, the characteristics of their family caregivers, and caregivers' reports of their experiences. These tables and figures appear in Chapters 2 through 4 and are labeled to reflect the source of the data. Appendix E describes the committee's methodology for generating these tables and figures. Additional information on the public use files is available at http://www.nhats.org. Published findings from other surveys are presented throughout the report.

In its NHATS analyses, the committee distinguishes between the survey's sample of older adults who need any type of assistance because of health or functioning reasons and "high-need" older adults. In these analyses, the term "high-need" is used for individuals who have probable dementia or who need help with at least two of the following activities: bathing, dressing, eating, toileting, or getting in and out of bed. These differences are important when considering potential policies and programs.

[10] See http://www.nationalacademies.org/hmd/Activities/Aging/FamilyCaregivingforOlderAdults.aspx (accessed August 22, 2016).

For example, LTSS may target family caregivers who provide intensive care in the home or in an assisted living facility while employment-based policies may focus on employed caregivers who may or may not be providing intensive levels of care.

Challenges in Studying Family Caregiving

The depth and breadth of issues involved in family caregiving are especially complex because caregiving touches so much of life—family composition and relationships; work; gender; race, culture, and ethnicity; the health care system; LTSS; income and education; location; and many other aspects of life in contemporary America. All these factors, in turn, affect the family caregivers and the older adults for whom they are caring. Moreover, none of these societal factors are static, making it difficult for programs and research to stay current.

So much of what is known about family caregivers of older adults is derived from population-based surveys. Unfortunately, no survey, including NHATS and NSOC, has a large enough sample to assess the needs and experiences of older adults or their caregivers by all of the varied subgroups of interest across dimensions of race and ethnicity, rural residence, or sexual orientation.

The vocabulary of caregiving is also challenging. Many fundamental terms in the caregiving literature lack consistent definition. This includes not only the term "family caregiver," as noted earlier, but also the types of supports that older adults need and the activities caregivers are engaged in, the services that caregivers need, and the effects of caregiving on caregivers themselves (e.g., depression or burden). Different terms are also used to describe family caregivers who are engaged in the most intensive and time-consuming tasks or who are supporting care recipients with significant, long-term impairments.

Outside the Scope of the Study

Family caregivers are essential to the well-being of many types of people with significant care needs, whether young or old. Their needs may be acute, progressively serious, and/or lifelong. Children with chronic illness and disability are typically cared for by young adult parents; adult children with developmental disabilities or mental illness are often cared for by their middle-aged and older parents; and returning veterans with physical and cognitive disability are cared for by their spouses or other family members. The reader should note that while this report focuses on care recipients age 65 and older, many of the conclusions and recommendations presented in this report apply to all family caregivers regardless of the care recipient's age.

ORIENTATION TO THE ORGANIZATION OF THIS REPORT

Chapter Objectives

This introductory chapter has described the background, scope, methods, and committee vision for this report.

Chapter 2, *Older Adults Who Need Caregiving and the Family Caregivers Who Help Them*, reviews what is known about the number and characteristics of older adults who need help *because of health or functional limitations* and the family caregivers who help them. It also describes the demographic and other societal trends that will affect the nation's capacity to care for older adults in the future.

Chapter 3, *Family Caregiving Roles and Impacts*, examines the multiple and evolving roles of caregivers of older adults as well as the impact of assuming these roles on caregivers' health and well-being (both positive and negative). It describes caregiver tasks, the dynamic nature of caregiving over time, the increasing complexity and scope of caregiver responsibilities, and issues involved in surrogate decision making.

Chapter 4, *Economic Impact of Family Caregiving*, examines the economic impact of unpaid caregiving on family caregivers of older adults *who need help because of health or functional limitations* and explores which caregivers are at greatest risk of severe consequences. Workplace and government policies and programs designed to support caregivers and/or mitigate these effects are also discussed.

Chapter 5, *Programs and Supports for Family Caregivers of Older Adults*, reviews the evidence on the effectiveness of interventions designed to support family caregivers of older adults, including educational and skills training, environmental modifications, care management, counseling, and multicomponent models. It also examines why promising interventions have not been disseminated and adopted in everyday settings.

Chapter 6, *Family Caregivers' Interactions with Health Care and Long-Term Services and Supports*, examines caregivers' experiences in health care and social services settings as they try to fulfill their roles and responsibilities described in the previous chapters. It reviews the challenges that caregivers encounter in helping older adults obtain needed services and outlines opportunities for advancing quality care and better recognition of and support for family caregivers.

Chapter 7, *Recommendations to Support Family Caregivers of Older Adults*, presents the committee's conclusions and recommendations drawing from and summarizing the evidence presented in the previous chapters.

REFERENCES

ACL (Administration for Community Living). 2016a. *Fiscal year 2016 justification of estimates for appropriations committees.* http://www.acl.gov/About_ACL/Budget/docs/FY_2016_ACL_CJ.pdf (accessed May 19, 2016).

ACL. 2016b. *Aging integrated database: Title VI services by tribal organization.* http://www.agid.acl.gov (accessed August 22, 2016).

Alzheimer's Association. 2015. *Alzheimer's Association annual report.* https://www.alz.org/annual_report/downloads/annual-report.pdf (accessed May 19, 2016).

Apesoa-Varano, E. C., T. F. Yajarayma, S. C. Reinhard, R. Choula, and H. M. Young. 2015. Multi-cultural caregiving and caregiver interventions: A look back and a call for future action. *Generations* 39(4):39-48.

Barretto, T., R. Varghese, S. Pedersen, L. Clark-Shirley, S. Shetty, M. Roy, S. Toor, M. Siers, R. Bertrand, and L. Buatti. 2014. *National Study of Aging and Disability Resource Centers process and outcome study report.* http://www.aoa.acl.gov/Program_Results/docs/ADRCs-final-study-report.pdf (accessed May 19, 2016).

BLS (Bureau of Labor Statistics). 2015. *Economic news release. Table 6. Selected paid leave benefits: Access.* http://data.bls.gov/cgi-bin/print.pl/news.release/ebs2.t06.htm (accessed August 3, 2015).

Brody, E. M. 1966. The aging family. *The Gerontologist* 6(4):201-206.

Colello, K. J. 2007. *Family caregiving to the older population: Background, federal programs, and issues for Congress.* Washington, DC: Congressional Research Service.

CMS (Centers for Medicare & Medicaid Services). 2015. *CMS quality measure development plan: Supporting the transition to the Merit-based Incentive Payment System (MIPS) and Alternative Payment Models (APMs) (DRAFT).* https://www.cms.gov/Medicare/Quality-Initiatives-Patient-Assessment-Instruments/Value-Based-Programs/MACRA-MIPS-and-APMs/Draft-CMS-Quality-Measure-Development-Plan-MDP.pdf (accessed April 11, 2016).

CMS. 2016a. *Health care innovation awards round two.* https://innovation.cms.gov/initiatives/Health-Care-Innovation-Awards/Round-2.html (accessed August 15, 2016).

CMS. 2016b. State Innovation Models Initiative: General information. https://innovation.cms.gov/initiatives/state-innovations (accessed July 18, 2016).

CMS. 2016c. *Medicare-Medicaid Coordination Office fiscal year 2015 report to Congress.* https://www.cms.gov/Medicare-Medicaid-Coordination/Medicare-and-Medicaid-Coordination/Medicare-Medicaid-Coordination-Office/Downloads/MMCO_2015_RTC.pdf (accessed April 11, 2016).

Doty, P., and B. Spillman. 2015. Help for family caregivers available from government programs and policies. In *Family caregiving in the new normal*, edited by J. E. Gaugler and R. L. Kane. London, UK: Elsevier.

Draper, D. 2010. *Respite care: Grants and cooperative agreements awarded to implement the Lifespan Respite Care Act.* http://www.gao.gov/assets/100/97150.pdf (accessed August 15, 2016).

Dupke, N. J., K. L. Plant, and J. Kosteas. 2016. Supporting caregivers of veterans online: A partnership of the National Council on Aging and VA. *Federal Practitioner* 33(1):41-46.

Feinberg, L. 2004. *The state of the states in family caregiver support: A 50-state study.* San Francisco, CA: Family Caregiver Alliance. https://www.caregiver.org/sites/caregiver.org/files/pdfs/50_state_report_complete.pdf (accessed May 19, 2016).

Feinberg, L. F., and S. L. Newman. 2006. Preliminary experiences of the states in implementing the National Family Caregiver Support Program: A 50-state study. *Journal of Aging and Social Policy* 18(3-4):95-113.

Freedman, V. A., J. D. Kasper, J. C. Cornman, E. M. Agree, K. Bandeen-Roche, V. Mor, B. C. Spillman, R. Wallace, and D. A. Wolf. 2011. Validation of new measures of disability and functioning in the National Health and Aging Trend Study. *Journal of Gerontology* 66A(9):1013-1021.

Freedman, V. A., B. C. Spillman, P. M. Andreski, J. C. Cornman, E. M. Crimmins, E. Kramarow, J. Lubitz, L. G. Martin, S. S. Merkin, R. F. Schoeni, T. E. Seeman, and T. A. Waidmann. 2013. Trends in late-life activity limitations in the United States: An update from five national surveys. *Demography* 50(2):661-671.

FSRTC (Family Support Research & Training Center). 2016. *About the Family Support Research & Training Center.* http://fsrtc.ahslabs.uic.edu/about (accessed April 12, 2016).

Gould, E., S. Hughes, C. O'Keefe, and J. Weiner. 2014. *The Alzheimer's Disease Supportive Services Program: 2014 report on completed grants.* Washington, DC: Alzheimer's Association and RTI International. http://www.aoa.gov/AoA_Programs/HPW/ALz_Grants/docs/Closed-grant-aggregate.pdf (accessed May 19, 2016).

Grabowski, D. C., D. J. Caudry, K. M. Dean, and D. G. Stevenson. 2015. Integrated payment and delivery models offer opportunities and challenges for residential care facilities. *Health Affairs* 34(10):1650-1656.

HHS (U.S. Department of Health and Human Services). 2016. *Fiscal year 2017 justification of estimates for Appropriations Committees: Health Resources and Services Administration.* http://www.hrsa.gov/about/budget/budgetjustification2017.pdf (accessed March 7, 2016).

IOM (Institute of Medicine). 1991. *Extending life, enhancing life: A national research agenda on aging.* Washington, DC: National Academy Press.

IOM. 2001. *Crossing the quality chasm: A new health system for the 21st century.* Washington, DC: National Academy Press.

IOM. 2008. *Retooling for an aging America: Building the health care workforce.* Washington, DC: The National Academies Press.

IOM. 2012. *The mental health and substance use workforce for older adults: In whose hands?* Washington, DC: The National Academies Press.

Internal Revenue Service (IRS). 2014. *Publication 502—medical and dental expenses.* https://www.irs.gov/pub/irs-pdf/p502.pdf (accessed July 1, 2016).

IRS. 2015. *Questions and answers: Changes to the itemized deduction for 2015 medical expenses.* https://www.irs.gov/individuals/questions-and-answers-changes-to-the-itemized-deduction-for-medical-expenses (accessed August 9, 2016).

IRS. 2016. *Publication 14-B: Dependent care assistance.* https://www.irs.gov/publications/p15b/ar02.html#en_US_2016_publink1000193662 (accessed July 1, 2016).

Kabat, M. 2015. *Department of Veterans Affairs caregiver support program overview.* http://www.rosalynncarter.org/UserFiles/Kabat(1).pdf (accessed May 19, 2016).

Kasper, J. D., and V. A. Freedman. 2014. Findings from the 1st round of the National Health and Aging Trends Study (NHATS): Introduction to a special issue. *Journals of Gerontology, Series B: Psychological Sciences and Social Sciences* 69(7):S1-S7.

Kasper, J. D., V. A. Freedman, and B. Spillman. 2014. *Disability and care needs of older Americans by dementia status: An analysis of the 2011 National Health and Aging Trends Study.* http://aspe.hhs.gov/daltcp/reports/2014/NHATS-DS.pdf (accessed February 4, 2015).

Lewin Group and Administration for Community Living (ACL). 2016. *National Family Caregiver Support Program (NFCSP) process evaluation. Aging network webinar.* Paper presented at the Aging Network Webinar, March 14.

Link, G. 2015/2016. The Administration for Community Living: Programs and initiatives providing family caregiver support. *Generations* 39(4):58.

Lipson, 2015. The policy and political environment of family caregiving: A glass half full. In *Family caregiving in the new normal*, edited by J. E. Gaugler and R. L. Kane. London, UK: Elsevier.

Medicare Payment Advisory Commission (MedPAC). 2015. *The next generation of Medicare beneficiaries.* http://www.medpac.gov/documents/reports/chapter-2-the-next-generation-of-medicare-beneficiaries-(june-2015-report).pdf?sfvrsn=0 (accessed October 16, 2015).

Napili, A., and K. J. Colello. 2013. *Funding for the Older Americans Act and other aging services programs.* Washington, DC: Congressional Research Service.

National Association of Area Agencies on Aging. 2014. *2014 Eldercare Locator data report.* http://www.eldercare.gov/Eldercare.NET/Public/About/docs/data-report-locator-2015-06-29.pdf (accessed May 20, 2016).

National Association of Area Agencies on Aging, 2016. *Area Agencies on Aging: Local leaders in aging and community living.* Washington, DC. http://www.n4a.org/files/LocalLeaders AAA.pdf (accessed May 16, 2016).

National Association of States United for Aging and Disabilities. 2016. *About state agencies.* http://www.nasuad.org/about-nasuad/about-state-agencies (accessed May 16, 2016).

NQF (National Quality Forum). 2016. *CMS issues framework for future clinician-based quality measures.* http://www.qualityforum.org/CMS_Issues_Framework_for_Clinician-Based_Quality_Measures.aspx (accessed April 11, 2016).

NRC (National Research Council). 1988. *The aging population in the twenty-first century: Statistics for health policy.* Washington, DC: National Academy Press.

NRC. 1994. *Demography of aging.* Washington, DC: National Academy Press.

NRC. 2003. *Elder mistreatment: Abuse, neglect, and exploitation in an aging America.* Washington, DC: The National Academies Press.

NRC. 2012. *Aging and the macroeconomy: Long-term implications of an older population.* Washington, DC: The National Academies Press.

O'Shaughnessy, C. V. 2013. *Family caregivers: The primary providers of assistance to people with functional limitations and chronic impairments.* http://www.nhpf.org/library/background-papers/BP84_FamilyCaregiving_01-11-13.pdf (accessed February 5, 2015).

Ramchand, R., T. Tanielian, M. P. Fisher, C. A. Vaughan, T. E. Trail, and C. Epley. 2014. *Hidden heroes: America's military caregivers.* Santa Monica, CA: RAND Corporation.

VA (U.S. Department of Veterans Affairs). 2015a. *Medical programs and information technology programs congressional submission FY 2016 and FY 2017 advance appropriations.* http://www.va.gov/budget/docs/summary/Fy2017-VolumeII-MedicalProgramsAnd InformationTechnology.pdf (accessed May 20, 2016).

VA. 2015b. *VA caregiver support.* http://www.caregiver.va.gov/support/support_services.asp (accessed March 1, 2016).

VA. 2016a. *Geriatrics and Extended Care (GEC). GEC data reports.* http://www.va.gov/Geriatrics/GEC_Data_Reports.asp (accessed March 2, 2016).

VA. 2016b (unpublished). *GEC number of veterans served from VHA Service Support Center (VSSC), Non-Institutional Care Workload Reports. VHA intranet.*

VA. 2016c. *GEC expenditures from FY 2017 congressional budget submission. Link to volume II, medical care.* http://www.va.gov/budget/docs/summary/FY2017-VolumeII-MedicalProgramsAndInformationTechnology.pdf (accessed March 26, 2016).

Wright, P., C. Malcolm, B. Hicken, and R. Rupper. 2015. The VA Caregiver Support Line: A gateway of support for caregivers of veterans. *Journal of Gerontological Social Work* 58(4):386-398.

2

Older Adults Who Need Caregiving and the Family Caregivers Who Help Them

ABSTRACT: This chapter sets the stage for the remainder of the report and has two principal objectives. The first is to describe the older adult population with care needs because of health or functional limitations and the family caregivers who help them. The second is to review demographic and societal trends affecting the demand for and supply of family caregivers, including the marked growth in and aging of the older adult population; the increasing diversity of the older adult population; the changing nature of family relationships; women's growing participation in the workforce; and the declining size of American families.

Chapter 1 noted that millions of Americans in every walk of life are engaged in or affected by family caregiving for older adults. The faces and experiences of these individuals and the older adults they care for are as varied as the nation's population. American families are more diverse—ethnically, racially, economically, religiously, and in many other ways—than ever. So are their living arrangements and basic notions of what constitutes family. As the previous chapter reported, the committee approached its assessment of family caregiving with the view that family caregivers of older adults may be relatives, partners, friends, or neighbors whose caregiving is driven primarily by a personal relationship.

This chapter sets the stage for the remainder of the report by describing the estimated number and characteristics of older adults who need help with self-care, mobility, or household activities for health or functioning reasons, and the family caregivers who help them. It also reviews the demographic and other societal trends that will affect the nation's capacity to care for older adults in the future.

PREVALENCE OF THE NEED FOR A CAREGIVER

The need for help with everyday activities is not an inevitable consequence of aging (Feder, 2015; He and Larsen, 2014; NRC, 2012; Stone, 2015). Limitations in physical health and functioning, mental health, and/or cognitive functioning—not age—are the primary reasons why older adults need help from others. Living longer, however, often means living with impairments that may affect one's ability to perform daily activities. As people age, they are increasingly likely to develop a physical or cognitive impairment that impacts their ability to function independently (Adams et al., 2013; Anderson, 2010; CMS, 2012; Wolff and Jacobs, 2015). Between ages 85 and 89 years, for example, more than half of older adults (58.5 percent) receive a family caregiver's help because of health problems or functional limitations (Freedman and Spillman, 2014a). From age 90 years and onward, only a minority of individuals (24 percent) do *not* need some help from others.

Whether rates of disability among older adults will increase significantly in the future is uncertain. Although the prevalence of major chronic diseases—including cancer, diabetes, heart disease, hypertension, lung disease, and stroke—are expected to increase among older adults (Gaudette et al., 2015), research suggests that future disability rates may not (NIH, 2010). Numerous factors may lead to declines in disability including, for example, improvements in medical treatments, increases in health-improving behaviors, improvements in socioeconomic and education levels, as well as increased use of assistive technologies. Future research may also bring new therapies that can prevent or minimize disability from stroke, diabetes, and other conditions.

Understanding the Available Data

Examining the prevalence and nature of family caregiving of older adults is challenging because researchers use different assumptions and survey methods for identifying the older adults who need help and who their caregivers are. Estimates of the need for caregiving, for example, are highly sensitive to how disability is defined. A definition that includes older adults who need help with household activities will generate significantly larger estimates than one that is based on needs for help with self-care (Freedman and Spillman, 2014a). Surveys with long reference periods (e.g., 1 year) will generate larger estimates than surveys with short reference periods (e.g.,

1 month) because they are more likely to include individuals who have short-term, intensive needs during, for example, an acute illness or injury (Giovannetti and Wolff, 2010).

Due to resource constraints, all the surveys that are relevant to family caregiving are limited in size, which in turn limits subgroup analyses. No current survey has sufficient power to assess the needs and experiences of older adults and their caregivers by all of the varied subgroups of interest, including those defined by race and ethnicity, rural residence, or sexual orientation. It is also important to recognize that while data are available on older adults who need but do not have a family caregiver, it has not been analyzed. About 20 percent of the National Health and Aging Trends Study (NHATS) respondents report receiving no help despite having difficulty with self-care, mobility, or household activities. They are able to remain independent by using assistive devices, paid help, and/or restricting their activities. Comparisons between these individuals and older adults who receive help are not available (Freedman and Spillman, 2014a; Freedman et al., 2014).

Disability surveys typically identify older adults with functional limitations by asking respondents (or their proxies) about their ability, difficulty, or need for assistance in taking care of themselves. But no two surveys ask about the limitations in precisely the same way. The most common questions focus on self-care activities (often referred to as activities of daily living or ADLs) such as bathing, eating, dressing, and toileting; transferring (getting in and out of bed); mobility (getting around inside or outside one's home or building); and household activities (instrumental activities of daily living or IADLs) such as using the telephone, taking medications, managing money, doing housework and laundry, preparing meals, and shopping for groceries.[1]

Although difficulty performing household activities creates a need for assistance from others, difficulty with self-care suggests a need for more intensive help.

National Health and Aging Trends Study and the National Survey of Caregivers

The prevalence data presented in this chapter (and throughout this report) are derived primarily from NHATS and its companion National Study of Caregiving (NSOC). The federally-funded NHATS, a longitudinal survey first fielded in 2011, was specifically designed to document how functioning in daily life changes with age (Freedman et al., 2011). It draws

[1] Although ADLs and IADLs are commonly used to characterize levels of disability, neither is consistently defined in the literature.

from a nationally representative sample of Medicare beneficiaries (age 65 and older) in the continental United States who live independently or in a senior community, assisted living facility, nursing home, or other residential setting (Freedman et al., 2013; Kasper et al., 2014). NHATS employs a disability measurement protocol that includes activities characteristic of the traditional ADL and IADL measures as well as other contributing aspects of disability, such as physical, sensory, and cognitive capacity; the ability to carry out essential activities independently; and participation and restrictions in valued activities (Freedman et al., 2011). It also uses a protocol that has been assessed for sensitivity and specificity for identifying care recipients who have "probable dementia" relative to an actual diagnosis of dementia (Kasper et al., 2013, 2014).[2]

NSOC is a survey of the family and other unpaid caregivers named by NHATS respondents who reported receiving help for health or functioning reasons. NHATS asks older adults to name all the people who helped them; most identified only one person. NSOC estimates, which are reviewed later in the chapter, do not include family caregivers of nursing home residents. Thus, population-based estimates on the number of family caregivers assisting older adults in nursing homes are not available. It is not possible to use NSOC data to estimate the number of caregivers who are helping more than one older adult (e.g., an adult child caring for two parents with impairments). See Appendix E for a description of the committee's analyses of NHATS and NSOC.

What Kind of Assistance Do Older Adults Need?

Figure 2-1 provides an overall picture of the number and proportion of older adults who receive help. In 2011, the majority of older adults (71 percent) did not receive assistance for health or functioning reasons (Freedman and Spillman, 2014b). However, 17 percent or 6.3 million older adults received help with household tasks or self-care (defined here as bathing, dressing, eating, toileting, or mobility) due to health or functioning limitations other than dementia, while another 9 percent or 3.5 million older adults received help because they had dementia. Three percent (1.1 million) resided in a nursing home. Chapter 3 describes the full range of supports that family caregivers provide to older adults, including emotional support, help with medical/nursing tasks, and care coordination.

---

[2] NHATS respondents were considered to have "probable dementia," which includes individuals whose doctor said they had dementia or Alzheimer's disease and individuals classified as having probable dementia based on results from a proxy screening instrument and several cognitive tests. For details on the NHATS dementia protocol, see Kasper et al., 2013.

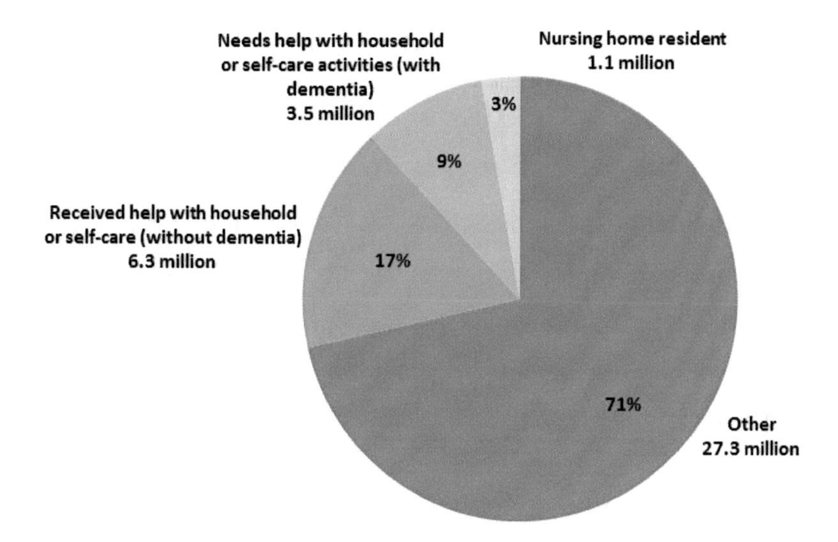

FIGURE 2-1 Number and percentage of older adults receiving assistance in the prior month by level of assistance, 2011.
NOTES: As reported by Medicare beneficiaries age 65 and older (or their proxy). Household help includes assistance (for health or functioning reasons only) with laundry, hot meals, shopping for personal items, paying bills/banking, and/or handling medications. "Self-care" refers to bathing, dressing, eating, toileting, or getting in and out of bed. "Other" refers primarily to individuals who receive no help, but also includes persons who may have had help with household activities from someone for reasons other than health or functioning.
SOURCE: Data from the 2011 NHATS.

Figure 2-2 further illustrates the huge impact of dementia on caregiving needs. Of the 4.9 million older adults who received help with self-care, 3.5 million (71.4 percent) were classified as having probable dementia. People with more advanced dementia may require constant supervision to protect themselves and others from harm—even if they are able to perform some self-care or household tasks. Individuals in the early stages of dementia may also require support, including assistance with paying bills, personal care, mobility tasks, and surrogacy (Black et al., 2013). With disease progression, people with dementia also experience a wide range of co-morbidities, including vision, hearing, and mobility limitations.

An important note is that estimates of average need, such as those in Figure 2-1 and Figure 2-2, mask substantial variation in the amount of time older adults need help due to an impairment. In a recent microsimulation, for example, Favreault and Dey (2016) projected the distribution in the

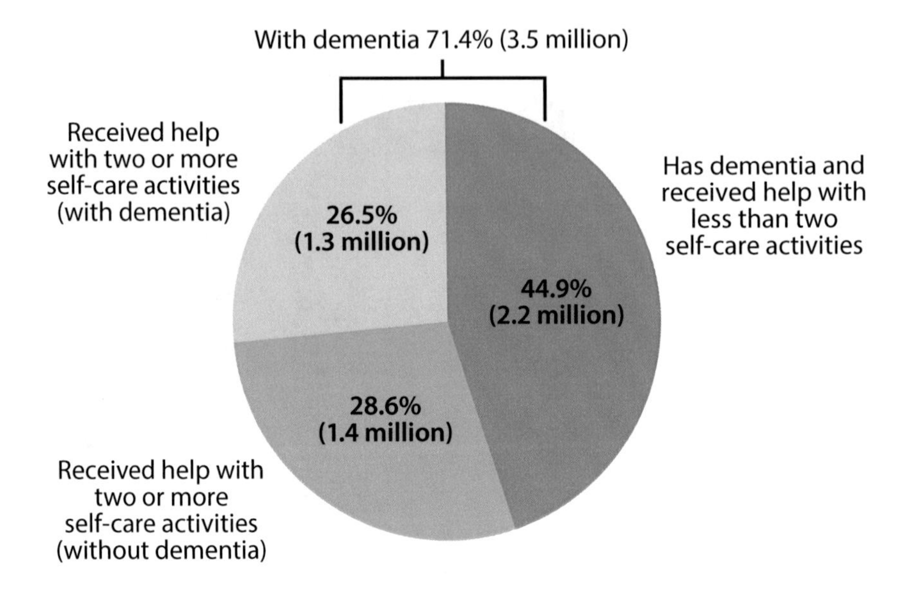

FIGURE 2-2 High-need older adults, by dementia status and self-care needs, 2011.
NOTES: As reported by Medicare beneficiaries age 65 and older (or their proxy) for the prior month. Self-care activities include bathing, dressing, eating, toileting, or getting in and out of bed. "Probable dementia" includes individuals whose doctor said they had dementia or Alzheimer's disease and individuals classified as having probable dementia based on results from a proxy screening instrument and several cognitive tests. Excludes nursing home residents.
SOURCE: Data from the 2011 NHATS.

number of years that an older adult could anticipate needing long-term services and supports (LTSS) (see Table 2-1). They estimated that upon turning age 65, more than half of individuals (52.3 percent) can expect some period of time when they will need help with at least two ADLs (i.e., eating, toileting, transferring, bathing, dressing, or continence) for at least 90 days or need supervision for health and safety threats due to severe cognitive impairment. However, the duration of such need is quite variable, less than 1 year for 18.9 percent of people and more than 5 years for 13.9 percent of people. The simulation also estimated substantial differences in need between men and women. Women (17.8 percent) are much more likely than men (9.8 percent) to need LTSS for 5 years or more.

TABLE 2-1 Projected Future Need for Long-Term Services and Supports at Age 65 in 2015-2019, by Gender

Number of Years Disabled	All (Percentage)	Men (Percentage)	Women (Percentage)
None	47.7	53.3	42.5
Less than 1 year	18.9	18.4	19.4
1-1.99 years	7.8	7.4	8.1
2-4.99 years	11.7	11.1	12.3
More than 5 years	13.9	9.8	17.8

NOTES: Includes persons needing assistance (including nursing home residents) with at least two activities of daily living (i.e., eating, toileting, transferring, bathing, dressing, or continence) for at least 90 days or needing supervision for health and safety threats due to severe cognitive impairment. Percentages may not total to 100 due to rounding.
SOURCE: Favreault and Dey, 2016.

WHO ARE THE FAMILY CAREGIVERS OF OLDER ADULTS?

The committee examined two subgroups of family caregivers: those who help an older adult with any need (see Figure 2-1) because of health or functioning reasons and those caregivers who help "high-need" older adults (see Figure 2-2 and Table 2-2). "High-need" is used to describe individuals with probable dementia or who need help with at least two self-care activities (i.e., bathing, dressing, eating, toileting, or getting in and out of bed).

According to NSOC, 17.7 million individuals were caregivers of an older adult in 2011 because of health or functioning reasons or approximately 7.7 percent of the total U.S. population age 20 and older (see Table 2-2). Nearly half of those caregivers (8.5 million) provided care to a high-need older adult. This estimate does not include caregivers of nursing home residents, and comparable information about the number of family caregivers assisting older adults in nursing homes is not available.

For most family caregivers, caregiving is not a short-term obligation. Only 15 percent of NSOC caregivers had provided care for 1 year or less at the time of the survey whereas nearly 70 percent were caregiving for 2 to 10 years, and 15 percent had already provided care for more than 10 years by the time of the survey (see Table 2-3). The median number of years of family care for older adults with high needs was 5 years.[3] This is an important finding because, as discussed in Chapter 3 and Chapter 4, family caregivers are more likely to suffer negative consequences (e.g.,

[3] Committee NSOC calculations.

TABLE 2-2 Family Caregivers of Older Adults, Number and Percentage by Care Recipient's Level of Need, 2011

Care Recipient's Level of Need	Number of Caregivers	Percentage of Adults Age 20+
Any need in mobility, self-care, or household activities due to health or functioning limitations	17.7 million	7.7
High-need: care recipient has probable dementia and/or needs assistance with two or more self-care activities	8.5 million	3.7

NOTES: Includes family caregivers of Medicare beneficiaries age 65 and older in the continental United States who resided in community or residential care settings (other than nursing homes) and received help with self-care, mobility, or household activities for health or functioning reasons. "Self-care" refers to bathing, dressing, eating, toileting, or getting in and out of bed. "Probable dementia" includes individuals whose doctor said they had dementia or Alzheimer's disease and individuals classified as having probable dementia based on results from a proxy screening instrument and several cognitive tests.
SOURCES: Data from the 2011 NHATS and the companion NSOC.

TABLE 2-3 Average Number of Years That Caregivers of Older Adults Spent Caregiving at the Time of the Survey

Average Number of Years	Percentage
1 year or less	15.3
2 to 4 years	34.7
5 to 10 years	34.9
More than 10 years	15.1

NOTES: Includes family caregivers of Medicare beneficiaries age 65 and older in the continental United States who resided in community or residential care settings (other than nursing homes) and received help with self-care, mobility, or household activities for health or functioning reasons. Respondents were asked "How many years have you been helping the care recipient?" Responses were given in whole numbers.
SOURCES: Data from the 2011 NHATS and the companion NSOC.

anxiety, depression, social isolation, and financial losses) the longer they are engaged in caregiving.

Some researchers distinguish between primary caregivers—individuals who self-identify as having primary responsibility for providing care and/or who spend the most time providing care—from secondary caregivers—individuals who provide intermittent supplementary or complementary help to the care recipient. Spouses and daughters are more likely to be primary caregivers and men and non-relatives are more likely to play a secondary caregiving role. Primary caregivers typically provide many more hours of care than secondary caregivers and make the majority of decisions regarding care provision to the care recipient (Chadiha et al., 2011; Tennstedt et al., 1989). Although it is widely recognized that caregiving may be distributed among multiple family members and friends, relatively little is known about the number of caregivers who play a secondary role, the types and amount of help they provide, and the extent to which relationships between primary and secondary caregivers are supportive or conflictual.

Anticipating Future Years as a Caregiver of an Older Adult

Adults may be called on to provide care to an older adult more than once in their lifetime. Young adults, for example, may participate in the care of their grandparents; adults in their 50s and 60s may care for one or both parents, parents-in-law, a spouse/partner, other relatives, or friends; and older adults may provide care to spouses, siblings, or friends and neighbors. The committee could not find published estimates of the likelihood of becoming a caregiver over a lifetime or for how long. To consider the latter question, the committee commissioned an analysis, by Vicki A. Freedman, Ph.D., to estimate the average number of years and percentage of remaining life that U.S. adults might expect to spend caring for an older adult who needs help with activities of daily living. Table 2-4 presents the key findings in this analysis. Appendix D contains the complete analysis and describes the methodology in detail.

Freedman's analysis drew from the 2011 Current Population Survey, life tables from the National Center for Health Statistics, and the 2011 NSOC and NHATS datasets to develop assumptions about future prevalence of disability, numbers of available caregivers, and mortality rates. The analysis assumed that current age-specific caregiving rates (based on NSOC data) and life expectancy (based on the life tables) would not change over the life of the hypothetical cohort. These assumptions—unavoidable because of the available data and time to conduct the analysis—are an important limitation of the analysis. Actual caregiving rates in the future may differ and will depend on numerous factors that are difficult to predict, such as rates of late-life disability, family size and composition, competing demands from work and family, the availability and affordability of paid caregivers, new technologies, and cultural norms (Kaye, 2013; Marks, 1996; Stone, 2015). Future mortality rates are similarly uncertain, reflecting demographers' differing views about future life expectancy (Social Security Trustees Report, 2015).

Another important note is that because these are estimates of an average for the overall adult population, they do not convey the considerable

TABLE 2-4 Estimated Average Number of Years and Percentage of Remaining Life Caring for an Older Adult, by Age Group

	Older Adults with One or More Activity Limitations						High-Need Older Adults	
	All Family Caregivers		Men		Women		All Family Caregivers	
Age Group	Average Number of Years Spent Caregiving	Percentage of Remaining Life	Average Number of Years Spent Caregiving	Percentage of Remaining Life	Average Number of Years Spent Caregiving	Percentage of Remaining Life	Average Number of Years Spent Caregiving	Percentage of Remaining Life
20-29	5.1	8.6	4.1	7.2	6.1	9.9	2.4	4.1
30-39	5.0	10.0	4.0	8.4	6.0	11.5	2.4	4.7
40-49	4.8	11.9	3.9	10.1	5.7	13.4	2.3	5.6
50-59	4.2	13.5	3.5	11.9	4.9	14.9	2.0	6.2
60-69	3.3	14.4	2.9	13.8	3.7	15.0	1.5	6.5
70-79	2.2	14.1	2.2	15.8	2.1	12.8	0.9	6.0
80+	1.0	11.5	1.3	15.7	0.8	8.8	0.5	6.1

NOTE: Estimates are averages that include people who never become caregivers, but exclude people who assist older adults who reside in nursing homes. Family caregivers are adults age 20 or older who assist an older adult who needs help because of health or functioning reasons. High-need older adults have probable dementia or need help with at least two self-care activities (bathing, dressing, eating, toileting, or getting in and out of bed). Excludes caregivers of nursing home residents.
SOURCE: Freedman, 2015 (see Appendix D).

variation in individual caregiving experiences. The average duration of caregiving is based on the experiences of individuals who will never be a caregiver and as well as individuals who will be a caregiver for many years, even decades. Estimates of the variation of lifetime caregiving as well as the proportion of people who never become caregivers unfortunately do not exist; however, other available evidence suggests that the variation is substantial (Miyawaki, 2016).

Table 2-4 provides Freedman's projections for U.S. adults in different age groups for two levels of need for caregiving: first, caring for older adults who need any help because of health or functioning reasons and, second, caring for high-need older adults (as defined by the committee above). The analysis estimates that adults in their 20s will, on average, spend 5.1 years—or 8.6 percent of their remaining lifetime—caring for an older adult with at least one activity limitation. Nearly half of these caregiving years (2.4 years) are estimated to be spent providing care to a high-need older adult. These estimates are averages that include those who will never become caregivers as well as those who will provide care—to one or more older adults and in varying durations. The average number of years spent caregiving by those who do become caregivers, of course, is higher than the overall average, but the methods used here cannot estimate that magnitude.

Women are estimated to spend more years caregiving than men—on average 6.1 years or nearly 10 percent of their adult life—whereas men are estimated to spend on average 4.1 years or just more than 7 percent of their adult life. The percentage of remaining life to be spent providing care peaks at different ages for men and women. For men, once they reach age 70, nearly 16 percent of their remaining lifetime—or 1 to 2 years—is spent caring for an older adult. For women, this figure peaks between ages 50 and 69, when about 15 percent of their remaining lifetime—or about 4 to 5 years—is spent caring.

Characteristics of Family Caregivers of Older Adults[4]

Tables 2-5 and 2-6 describe an array of factors that characterize the population of family caregivers helping older adults. Although caregiver surveys often produce differing estimates of the size of the caregiver population, national surveys consistently show that caregivers are predominantly middle-aged daughters or spouses (Johnson and Wiener, 2006; Spillman and Pezzin, 2000; Wolff and Kasper, 2006). Women have always made up

[4] This section draws primarily from the 2011 NSOC. As noted earlier, the family caregivers included in NSOC data are caregivers of Medicare beneficiaries age 65 and older in the continental United States who need help due to health or functioning. Caregivers of nursing home residents are excluded.

TABLE 2-5 Selected Demographic Characteristics of Family Caregivers, High-Need Family Caregivers, and the Overall U.S. Adult Population, by Percentage, 2011

Characteristic	Family Caregivers (percentage)	High-Need Caregivers (percentage)	U.S. Adults (percentage)
Age			
20-44	14.7	15.6	33.6
45-54	23.7	23.4	14.3
55-64	26.8	28.4	12.2
65-74	18.9	16.3	7.2
75+	13.4	13.0	6.1
Gender			
Male	38.3	36.2	48.5
Female	61.7	63.8	51.5
Race/ethnicity			
White, non-Hispanic	70.9	66.4	67.0
Black, non-Hispanic	12.6	12.4	12.0
Other, non-Hispanic	4.8	5.7	6.0
Hispanic	11.6	15.2	15.0
Education			
Less than high school	12.9	13.1	14.1
High school graduate or equivalent	25.5	24.8	28.4
More than high school/less than bachelor's degree	33.2	35.4	29.0
Bachelor's degree or higher	26.9	24.9	28.5

NOTES: Includes family caregivers of Medicare beneficiaries age 65 and older in the continental United States who resided in community or residential care settings (other than nursing homes) and received help with self-care, mobility, or household activities for health or functioning reasons. "High-need" refers to caregivers of older adults who have probable dementia or need assistance with two or more self-care activities (bathing, dressing, eating, toileting, or getting in and out of bed). Percentages are for adults age 20 and older except for race/ethnicity of the overall U.S. population (18 and older) and the education level of the overall U.S. population (25 and older). Percentages for caregivers may not total 100 due to missing data.
SOURCES: Family caregiver data, 2011 NHATS/NSOC; overall U.S. data, Kids Count Data Center, 2015; and U.S. Census Bureau, 2016a,b.

the majority of the nation's caregivers (NAC and AARP Public Policy Institute, 1997, 2004, 2009, 2015a; Penrod et al., 1995; Pinquart and Sörensen, 2006; Yee and Schulz, 2000), although some evidence shows that men are assuming increasing roles in caregiving (NAC and AARP Public Policy Institute, 2015a; Spillman et al., 2000), especially in the lesbian, gay, bisexual, and transgender (LGBT) community (Grossman et al., 2007; Hughes and

Kentlyn, 2011). In 2011, roughly 62 percent of NSOC caregivers were female (see Table 2-5) and more than one-third were daughters, daughters-in-law, or stepdaughters of the care recipient (see Table 2-6). Those three groups may play an even greater role in caring for high-need individuals; 38 percent of family caregivers for high-need older adults were daughters, daughters-in-law, or stepdaughters compared to 33.6 percent of all caregivers. Women also make up a majority of NSOC care recipients, as 70 percent of both all-need and high-need NSOC care recipients were female. Half of the NSOC caregivers were between the ages of 45 and 64 (50.5 percent), but nearly one-third (32.3 percent) were older adults themselves.

Caregivers' family ties to care recipients are an important policy consideration because the nature of these relationships can determine the caregiver's access to family and medical leave or paid sick days to care for a seriously ill relative or access to their health information. For example, in most states the Family and Medical Leave Act (FMLA) pertains only to workers caring for spouses, domestic partners, children, and parents (Mayer, 2013)—omitting nearly one in four caregivers (23.7 percent) and

TABLE 2-6 Family Relationships of Caregivers of Older Adults, by Care Recipient's Level of Need, by Percentage, 2011

Family Relationship	All Caregivers (percentage)	High-Need Caregivers (percentage)
Relationship to recipient		
Spouse	21.5	18.1
Daughter, daughter-in-law, stepdaughter	33.6	38.0
Son, son-in-law, stepson	21.2	21.8
Other	23.7	22.1
Marital status		
Married/partnered	66.6	66.1
Separated/divorced	11.6	12.0
Widowed	5.9	6.0
Never married	14.3	13.7
Lives with the care recipient		
Yes	43.8	42.2
Children younger than 18		
None	82.9	81.0
Any	15.7	17.1

NOTES: Includes family caregivers of Medicare beneficiaries age 65 and older in the continental United States who resided in community or residential care settings (other than nursing homes) and received help with self-care, mobility, or household activities for health or functioning reasons. "High-need" refers to caregivers of older adults who have probable dementia or need assistance with two or more self-care activities (bathing, dressing, eating, toileting, or getting in and out of bed). Percentages may not total 100 due to missing data.
SOURCES: Data from the 2011 NHATS and the companion NSOC.

likely many others because stepchildren and sons- and daughters-in-law are not eligible for FMLA benefits (see Table 2-6).[5,6] Half of the NSOC caregivers (50.3 percent) were employed.

Same-generation caregivers (usually an older adult's spouse) have different physical and cognitive capabilities and commitment to caregiving than next-generation caregivers (usually an older adult's children). Because same-generation caregivers of older adults are older than next-generation caregivers, they are at a higher risk of age-related physical and cognitive declines including chronic illness and some level of disability. Same-generation caregivers are also more likely to feel that caregiving is an obligation. A recent study found that 60 percent of spousal caregivers reported having no choice in taking on the caregiving role while 51 percent of adult children reported having no choice (Schulz et al., 2012).

Concern is growing about the impact of caregiving on those who live far from care recipients because of the expense of travel, difficulties in communication about care recipients' health and LTSS needs, and other logistical challenges in meeting someone's needs from a distance (Bevan et al., 2012; Cagle and Munn, 2012; Wolf and Longino, 2005). Nevertheless, evidence suggests that most family caregivers live near the care recipient if they do not live together (Johnson and Wiener, 2006; NAC and AARP Public Policy Institute, 2015b; Spillman and Pezzin, 2000; Wolff and Kasper, 2006). A large proportion of NSOC respondents (43.8 percent) live with the care recipient (also known as co-residents), including high-need individuals (see Table 2-6). This is an important group because, as Chapter 3 will discuss, co-resident caregivers are at increased risk of adverse physical and psychological outcomes (Monin and Schulz, 2009; Schulz et al., 2007, 2009). Spouses who are caregivers of older adults are especially vulnerable to such adverse outcomes (Capistrant et al., 2012; Dassel and Carr, 2014; Ji et al., 2012; Schulz et al., 2009). More than one in five (21.5 percent) NSOC caregivers were spouses.

The racial and ethnic makeup of the caregiver population in 2011 largely reflected the overall U.S. population, including the racial and ethnic makeup of the high-need caregiver group (see Table 2-5). One important gap in nationally representative survey data, such as NSOC, is the incompleteness of data about the prevalence and characteristics among diverse subgroups of caregivers. Data from non-representative samples suggests that important differences may exist. For example, a meta-analysis of 116

[5] FMLA requires certain employers to provide job-protected, unpaid leave to employees caring for certain seriously ill family members. See Chapter 4 for a review of FMLA and other workplace issues affecting family caregivers.

[6] The number of caregivers who are stepchildren or in-laws of care recipients cannot be calculated from NSOC data.

caregiving studies in the gerontological literature found that multicultural caregivers were more likely to be younger, non-spouses and to be less well-off economically compared with white non-Hispanic caregivers, though the effect sizes were modest (Pinquart and Sörensen, 2005). Trends in the racial and ethnic makeup of the United States are reviewed below.

SOCIAL AND DEMOGRAPHIC TRENDS AFFECTING CAREGIVING

A number of current and future social and demographic trends will likely affect both the need for eldercare and the availability of potential family caregivers for older adults in the future. In 2012, 43.1 million or 13.7 percent of U.S. residents were age 65 and older (see Table 2-7). At

TABLE 2-7 Age, Race, and Hispanic Origin of the Older Adult Population, by Number and Percentage, 2012

	Number (in 1,000s)	Percentage of U.S. Population
Total U.S. population	313,914	100.0
65+	43,145	13.7
Age cohorts		Percentage of 65+ population
65-69	13,977	32.4
70-74	10,008	23.2
75-79	7,490	17.4
80-84	5,783	13.4
85+	5,887	13.6
Race		
White	37,095	86.0
Black	3,781	8.8
American Indian or Alaska Native	266	.6
Asian	1,628	3.8
Pacific Islander	42	.1
Two or more races	333	.8
Hispanic origin		
Hispanic	3,144	7.3
Non-Hispanic	40,002	92.7

NOTE: The above U.S. Census racial categories are defined as white (with origins in Europe, the Middle East, or North Africa), Black or African American (with origins in the black racial groups of Africa), Asian (with origins in the Far East, Southeast Asia, or the Indian subcontinent), Native Hawaiian or other Pacific Islander, American Indians or Alaska Natives, and "some other race."
SOURCE: Ortman et al., 2014.

that time, 86 percent of the older adult population was white; 8.8 percent, African American; 7.3 percent, of Hispanic origin (any race); 3.8 percent, Asian; and 1.5 percent, others (American Indian, Alaska Native, Pacific Islander, or multiracial). This one-time snapshot, however, belies an older population that is rapidly changing not only in numbers and racial and ethnic makeup, but in numerous other ways. The nation is in the midst of historic demographic change that has substantial implications for older adults and their families, providers of health care services and LTSS, the national economy, and society overall (Colby and Ortman, 2014; Frey, 2014; IOM, 2008; Mather et al., 2015; NRC, 2012). These trends, described below, make clear that in the future, if not now, the older adult population needing help is likely to exceed the capacity of family caregivers to provide it. The effects of these unprecedented demographic trends will depend, in part, on the actions that public and private decision makers take in the coming years to lessen the strain on the daily lives of caregiving families.

Rapidly Increasing Numbers Especially Among the Oldest Old

Much has been written about the aging of the baby boomer population (Colby and Ortman, 2014; IOM, 2008; Frey, 2014; Mather et al., 2015). According to the U.S. Census, by 2030—just 14 years after the publication of this report—more than one in five of U.S. residents will be age 65 or older (see Figure 2-3) (Ortman et al., 2014). This represents a 40.7 percent increase in the size of the older population between 2012 and 2030. By contrast, the overall U.S. population is expected to grow only 12.4 percent—from 313.9 million to 358.5 million—during the same time period.

The dramatic rise in the total number of older Americans is not due solely to the increasing numbers of baby boomers turning 65. Older adults—whether male or female, white or African American, Hispanic or non-Hispanic—are expected to live increasingly longer lives in future decades (Ortman et al., 2014). With increasing life spans and the growing older adult boomer population, the U.S. Census Bureau projects significant growth in the number of the oldest of the older age groups. For example, the projection for 2030 is that more than 19 million U.S. residents will be age 80 or older; by 2050, this population is forecast to grow to more than 30 million (Ortman et al., 2014). The impact of the age distribution of the older adult population on the need for family caregiving is likely to be substantial. The number of individuals most likely to need intensive support from family caregivers—people in their 80s and beyond—is growing the fastest among the older age cohorts. From 2012 to 2050, the proportion of the U.S. older adult population, age 80 and older, is projected to climb from 27 to 37 percent (Ortman et al., 2014).

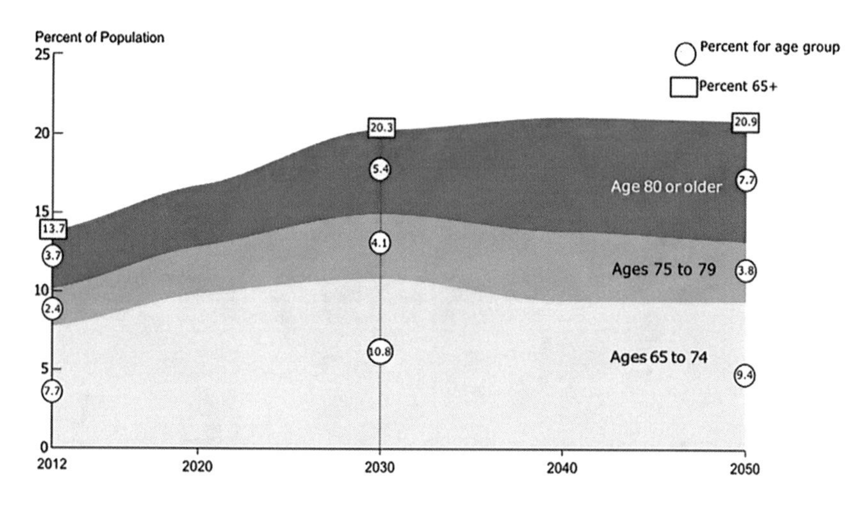

FIGURE 2-3 Older adults as a share of the U.S. population by percentage, 2012 to 2050.
SOURCE: Data drawn from Ortman et al., 2014.

Increasing Diversity

The U.S. population is becoming older, and while non-Hispanic whites today remain the largest single group of older adults, the nation is experiencing a historic shift in the diversity of older racial and ethnic groups (Frey, 2014). Sometime after 2040, no racial or ethnic group will make up the majority of the U.S. population (Frey, 2014). These changes will bring an evolution in the values, preferences, and meanings that individuals bring to family caregiving. Over the coming decades, America's Hispanic, Asian, and multiracial populations are each expected to more than double in number. Figure 2-4 illustrates the impact of this trend on the makeup of the population older than 65. In 2030, 20.2 million of the 72.8 million older Americans will identify as a member of a minority group. The older Hispanic population is growing faster than any other older age group. In 2030, there will be more than 8 million older Hispanic adults—nearly triple the number 30 years earlier and surpassing the number of African American older adults (7.5 million) (PRB, 2013). During the same period, the number of older, non-Hispanic Asians is forecast to increase from 1.5 million to 3.5 million. By the year 2060, 56 percent of adults ages 65 and older are expected to be non-Hispanic whites (U.S. Census Bureau, 2012).

The literature on caregiving across sexual minorities is sparse. What

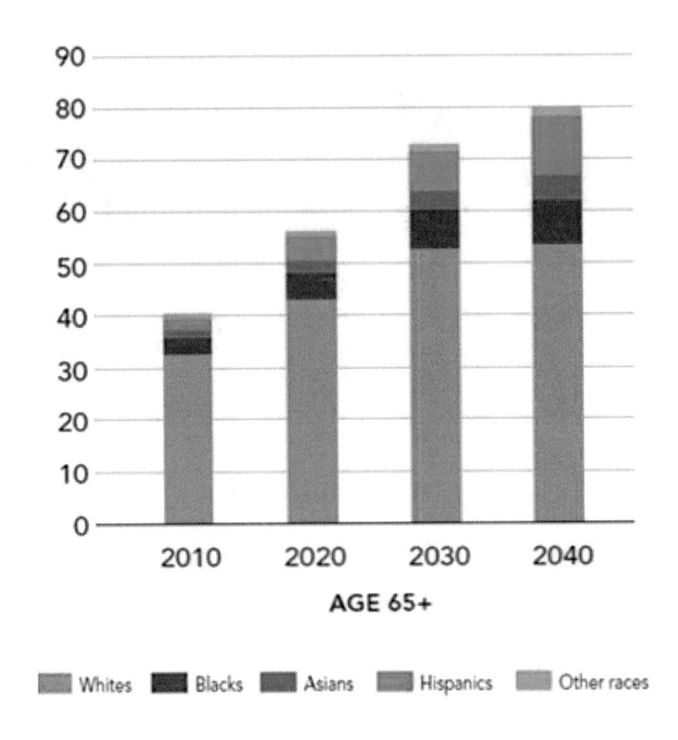

FIGURE 2-4 The changing racial and ethnic diversity of the older adult population, 2010 to 2040 (in millions).
SOURCE: Adapted from Frey, 2014 (Figure 1.3).

does exist indicates that the caregiving experience for persons who identify with the LGBT community is similar to non-LGBT persons. LGBT individuals are more likely to provide care, or receive care, for or from a non-relative than non-LGBT individuals (Fredriksen-Goldsen et al., 2011). How much of this is due to the differing definition of spouse/partner than in the heterosexual community is not known. A recurring problem in empirical studies is the lack of rigorous sampling designs: most samples are small, regional, and lack generalizability, and do not focus on the heterogeneity across specific groups of sexual minorities (Fredriksen-Goldsen and Hooyman, 2007).

Changes in diversity are important for several reasons. First, the nation is moving toward person- and family-centered care as major tenets of quality health care and LTSS. Included in this quality improvement strategy is the idea that respecting the person's and family's values, beliefs, and preferences can improve individual and population health (NQF, 2014). Second, this has far-reaching implications for the provider workforce. Studies show that people often prefer to be treated by health care professionals of the same racial or ethnic background (Acosta and Olsen, 2006; IOM, 2004; Mitchell and Lassiter, 2006; Tarn et al., 2005). Also, a provider from a person's own background may have a better understanding of culturally appropriate demonstrations of respect for older adults and may also be more likely to speak the same language (Yeo, 2009). For LGBT persons, discrimination by service providers is a major concern; another issue is the lack of culturally appropriate resources for both caregivers and older individuals (Fredriksen-Goldsen and Hooyman, 2007; Fredriksen-Goldsen et al., 2011). Family or surrogate family caregivers are likely to be the best able to provide culturally appropriate care according to the preferences of individual older adults.

Developing programs and services that are both accessible and tailored to the needs of diverse communities of caregivers presents significant challenges. Functional impairments tend to be more prevalent in older minority groups (Schoeni et al., 2009). Moreover, while older adults, in general, are expected to live longer lives in the future, persistent disparities in life expectancy are likely to widen (Olshansky et al., 2012). Much of this difference is associated with disparities in income, education, neighborhood environments, lifetime access to health care, and occupational hazards (PRB, 2013).

Yet, as noted earlier, caregiving research is greatly hampered by the lack of robust data on important differences among subgroups. In the future, federal and other sponsors of population surveys should make the necessary investment to increase sampling of older adults and caregivers to enable meaningful subgroup analyses. Consistent, reliable investment in longitudinal tracking of older adults and their caregivers is also needed.

Changing Family Structures

Caregiving for older adults in the future will depend, in part, on the availability and capacity of their family members to assist them. In previous generations, older adults could often count on large, extended families for help with health and functioning needs—although in most cases the caregiver was either a wife or adult daughter as they are today (Wolff and Kasper, 2006). Current trends in family patterns—including lower fertility, higher rates of childlessness, changes in traditional family structures, and increases in divorce and never-married status—lead to smaller families (especially available children and spouses), which portends a shrinking pool of potential caregivers (Redfoot et al., 2013).

The size of American families continues to drop and, as a consequence, the number of adult children available to help an older parent is declining (see Figure 2-5). Moreover, adult daughters, the backbone of caregiving, are far more likely to be in the workforce and also geographically distant. In addition, as older adults live into their 80s, 90s, and older, their aging children themselves may be living with chronic health problems and limitations in functioning.

Childlessness has also risen across racial and ethnic groups. In the 1970s, 10 percent of American women ended their childbearing years without having a child (Livingston and Cohn, 2010). By 2008, this proportion had doubled to nearly 20 percent. Johnson and colleagues estimate that, from 2010 to 2040, the percentage of frail older adults without a living child will increase from 14 to 21 percent and the percentage with only one or two children will increase from 38 to 49 percent (Johnson et al., 2007) (see Figure 2-5).

Marital status is closely associated with the availability of caregivers and social supports as well as overall economic well-being (Federal Interagency Forum on Aging-Related Statistics, 2012; PRB, 2013). Older adults—particularly women—are less likely to be widowed than in the past (West et al., 2014). Although this may suggest that spouses can be expected to play a greater role in caregiving, other factors suggest otherwise. Between

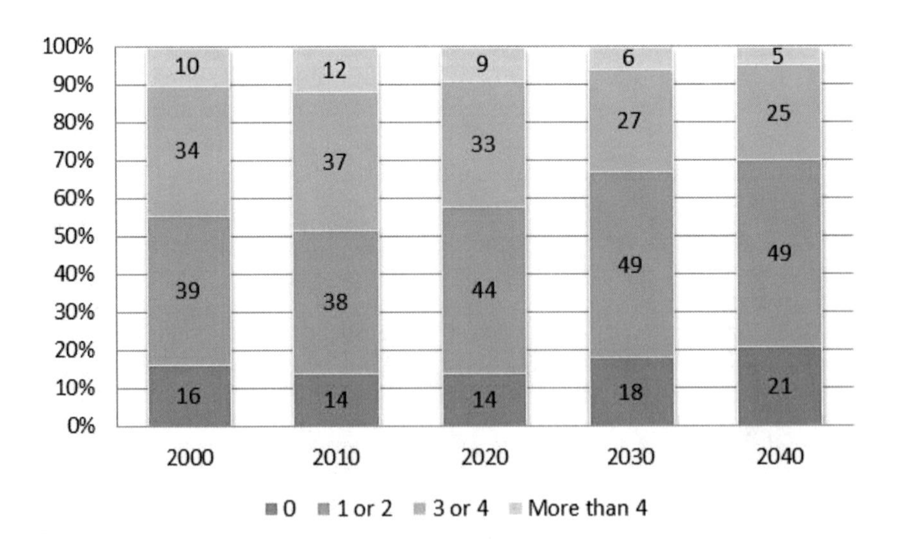

FIGURE 2-5 Projected distribution of the number of adult children for the frail older population, 2000 to 2040.
SOURCE: Johnson et al., 2007.

1990 and 2010, the divorce rates among adults ages 50 and older doubled (Brown and Lin, 2012) and an increasing proportion of women never marry (Jacobsen et al., 2011). Between 1986 and 2009, for example, the percentage of never-married, 50- to 54-year-old non-Hispanic white women tripled from 2.6 to 7.8 percent (Kreider and Ellis, 2011). Among African American women of the same age, the percentage increased fourfold from 6.3 to 24.5 percent. Additionally, LGBT older adults often do not have the same family support systems as heterosexual older adults, particularly because LGBT older adults are less likely to have children and are more likely to live alone (Cahill et al., 2000).

Non-traditional households and complex family structures are far more common than in the past. This change has important implications for family caregiving because adult stepchildren may have weaker feelings of obligation and provide less care to their aging stepparents than their parents (Pew Research Center, 2010; Silverstein and Giarrusso, 2010; van der Pas et al., 2013). Research also shows that divorce negatively impacts the quality of intergenerational relationships between older parents and their adult children and reduces resource transfers from parents to children (Wolf, 2001). Additional research is needed to fully understand how these trends in family structures affect the care of aging adults (Silverstein and Giarrusso, 2010; van der Pas et al., 2013).

In combination, race/ethnicity, low income, and limited education are strongly associated with poor health status and increased functional limitations among older persons (Crimmins and Saito, 2001; Molla et al., 2004; Olshansky et al., 2012). Gender and living arrangement are also important correlates of poverty in old age. Compared to men of the same age in every racial and ethnic group, older women have much higher levels of poverty. They are also more likely to be living alone. In 2014, more than one-third of women (35 percent) older than age 64 lived alone compared to 19 percent of men of the same age (ACL, 2015). The share of older women living alone is substantially higher: 42 percent among women ages 75 to 84 and more than half (56 percent) of women ages 85 and older (U.S. Census Bureau, 2014). The risk of poor health status and poverty that is associated with living alone is particularly worrisome in light of current trends in marriage, divorce, and family size.

Women in the Workforce

As discussed in Chapter 4, more than half of family caregivers of older adults are employed. This proportion is increasing, largely driven by the growing numbers of adult daughters and wives who work (Stone, 2015). In the four decades leading to 2012, women's participation in the workforce grew by 19 percent, from about one in three women to more than half of women (Toossi, 2013). The U.S. Bureau of Labor Statistics projects that women's participation in the workforce will continue to increase during the same years that they are most likely to be caregiving (Toossi, 2013). The percentage of women older than age 54 who work, for example, is expected to increase from 35.1 percent in 2012 to 37.5 percent in 2022. During the same period, the percentage of working women older than age 64—those most likely to be caring for a spouse—is expected to increase from 14.4 to 19.5 percent (Toossi, 2013). This trend is likely to contribute to the widening gap between the supply and demand for family caregivers of older adults.

BOX 2-1
Key Findings and Conclusions: Regarding the Older Adult Population That Needs Caregiving and the Family Caregivers Who Help Them

Markedly growing numbers of older adults need a caregiver's help:

- Many older adults never need a family caregiver's help. However, as older people age, they are increasingly likely to have a physical and/or cognitive impairment that affects their ability to function independently.
- The committee estimates that 6.3 million older adults received a family caregiver's help with household tasks or self-care for health or functioning reasons in 2011. An additional 3.5 million older adults received caregiving help because they had dementia and 1.1 million resided in nursing homes.
    - o Population estimates from other surveys vary widely because researchers use different definitions of caregiving and sampling designs to develop estimates of older adults' need for help with *self-care* (e.g., bathing, dressing, eating, and toileting), *mobility*, and *household activities* (e.g., using the telephone, taking medications, managing money, doing housework and laundry, preparing meals, and shopping for groceries).
- The demand for caregivers is increasing significantly not only because of the rapid growth in the number of older adults, but also because the faster growing cohort of older adults are those age 80 and older—the age when people are most likely to have a significant physical or cognitive impairment or both.
    - o More than half of 85- to 89-year-olds (59 percent) need caregiving because of health or functioning reasons.
    - o From age 90 on, only a minority of individuals (24 percent) do *not* need help from others.
- Dementia is an important factor in the prevalence of need for a family caregiver. In 2011, 3.5 million of the 4.9 million older adults who received

CONCLUSIONS

The committee's key findings and conclusions are described in detail in Box 2-1. In summary, this chapter raises profound concerns about the nation's capacity to meet the needs of its elders. The United States is undergoing historic demographic changes that have significant implications for current and future policy regarding family caregivers of older adults. By 2030, more than one in five U.S. residents will be age 65 or older. Much of the growth in the older population will be among those most likely to need intensive support—people age 80 and older.

help for health or functioning reasons were classified as having probable dementia.

The intensity and duration of need for help varies markedly:

- The need for a family caregiver among older adults is highly variable in both intensity and duration. Some older adults need daily help with self-care for decades. Others have short-term, intensive needs for help with medical and nursing tasks during an acute illness or injury.

Caregivers are as diverse as the American population:

- The nation is undergoing a historic shift in its racial, ethnic, and cultural composition. These changes will affect public attitudes, values, preferences, and expectations regarding family caregiving.
- Resource constraints have limited the sample size and design of current surveys relevant to family caregiving. As a result, little is known about important subgroups such as those defined by race and ethnicity, rural residence, or sexual orientation.

Social and demographic trends are driving a growing gap between the demand for and supply of family caregivers:

- The size of American families continues to decline because of lower fertility and higher rates of childlessness, divorce, and people never marrying.
- American families are more complex and non-traditional than the households of past generations with potentially important implications for family caregiving. Adult stepchildren may have weaker feelings of obligation and provide less care to their aging stepparents than their parents.
- Women have always been the nation's primary caregivers of older adults, but they are participating in the workforce in increasing numbers and are thus less available for caregiving.

While the need for caregiving is rapidly increasing, the size of the potential family caregiver "workforce" is shrinking. Current trends in family patterns, including lower fertility, higher rates of childlessness, and increases in divorce and never-married status, portend a shrinking pool of potential caregivers in the near future. Unlike in the past, older adults will have fewer family members to rely on, may be geographically distant from their children and live alone, and are more likely to be unmarried or divorced.

The committee has relied heavily on national data on older adults and their family caregivers and projections made by others who have used these data to identify the scope of problems related to family caregiving. National data on family caregiving and caregivers will be important in monitoring future progress and challenges in family caregiving. As the population of older adults and their caregivers change in diversity, gender, identity, living arrangements, reliance on new technology, and other ways, national data collection needs to change correspondingly. Without adequate data on family caregivers and caregiving, public and private decision makers will not have the evidence base on which to make sound decisions. Despite the limitations in the available data, the NHATS and NSOC findings presented in this chapter have important implications for individuals and families, as well as policy makers, health and social service providers, employers, and others—particularly in light of the consequences of family caregiving reviewed later in this report. At a minimum, they underscore the enormous commitment of time that family caregivers contribute to the well-being of the large and growing numbers of older Americans with physical and/or cognitive limitations. Yet it is not clear that Americans understand and appreciate the amount of time and the likely demands of being a caregiver sometime in the future. Raising awareness and public education about the needs and challenges of family caregiving of older adults will be a critical step toward preparing the nation as a whole.

REFERENCES

ACL (Administration for Community Living). 2015. *A profile of older Americans: 2014*. http://www.aoa.acl.gov/Aging_Statistics/Profile/2014/docs/2014-Profile.pdf (accessed May 12, 2015).

Acosta, D., and P. Olsen. 2006. Meeting the needs of regional minority groups: The University of Washington's programs to increase the American Indian and Alaskan Native physician workforce. *Academic Medicine* 81(10):863-870.

Adams, P. F., W. K. Kirzinger, and M. E. Martinez. 2013. Summary health statistics for the U.S. population: National Health Interview Survey, 2012. *Vital Health Statistics* 10(259).

Anderson, G. 2010. *Chronic care: Making the case for ongoing care*. http://www.rwjf.org/content/dam/farm/reports/reports/2010/rwjf54583 (accessed May 25, 2015).

Bevan, J. L., S. K. Vreeburg, S. Verdugo, and L. Sparks. 2012. Interpersonal conflict and health perceptions in long-distance caregiving relationships. *Journal of Health Communication* 17(7):747-761.

Black, B. S., D. Johnston, P. V. Rabins, A. Morrison, C. Lyketsos, and Q. M. Samus. 2013. Unmet needs of community-residing persons with dementia and their informal caregivers: Findings from the Maximizing Independence at Home Study. *Journal of the American Geriatrics Society* 61(12):2087-2095.

Brown, S. L., and I.-F. Lin. 2012. The gray divorce revolution: Rising divorce among middle-aged and older adults, 1990-2010. *Journals of Gerontology Series B: Psychological Sciences and Social Sciences* 67(6):731-741.

Cagle, J. G., and J. C. Munn. 2012. Long-distance caregiving: A systematic review of the literature. *Journal of Gerontological Social Work* 55(8):682-707.

Cahill, S., K. South, and J. Spade. 2000. *Outing age: Public policy issues affecting gay, lesbian, bisexual, and transgender elders.* New York: Policy Institute of the National Gay and Lesbian Taskforce.

Capistrant, B. D., J. R. Moon, L. F. Berkman, and M. M. Glymour. 2012. Current and long-term spousal caregiving and onset of cardiovascular disease. *Journal of Epidemiology and Community Health* 66(10):951-956.

Chadiha, L. A., S. Feld, and J. Rafferty. 2011. Likelihood of African American primary caregivers and care recipients receiving assistance from secondary caregivers: A rural-urban comparison. *Journal of Applied Gerontology* 30(4):422-442.

CMS (Centers for Medicare & Medicaid Services). 2012. *Chronic conditions among Medicare beneficiaries, Chartbook,* 2012 ed. http://www.cms.gov/Research-Statistics-Data-and-Systems/Statistics-Trends-and-Reports/Chronic-Conditions/Downloads/2012Chartbook.pdf (accessed April 23, 2015).

Colby, S. L., and J. M. Ortman. 2014. *The baby boom cohort in the United States: 2012 to 2060. Current Population Reports, P25-1141.* https://www.census.gov/prod/2014pubs/p25-1141.pdf (accessed April 30, 2015).

Crimmins, E. M., and Y. Saito. 2001. Trends in healthy life expectancy in the United States, 1970-1990: Gender, racial, and educational differences. *Social Science & Medicine* 52(11):1629-1641.

Dassel, K. B., and D. C. Carr. 2014. Does dementia caregiving accelerate frailty? Findings from the Health and Retirement Study. *The Gerontologist* 56(3):444-450.

Favreault, M., and J. Dey. 2015. *ASPE issue brief. Long-term services and supports for older Americans: Risks and financing research brief. Revised February 2016.* http://aspe.hhs.gov/basic-report/long-term-services-and-supports-older-americans-risks-and-financing-research-brief (accessed March 24, 2016).

Feder, J. 2015. The challenge of financing long-term care. *St. Louis University Journal of Health Law and Policy* 8(1):47-60.

Federal Interagency Forum on Aging-Related Statistics. 2012. *Older Americans 2012: Key indicators of well-being.* http://www.agingstats.gov/agingstatsdotnet/Main_Site/Data/2012_Documents/Docs/EntireChartbook.pdf (accessed April 29, 2015).

Fredriksen-Goldsen, K. I., and N. R. Hooyman. 2007. Caregiving research, services, and policies in historically marginalized communities. *Journal of Gay & Lesbian Social Services* 18(3-4):129-145.

Fredriksen-Goldsen, K., H. Kim, C. Emlet, A. Muraco, E. Erosheva, C. Hoy-Ellis, J. Goldsen, and H. Petry. 2011. *The aging and health report: Disparities and resilience among lesbian, gay, bisexual, and transgender older adults.* http://caringandaging.org/wordpress/wp-content/uploads/2011/05/Full-Report-FINAL-11-16-11.pdf (accessed July 1, 2016).

Freedman, V. A., and B. C. Spillman. 2014a. Disability and care needs among older Americans. *Milbank Quarterly* 92(3):509-541.

Freedman, V. A., and B. C. Spillman. 2014b. The residential continuum from home to nursing home: Size, characteristics and unmet needs of older adults. *Journals of Gerontology Series B: Psychological Sciences and Social Sciences* 69(Suppl 1):S42-S50.

Freedman, V. A., J. D. Kasper, J. C. Cornman, E. M. Agree, K. Bandeen-Roche, V. Mor, B. C. Spillman, R. Wallace, and D. A. Wolf. 2011. Validation of new measures of disability and functioning in the National Health and Aging Trends Study. *Journal of Gerontology* 66A(9):1013-1021.

Freedman, V. A., B. C. Spillman, P. M. Andreski, J. C. Cornman, E. M. Crimmins, E. Kramarow, J. Lubitz, L. G. Martin, S. S. Merkin, R. F. Schoeni, T. E. Seeman, and T. A. Waidmann. 2013. Trends in late-life activity limitations in the United States: An update from five national surveys. *Demography* 50(2):661-671.

Freedman, V. A., J. D. Kasper, B. C. Spillman, E. M. Agree, V. Mor, R. B. Wallace, and D. A. Wolf. 2014. Behavioral adaptation and late-life disability: A new spectrum for assessing public health impacts. *American Journal of Public Health* 104(2):e88-e94.

Frey, W. 2014. A pivotal period for race in America. In *Diversity explosion: How new racial demographics are remaking America*. Washington, DC: Brookings Institution Press.

Gaudette, E., B. Tysinger, A. Cassil, and D. Goldman. 2015. *Strengthening Medicare for 2030: Health and health care of Medicare beneficiaries in 2030.* http://www.brookings.edu/~/media/Research/Files/Papers/2015/06/04-medicare-2030-paper-series/Medicare2030_Chartbook.pdf (accessed April 5, 2016).

Giovannetti, E. R., and J. L. Wolff. 2010. Cross-survey differences in national estimates of numbers of caregivers of disabled older adults. *The Milbank Quarterly* 88(3):310-349.

Grossman, A., A. D'Augelli, and E. Dragowski. 2007. Caregiving and care receiving among older lesbian, gay, and bisexual adults. *Journal of Gay & Lesbian Social Services* 18(3/4):15-38.

He, W., and L. J. Larsen. 2014. Older Americans with a disability: 2008-2012. *U.S. Census Bureau. American Community Survey Reports (ACS-29).* https://www.census.gov/content/dam/Census/library/publications/2014/acs/acs-29.pdf (accessed May 14, 2015).

Hughes, M., and S. Kentlyn. 2011. Older LGBT people's care networks and communities of practice: A brief note. *International Social Work* 54(3):436-444.

IOM (Institute of Medicine). 2004. *In the nation's compelling interest: Ensuring diversity in the health care workforce.* Washington, DC: The National Academies Press.

IOM. 2008. *Retooling for an aging America: Building the health care workforce.* Washington, DC: The National Academies Press.

Jacobsen, L. A., M. Mather, and M. Lee. 2011. *America's aging population. Population bulletin 66, no. 1.* http://www.prb.org/pdf11/aging-in-america.pdf (accessed May 26, 2015).

Ji, J., B. Zoller, K. Sundquist, and J. Sundquist. 2012. Increased risks of coronary heart disease and stroke among spousal caregivers of cancer patients. *Circulation* 125(14):1742-1747.

Johnson, R. W., and J. M. Wiener. 2006. *A profile of frail older Americans and their caregivers.* Washington, DC: Urban Institute.

Johnson, R. W., D. Toohey, and J. M. Wiener. 2007. *Meeting the long-term care needs of the baby boomers: How changing families will affect paid helpers and institutions.* http://www.urban.org/UploadedPDF/311451_Meeting_Care.pdf (accessed April 9, 2015).

Kasper, J. D., V. A. Freedman, and B. C. Spillman. 2013. *Classification of persons by dementia status in the National Health and Aging Trends Study.* https://www.nhats.org/scripts/documents/NHATS_Dementia_Technical_Paper_5_Jul2013.pdf (accessed May 20, 2015).

Kasper, J. D., V. A. Freedman, and B. Spillman. 2014. *Disability and care needs of older Americans by dementia status: An analysis of the 2011 National Health and Aging Trends Study.* http://aspe.hhs.gov/daltcp/reports/2014/NHATS-DS.pdf (accessed February 4, 2015).

Kaye, H. S. 2013. Disability rates for working-age adults and for the elderly have stabilized, but trends for each mean different results for costs. *Health Affairs* 32(1):127-134.

Kids Count Data Center. 2015. *Adult population by race.* http://datacenter.kidscount.org/data/Tables/6539-adult-population-by-race?loc=1&loct=1#detailed/1/any/false/869,36,868,867,133/68,69,67,12,70,66,71,2800/13517,13518 (accessed March 7, 2016).

Kreider, R. M., and R. Ellis. 2011. *Number, timing and duration of marriages and divorces: 2009. U.S. Census Bureau Current Population Reports.* https://www.census.gov/prod/2011pubs/p70-125.pdf (accessed May 29, 2015).

Livingston, G., and D. Cohn. 2010. *Childlessness up among all women; down among women with advanced degrees. Pew Research Social and Demographic Trends.* http://www.pewsocialtrends.org/files/2010/11/758-childless.pdf (accessed May 28, 2015).

Marks, N. F. 1996. Caregiving across the lifespan: National prevalence and predictors. *Family Relations* 45(1):27-36.

Mather, M., L. A. Jacobsen, and K. M. Pollard. 2015. Aging in the United States. *Population Bulletin* 70(2):1-18.

Mayer, G. 2013. *The Family and Medical Leave Act (FMLA): Policy issues.* http://digitalcommons.ilr.cornell.edu/cgi/viewcontent.cgi?article=2316&context=key_workplace (accessed July 18, 2016).

Mitchell, D. A., and S. L. Lassiter. 2006. Addressing health care disparities and increasing workforce diversity: The next step for the dental, medical, and public health professions. *American Journal of Public Health* 96(12):2093-2097.

Miyawaki, C. E. 2016. Caregiving practice patterns of Asian, Hispanic, and non-Hispanic white American family caregivers of older adults across generations. *Journal of Cross-Cultural Gerontology* 31(1):35-55.

Molla, M. T., J. H. Madans, and D. K. Wagener. 2004. Differentials in adult mortality and activity limitation by years of education in the United States at the end of the 1990s. *Population and Development Review* 30(4):625-646.

Monin, J. K., and R. Schulz. 2009. Interpersonal effects of suffering in older adult caregiving relationships. *Psychology and Aging* 24(3):681-695.

NAC (National Alliance for Caregiving) and AARP Institute. 1997. *Family caregiving in the U.S.: Findings from a national survey.* http://www.caregiving.org/data/04finalreport.pdf (accessed July 18, 2016).

NAC and AARP Institute. 2004. *Caregiving in the U.S.* http://www.caregiving.org/data/04finalreport.pdf (accessed July 18, 2016).

NAC and AARP Institute. 2009. *Caregiving in the U.S.: A focused look at those caring for someone age 50 or older.* http://www.caregiving.org/pdf/research/FINALRegularExSum50plus.pdf (accessed April 14, 2015).

NAC and AARP Public Policy Institute. 2015a. *2015 report: Caregiving in the U.S.* http://www.caregiving.org/wp-content/uploads/2015/05/2015_CaregivingintheUS_Final-Report-June-4_WEB.pdf (accessed August 4, 2015).

NAC and AARP Public Policy Institute. 2015b. *Caregivers of older adults: A focused look at those caring for someone age 50+.* http://www.aarp.org/content/dam/aarp/ppi/2015/caregivers-of-older-adults-focused-look.pdf (accessed August 5, 2015).

NIH (National Institutes for Health). 2010. *Fact sheet—disability in older adults.* http://report.nih.gov/nihfactsheets/Pdfs/DisabilityinOlderAdults(NIA).pdf (accessed May 19, 2015).

NQF (National Quality Forum). 2014. *Final report: Addressing performance measure gaps in person-centered care and outcomes.* http://www.qualityforum.org/Publications/2014/08/Priority_Setting_for_Healthcare_Performance_Measurement__Addressing_Performance_Measure_Gaps_in_Person-Centered_Care_and_Outcomes.aspx (accessed December 4, 2015).

NRC (National Research Council). 2012. *Aging and the macroeconomy: Long-term implications of an older population.* Washington, DC: The National Academies Press.

Olshansky, S. J., T. Antonucci, L. Berkman, R. H. Binstock, A. Boersch-Supan, J. T. Cacioppo, B. A. Carnes, L. L. Carstensen, L. P. Fried, D. P. Goldman, J. Jackson, M. Kohli, J. Rother, Y. H. Zheng, and J. Rowe. 2012. Differences in life expectancy due to race and educational differences are widening, and many may not catch up. *Health Affairs* 31(8):1803-1813.

Ortman, J. M., V. A. Velkoff, and H. Hogan. 2014. *An aging nation: The older population in the United States.* http://www.census.gov/prod/2014pubs/p25-1140.pdf (accessed April 15, 2015).

Penrod, J. D., R. Kane, R. A. Kane, R. L. Kane, and M. D. Finch. 1995. Who cares? The size, scope and composition of the caregiver support system. *The Gerontologist* 35(4):489-497.

Pew Research Center. 2010. *The decline of marriage and the rise of new families.* Washington, DC: Pew Research Center. http://www.pewsocialtrends.org/files/2010/11/pew-social-trends-2010-families.pdf (accessed July 1, 2016).

Pinquart, M., and S. Sörensen. 2005. Ethnic differences in stressors, resources, and psychological outcomes of family caregiving: A meta-analysis. *The Gerontologist* 45(1):90-106.

Pinquart, M., and S. Sörensen. 2006. Gender differences in caregivers' stressors, social resources, and health: An updated meta-analysis. *The Journals of Gerontology Series B: Psychological Sciences* 61(1):33-45.

PRB (Population Reference Bureau). 2013. *The health and life expectancy of older blacks and Hispanics in the United States.* http://www.prb.org/pdf13/TodaysResearchAging28.pdf (accessed May 25, 2015).

Redfoot, D., L. Feinberg, and A. Houser. 2013. *The aging of the baby boom and the growing care gap: A look at future declines in the availability of family caregivers.* http://www.aarp.org/content/dam/aarp/research/public_policy_institute/ltc/2013/baby-boom-and-the-growing-care-gap-insight-AARP-ppi-ltc.pdf (accessed August 7, 2015).

Schoeni, R. F., V. A. Freedman, and L. G. Martin. 2009. Socioeconomic and demographic disparities in trends in old-age disability. In *Health at older ages: The causes and consequences of declining disability among the elderly*, edited by D. Cutler and D. A. Wise. Chicago, IL: University of Chicago Press.

Schulz, R., R. S. Hebert, M. A. Dew, S. L. Brown, M. F. Scheier, S. R. Beach, S. J. Czaja, L. M. Martire, D. Coon, K. M. Langa, L. N. Gitlin, A. B. Stevens, and L. Nichols. 2007. Patient suffering and caregiver compassion: New opportunities for research, practice, and policy. *The Gerontologist* 47(1):4-13.

Schulz, R., S. R. Beach, R. S. Hebert, L. M. Martire, J. K. Monin, C. A. Tompkins, and S. M. Albert. 2009. Spousal suffering and partner's depression and cardiovascular disease: The Cardiovascular Health Study. *The American Journal of Geriatric Psychiatry* 17(3):246-254.

Schulz, R., S. R. Beach, T. B. Cook, L. M. Martire, J. M. Tomlinson, and J. K. Monin. 2012. Predictors and consequences of perceived lack of choice in becoming an informal caregiver. *Aging & Mental Health* 16(6):712-721.

Social Security Trustees Report. 2015. *The 2015 annual report of the Board of Trustees of the Federal Old-Age and Survivors Insurance and Federal Disability Insurance Trust Funds.* https://www.ssa.gov/oact/tr/2015/tr2015.pdf (accessed July 18, 2016).

Spillman, B. C., and L. E. Pezzin. 2000. Potential and active family caregivers: Changing networks and the "Sandwich Generation." *Milbank Quarterly* 78(3):347-374.

Stone, R. I. 2015. Factors affecting the future of family caregiving in the United States. In *Family caregiving in the new normal*, edited by J. E. Gaugler and R. L. Kane. London, UK: Elsevier.

Silverstein, M. and R. Giarrusso. 2010. Aging and family life: A decade review. *Journal of Marriage and Family* 72(5):1039-1058.

Tarn, D. M., L. S. Meredith, M. Kagawa-Singer, S. Matsumura, S. Bito, R. K. Oye, H. Liu, K. L. Kahn, S. Fukuhara, and N. S. Wenger. 2005. Trust in one's physician: The role of ethnic match, autonomy, acculturation, and religiosity among Japanese and Japanese Americans. *The Annals of Family Medicine* 3(4):339-347.

Tennstedt, S. L., J. B. McKinlay, L. M. Sullivan. 1989. Informal care for frail elders: The role of secondary caregiver. *The Gerontologist* 29(5):677-683.

Toossi, M. 2013. *Monthly labor review. Labor force projection to 2022: The labor force participation rate continues to fall.* http://www.bls.gov/opub/mlr/2013/article/labor-force-projections-to-2022-the-labor-force-participation-rate-continues-to-fall.htm (accessed September 10, 2015).

U.S. Census Bureau. 2012. *U.S. Census Bureau projections show a slower growing, older, more diverse nation a half century from now*. https://www.census.gov/newsroom/releases/archives/population/cb12-243.html (accessed April 12, 2016).

U.S. Census Bureau. 2014. 2014 *Current Population Survey, Annual Social and Economic Supplement.* http://ceprdata.org/wp-content/cps/CPS_March_Codebook_2014_traditional.pdf (accessed August 22, 2016).

U.S. Census Bureau. 2016a. *American FactFinder.* http://factfinder.census.gov/faces/nav/jsf/pages/index.xhtml (accessed March 29, 2016)

U.S. Census Bureau. 2016b. *Table HINC-01. Selected characteristics of households, by total money income in 2014.* http://www.census.gov/hhes/www/cpstables/032015/hhinc/hinc01_000.htm (accessed January 12, 2016).

van der Pas, S., T. G. Van Tilburg, and M. Silverstein. 2013. Stepfamilies in later life. *Journal of Marriage and Family* 75(5):1065-1069.

West, L. A., S. Cole, D. Goodkind, and W. He. 2014. *65+ in the United States: 2010.* Washington, DC: U.S. Government Printing Office.

Wolf, D. A. 2001. Population change: Friend or foe of the chronic care system? *Health Affairs* 20(6):28-42.

Wolf, D. A., and C. F. Longino. 2005. "Our increasingly mobile society"? The curious persistence of a false belief. *The Gerontologist* 45(1):5-11.

Wolff, J. L., and B. J. Jacobs. 2015. Chronic illness trends and the challenges to family caregivers: Organizational and health system barriers. In *Family caregiving in the new normal*, edited by J. E. Gaugler and R. L. Kane. Oxford, UK: Elsevier. Pp. 79-104.

Wolff, J. L., and J. D. Kasper. 2006. Caregivers of frail elders: Updating a national profile. *The Gerontologist* 46(3):344-356.

Yee, J. L., and R. Schulz. 2000. Gender differences in psychiatric morbidity among family caregivers: A review and analysis. *The Gerontologist* 40(2):147-164.

Yeo, G. 2009. How will the U.S. healthcare system meet the challenge of the ethnogeriatric imperative? *Journal of the American Geriatrics Society* 57(7):1278-1285.

3

Family Caregiving Roles and Impacts

ABSTRACT: This chapter examines the multiple and evolving roles of caregivers of older adults and the impact of assuming these roles on caregivers' health and well-being. It describes caregiver tasks, the dynamic nature of caregiving over time, the increasing complexity and scope of caregiver responsibilities, and issues involved in surrogate decision making. Family caregiving is more intensive, complex, and long lasting than in the past and caregivers rarely receive adequate preparation for their role. A compelling body of evidence suggests that many caregivers experience negative psychological effects. Some caregivers are at higher risk than others, especially those who spend long hours caring for older adults with advanced dementia. Caregivers should have access to high-quality, evidence-based interventions designed to mitigate or prevent adverse health effects.

As a society, we have always depended on families to provide emotional support, and to assist their older parents, grandparents, and other family members when they can no longer function independently. This chapter examines the multiple and evolving roles of family caregivers of older adults and the impact of assuming these roles on caregivers' health and well-being. It describes the trajectory and dynamic nature of caregiving over time, the increasing complexity and scope of caregiver responsibilities including the issues involved in family caregivers' role as surrogate decision makers, and the evidence on the impact of caregiving on the health and well-being of caregivers of older adults.

The chapter reviews an extensive literature on family caregiving of older adults. It also draws from the National Health and Aging Trends Study (NHATS) and its companion the National Study of Caregiving (NSOC), two linked federally funded surveys designed to document how functioning changes with age, the role of the family caregivers identified by the NHATS respondents who live independently or in a senior community, assisted living facility, or other residential setting (Kasper et al., 2014). Family caregivers of nursing home residents are not included in NSOC. The committee distinguished between two subgroups of NSOC family caregivers: those who help an older adult because of health or functioning reasons and those caregivers who help "high-need" older adults. "High-need" refers to family caregivers of individuals who have probable dementia or who need help with at least two self-care activities (i.e., bathing, dressing, eating, toileting, or getting in and out of bed). See Chapter 2 and Appendix E for further information about the surveys and the committee's analyses of the publicly available survey datasets.

CAREGIVING TRAJECTORIES

Despite many common experiences, caregivers' roles are highly variable across the course of caregiving. The diversity of families, the timing of entry into the caregiving role, the duration of the role in relation to the overall life course of the caregiver, and transitions in care experienced over time all shape the nature of the caregiving role. The committee conceptualized caregiving over time as "caregiving trajectories" to highlight the dynamic nature of the role and the different directions it can take. Caregiving trajectories include transitions in both the care needs of the older adult and in the settings in which care is provided (Gitlin and Wolff, 2012).

In populations in which the care recipients become increasingly impaired over time, such as with increasing frailty, dementia, Parkinson's disease, or advanced cancer, the caregiving role expands accordingly. In populations in which care recipients experience short-term or episodic periods of disability, such as early-stage cancer and heart failure, the caregiving role may be short term but intense or it may wax and wane over time. Entry into the caregiving role is similarly variable. Individuals may take on the caregiving role as they gradually recognize a care recipient's need for assistance—when an individual has difficulty balancing a checkbook, for example—or they may suddenly plunge into the caregiving role in the context of a crisis such as an unexpected life-threatening diagnosis, stroke, hip fracture, or other catastrophic event.

Caregiving for older adults occurs across all the settings in which care is delivered and often involves interacting with numerous providers, back-and-forth transitions from hospital to home or rehabilitation facility, move to a senior residence or assisted living facility, placement in a nursing home, and ultimately end-of-life care. These transitions and role changes, along with the health and functional status of the care recipient, affect the social, physical, and emotional health of the caregiver over time (Carpentier et al., 2010; Cavaye, 2008; Gibbons et al., 2014; Peacock et al., 2014; Penrod et al., 2011, 2012; Schulz and Tompkins, 2010).

A caregiving episode can be defined both in terms of duration and intensity (i.e., the number of hours spent daily, weekly, or monthly to provide needed care to an older adult). As noted in Chapter 2, 15 percent of caregivers had provided care for 1 year or less by the time of the survey, and an equal percentage had provided care for more than 10 years.[1] The remaining 70 percent fell between these two extremes. The median number of years of caregiving for high-need older adults (i.e., who had probable dementia or needed help with two or more self-care activities) was 4 years;[2] it was 5 years if the care recipient had dementia *and* also needed help with two or more self-care activities. As might be expected, the intensity of caregiving varies with the older adult's level of impairment. Caregivers providing assistance only with household activities spend an average of 85 hours per month providing care while those who care for an older adult with three or more self-care or mobility needs spend 253 hours per month (Freedman and Spillman, 2014), equivalent to nearly two full-time jobs.

Individuals do not provide caregiving in isolation from the other roles and responsibilities in their lives. Their personal lives—as spouse or partner, parent, employee, business owner, community member—intersect with caregiving in different ways at different times. Under ideal circumstances, the caregiver is able to balance the responsibilities and rewards of competing roles such as caring for a child or working for pay and their caregiving responsibilities. However, accumulating caregiving demands and the costs of long-term services and supports (LTSS) can overwhelm and undermine other dimensions of one's life. Additional complexity in trajectories arises when family members disagree about the type of care needed and how it should be provided (Dilworth-Anderson et al., 2002), or when family roles and responsibilities shift over time. Appendixes F and G relate the experiences of several family caregivers: a husband, daughter, and family caring for older adults with advanced Alzheimer's disease and a wife helping to provide complex cancer treatment to her husband in a rural area.

---

[1] See Chapter 2, Table 2-3.

[2] Committee calculations.

Phases in the Caregiving Trajectory

Although the caregiving role is highly variable over time, different phases in the caregiving trajectory can be discerned when the role is considered longitudinally. For example, caregiving may follow a trajectory reflecting increasing care responsibilities punctuated by episodic events such as hospitalizations and placement in rehabilitation or long-term care facilities. Figure 3-1 shows how caregiving for persons with dementia typically follows a relatively linear trajectory driven by the progressive cognitive and functional decline of the care recipient. The trajectory begins with emerging awareness of the caregiver that there is a problem. Over time this evolves into increasing care needs as the care recipient requires assistance with household tasks and then self-care tasks. End-of-life care may involve placement into a long-term care facility or enrollment in a hospice program. Note that the tasks required of the caregiver are cumulative over time. Each phase of the trajectory brings with it new challenges that the caregiver must confront.

For stroke caregivers, the trajectory may begin with sudden intensity, gradually decrease as the older adult regains function, and then remain relatively stable over a long period of time (perhaps punctuated by short-term acute illnesses or set-backs). Alternatively, caregiving may gradually increase with stroke complications, recurrence, or new comorbid conditions. Transitions in the caregiving trajectory may be planned, as in the transitions from hospital to skilled rehabilitation facility to home, or they may be unplanned, as in an emergency room visit and rehospitalization (McLennon et al., 2014).

The caregiving trajectory in the cancer population tends to be nonlinear. It is often characterized by the rapidity with which caregivers have to take on the role as treatment decisions are made and treatment begins. As the cancer experience unfolds, caregiving transitions may occur in rapid succession, each having its own learning curve in movement from one treatment modality to the next (e.g., from post-operative recovery at home to beginning radiation or chemotherapy). Transitions among care settings also occur unpredictably. For example, transitions from home to emergency room to hospital are unpredictable but not uncommon. Moreover, the functional abilities of older adults with cancer may fluctuate rapidly, resulting in intense but short periods of caregiving. Rapid transitions in the caregiving role may occur in the context of advanced cancer as well, as the care recipient moves from management of advanced cancer symptoms (e.g., pain, sleep disturbance, and lack of appetite) through a succession of changes in functional status and self-care ability, leading ultimately to end-of-life care and bereavement. The rapid succession of caregiving transitions, some of

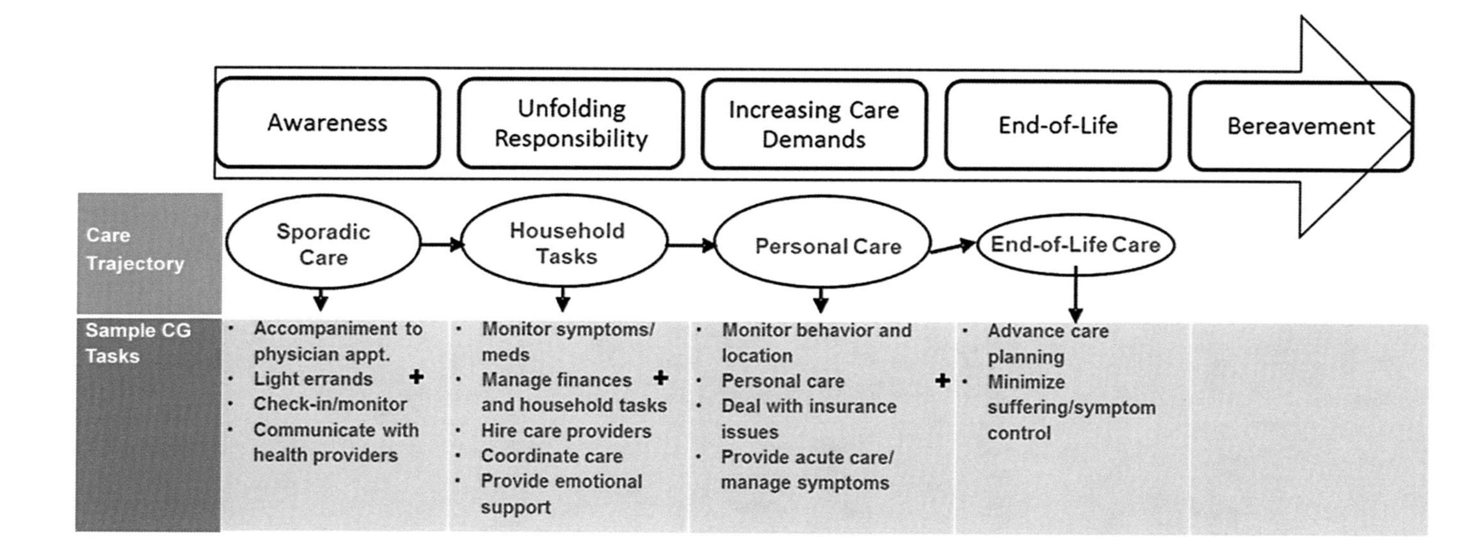

FIGURE 3-1 An example of a dementia care trajectory.
NOTE: CG = caregiving.
SOURCES: Adapted from Gitlin and Schulz (2012) and Schulz and Tompkins (2010).

which may occur with little warning, challenge caregivers' ability to provide care, as ability during one phase of the caregiving trajectory may or may not be sufficient to meet the demands of the next phase.

These are just a few of the varied trajectories associated with three common late-life illnesses. Each disease brings with it a unique pattern of unfolding needs that the caregiver must address. However, when considered over the long term, typical phases in caregiving trajectories can be discerned, as depicted in Figure 3-1. These phases are described below, with the caveat that they are not necessarily linear (Gitlin and Schulz, 2012; Gitlin and Wolff, 2012; Schulz and Tompkins, 2010).

Awareness

This phase includes recognition and increasing awareness within the older adult's social network of disabilities, changes in health, and/or behavioral change that signal the need for some level of caregiving. The older adult may downplay the need for care during this phase because of their concerns about becoming a burden to others (Cahill et al., 2009). Awareness of functional impairment can come on gradually, as in the case of someone with slowly progressive dementia, or suddenly as in the case of someone who has suffered a stroke or traumatic brain injury. With awareness that one is becoming a caregiver comes an array of daunting questions about how to meet the needs of the care recipient. How long will these needs, which may become increasingly more complex, have to be met and what will it take to meet these needs? How much family involvement will be necessary and how will caregiving roles within the family or broader social network be negotiated? What are the risks, costs, and benefits to whom over time? How much time will be involved in meeting these needs and how much involvement will be necessary? If paid help is needed to supplement family care, how much will it cost and can the family afford it? How can care needs be met in relationship to cultural norms and expectation?

In response to this awareness of need for caregiving on the part of the older adult and/or family members, one or more family members typically emerge as the caregivers. Who ends up being a caregiver within a family is often shaped by existing relationships, gender roles, cultural norms and expectations, and geographic proximity as well as a host of other factors (Cavaye, 2008). For example, African American caregivers are more likely to be non-spouses compared with white, non-Hispanic caregivers (NAC and AARP Public Policy Institute, 2009; Pinquart and Sörenson, 2005). Lesbian, gay, bisexual, and transgender (LGBT) individuals are more likely to care or be cared for by a non-relative than non-LGBT individuals (Fredriksen-Goldsen et al., 2011). Ultimately, one or more family members may take on the caregiving role and its varied responsibilities.

Unfolding Responsibility

As caregivers move into their role, they may experience role ambiguity, a redefining of their relationships with the care recipient and others, and may perceive stigma and/or experience discrimination as a result of the care recipient's condition (Gibbons et al., 2014). There are social changes with a shift from usual participation in life activities to a focus on the challenge of being a caregiver. The unpredictability of the illness experience of the care recipient may lead to uncertainty about the future. The confidence of the caregiver with respect to their caregiving role is linked to the illness status of the care recipient and the caregiver's knowledge and skills in addressing care recipient needs (Gibbons et al., 2014). Along with awareness of caregiving responsibilities, caregivers may also be engaged in trying to make sense of the older adult's impairments. For example, there is considerable variability in conceptions of dementia depending on the culture and educational level and socioeconomic status of the family caregivers (Hinton, 2002).

Increasing Care Demands

Schulz and Tompkins (2010) illustrate the caregiving trajectory for a typical older individual with functional decline who lives in the community and who over time experiences increasing reliance on the caregiver for assistance. The initial tasks may involve monitoring clinical symptoms and medications, as well as managing household tasks, communicating with health professionals, and providing emotional support to the care recipient. Over time, caregiving tasks often expand to include providing self-care tasks, becoming a surrogate decision maker for the care recipient, and providing specialized medical care such as giving injections. The diversity of tasks performed by caregivers is described in detail below. The common factor in the middle to late stages of a caregiving trajectory is the expansion and increased complexity and intensity of the caregiver's roles and responsibilities.

End of Life

This phase along the care trajectory may also involve nursing home care and repeated hospitalizations as the care recipient declines and ultimately dies. Although many caregivers become involved in end-of-life caregiving, few studies make explicit distinctions among the needs and experiences of family caregivers during disease-directed treatment, palliative or supportive care, and end-of-life phases (Schulz, 2013). The few studies that do focus on caregivers during the end-of-life phase suggest that caregiving demands become more urgent and intensive (Gibbons et al., 2014; Penrod et al., 2012). Caregivers continue to report high levels of burden and stress, but also find greater meaning and purpose in the experience of caregiving at the end of life (Emanuel et al., 2000; Gibbons et al., 2014; Wolff et al., 2007). To better understand caregiving during this critical phase in the trajectory, more fine-grained prospective studies are needed that clearly delineate the transition from disease management to supportive care to end-of-life care, and how these transitions affect the caregiver and formal care provided to the care recipient.

In summary, the caregiving role changes over time in concert with changes in the older adult's care needs, transitions from one care setting to another, and changes in the familial, social, and geographic contexts for caregiving. Diversity in family structures, norms, values, and relationships shape how the caregiving trajectory unfolds. Although typical phases in the caregiving trajectory can be identified, they are not necessarily linear and some degree of unpredictability always exists. Thus, caregivers' needs can be expected to change over time, indicating the need for assessment and periodic reassessment, as discussed below. Reassessment is especially important during transitional periods.

ROLES OF FAMILY CAREGIVERS

Despite the unique nature of any given caregiver's role over time, broad domains of activity characterize family caregiving. Caregiving ranges from assistance with daily activities and providing direct care to the care recipient to navigating complex health care and social services systems. The domains of the caregiving role include: assistance with household tasks, self-care tasks, and mobility; provision of emotional and social support; health and medical care; advocacy and care coordination; and surrogacy. Each domain has multiple tasks and activities (see Table 3-1). Cutting across

TABLE 3-1 What Family Caregivers Do for Older Adults

Domain	Caregivers' Activities and Tasks
Household tasks	• Help with bills, deal with insurance claims, and manage money • Home maintenance (e.g., install grab bars, ramps, and other safety modifications; repairs, yardwork) • Laundry and other housework • Prepare meals • Shopping • Transportation

TABLE 3-1 Continued

Domain	Caregivers' Activities and Tasks
Self-care, supervision, and mobility	• Bathing and grooming • Dressing • Feeding • Supervision • Management of behavioral symptoms • Toileting (e.g., getting to and from the toilet, maintaining continence, dealing with incontinence) • Transferring (e.g., getting in and out of bed and chairs, moving from bed to wheelchair) • Help getting around inside or outside
Emotional and social support	• Provide companionship • Discuss ongoing life challenges with care recipient • Facilitate and participate in leisure activities • Help care recipient manage emotional responses • Manage family conflict • Troubleshoot problems
Health and medical care	• Encourage healthy lifestyle • Encourage self-care • Encourage treatment adherence • Manage and give medications, pills, or injections • Operate medical equipment • Prepare food for special diets • Respond to acute needs and emergencies • Provide wound care
Advocacy and care coordination	• Seek information • Facilitate person and family understanding • Communicate with doctors, nurses, social workers, pharmacists, and other health care and long-term services and supports (LTSS) providers • Facilitate provider understanding • Locate, arrange, and supervise nurses, social workers, home care aides, home-delivered meals, and other LTSS (e.g., adult day services) • Make appointments • Negotiate with other family member(s) regarding respective roles • Order prescription medicines • Deal with insurance issues
Surrogacy	• Handle financial and legal matters • Manage personal property • Participate in advanced planning • Participate in treatment decisions

SOURCES: Spillman et al., 2014; Wolff, 2007.

these domains are ongoing cognitive and interpersonal processes in which caregivers engage including, for example, continual problem solving, decision making, communicating with others (family members and health and human service professionals), and constant vigilance over the care recipient's well-being (Gitlin and Wolff, 2012). How caregivers manage these tasks depends on their values, preferences, knowledge, and skills, as well as the accessibility, affordability, and adequacy of health care, LTSS, and other resources, as described further in Chapter 6.

The particular mix of caregiving activities and time commitments varies. In multiple studies, caregiving for persons with dementia has been shown consistently to be one of the most demanding types of caregiving (Ory et al., 1999; Pinquart and Sörenson, 2007). However, a 2004 survey found that the amount of care and level of burden experienced by cancer and dementia caregivers were nearly equivalent, but that specific tasks varied (Kim and Schulz, 2008). For example, cancer caregivers were more likely than dementia caregivers to provide help in getting in and out of bed, whereas dementia caregivers were more likely to deal with incontinence.

The caregiving experience also varies by distance. Long-distance caregivers who live at least 1 hour from the care recipient are typically involved in providing social and emotional support, advanced care planning, financial assistance, and care-coordination. They often share these responsibilities with a more proximal caregiver who provides assistance with personal care. Being separated from the care recipient complicates communication about the care recipient's health and care needs, and poses formidable challenges to address those needs through service providers. Because virtually all of the data on distance caregivers are based on small and/or nonrepresentative samples, caution is warranted in drawing firm conclusions based on these findings (Cagle and Munn, 2012). Better data are needed on the prevalence of long-distance caregiving, identifying who they are, the tasks they perform, and the impact caregiving has on their lives.

Assisting with Household Tasks, Self-Care, Mobility, and Supervision

Nearly all caregivers help older adults in need of care with household tasks such as shopping, laundry, housework, meals, transportation, bills, money management, and home maintenance (NAC and AARP Public Policy Institute, 2015; Spillman et al., 2014; Wolff et al., 2016). As indicated in Figure 3-2, these responsibilities are often daily ones if the older adult needs help because of health or functional limitations: 44 percent of caregivers reported helping with chores every day or most days.

Self-care and mobility tasks include walking, transferring (e.g., getting in and out of bed and chairs, moving from bed to wheelchair), bathing or showering, grooming, dressing, feeding, and toileting (e.g., getting to and

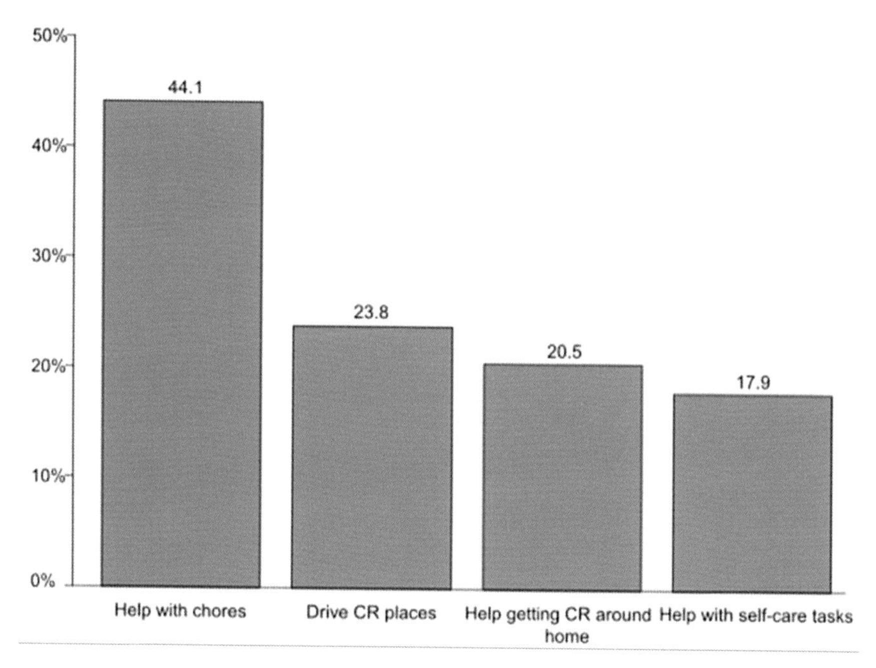

FIGURE 3-2 Percentage of caregivers who helped every day or most days during the past month, by type of help, 2011.
NOTES: Includes family caregivers of Medicare beneficiaries age 65 and older in the continental United States who resided in community or residential care settings (other than nursing homes) and received help with self-care, mobility, or household activities for health or functioning reasons. CR = care recipient.
SOURCES: Data from the 2011 NHATS and the companion NSOC.

from the toilet, maintaining continence, dealing with incontinence). Help with self-care tasks is a frequent and sometimes daily role for some caregivers; 17.9 percent of caregivers reported helping with self-care every day or most days.

Caregivers providing care to "high-need" older adults—those who have at least two self-care needs or dementia—are more likely to help with a wide variety of tasks, including helping with chores, helping the older adult get around the house, keeping track of medications, and making medical appointments. Older adults with both dementia and two or more self-care needs receive the highest levels of help from caregivers: 42 percent of their caregivers provide help with self-care tasks every day or most days. In addition, caregivers of high-need older adults also help with medication management (65 percent), medical tasks (20 percent), and with skin care

TABLE 3-2 Type and Frequency of Family Caregiver Tasks in the Past Month, by Care Recipient's Dementia Status and Need for Help with Self-Care, by Percentage, 2011

	Care Recipient's Dementia Status and Need for Help			
Tasks	Dementia Only	No Dementia; Has Two or More Self-Care Needs	Dementia; Has Two or More Self-Care Needs	No Dementia; Has Less Than Two Self-Care Needs
How often did you help . . .	Every day or most days (percentage)			
With chores	44.6	55.6	49.7	38.7
With self-care	10.5	32.0	42.0	8.6
Drive care recipient places	24.8	25.8	19.2	24.2
Help care recipient get around his/her home	14.8	35.7	37.4	12.4
Did you help . . .	Yes (percentage)			
Keep track of meds	61.2	57.4	65.4	36.8
Care recipient take shots or injections	6.3	13.3	12.0	5.3
Manage medical tasks	9.2	17.2	20.5	6.0
With special diet	25.8	40.5	30.9	22.9
With skin care wounds	17.0	34.0	35.2	18.2
Make medical appointments	74.6	59.1	75.0	52.0
Speak to medical provider	65.9	52.1	71.6	47.2
Add/change health insurance	29.3	24.1	30.9	22.5
With other insurance matters	37.7	35.5	47.0	27.6
Population represented (in 1,000s)	2,931	2,745	2,828	9,190

NOTES: Includes family caregivers of Medicare beneficiaries age 65 and older in the continental United States who resided in community or residential care settings (other than nursing homes) and received help with self-care, mobility, or household activities for health or functioning reasons. Self-care activities are bathing, dressing, eating, toileting, or getting in and out of bed. "Probable dementia" includes individuals whose doctor said they had dementia or Alzheimer's disease and individuals classified as having probable dementia based on results from a proxy screening instrument and several cognitive tests.
SOURCES: Data from the 2011 NHATS and the companion NSOC.

wounds (35 percent) (see Table 3-2). Older adults with dementia or other conditions that severely impair cognitive function may also require constant supervision and hands-on assistance because of their functional limitations and behavioral symptoms.

Providing Emotional and Social Support

When older adults first need caregiving because of increasing frailty or onset of a debilitating disease, they need emotional and social supports that are different from the usual exchanges among family members (Brody, 1985). One important change is in the balance of reciprocity in the caregiver–care recipient relationship. With increasing needs, the care recipient may be able to give less to the relationship while needing more from it, despite efforts to maintain some reciprocity (Pearlin et al., 1990). In addition, the care recipient's own emotional response to his or her changing circumstances may require a higher level of emotional support from the caregiver. Caregivers may find themselves dealing with unfamiliar depressive symptoms, anxiety, irritability, or anger in the care recipient.

These changes may be so subtle as to be nearly imperceptible at first. With advancing frailty, changes in the relationship may be recognized only retrospectively after they have been underway for some time. Conversely, relationship changes may occur suddenly, as with a stroke. For example, among stroke caregivers, the most stressful problems are in the caregiver–stroke survivor relationship (including poor communication, frustration with role reversal, and intimacy issues) (King et al., 2010). The task perceived as most time consuming by caregivers was providing emotional support (Bakas et al., 2004). In a study focused on the first year of caregiving after a stroke, caregivers surveyed 8 to 12 months after the stroke event reported that the problems perceived as most stressful were that the care recipient appeared sad or depressed, talked about feeling lonely, had problem controlling bowels, felt worthless or like a burden, and/or appeared anxious or worried (Haley et al., 2009).

Health and Medical Care

Family involvement in health and medical tasks at home is not new, but it has become more common, and is often far more complex than in the past. Older adults' homes have become *de facto* clinical care settings where caregivers are performing an array of nursing or medical tasks once provided only by licensed or certified professionals in hospitals and nursing homes (Reinhard and Feinberg, 2015; Reinhard et al., 2012). This is, in part, the result of ongoing efforts to shorten lengths of hospitalizations and reduce nursing home placements, coupled with increasingly complex options for the medical treatment of chronic and acute conditions in noninstitutional settings. The "Home Alone" study by the AARP Public Policy Institute and the United Hospital Fund documented the marked impact of this trend on the roles of caregivers. More recent caregiver surveys continue to find similar results (Kasper et al., 2014; Reinhard and Feinberg, 2015; Spillman et al., 2014; Wolff et al., 2016).

The health and medical care domain of the caregiving role is increasingly complex. Medications were once simply administered. Today, medications prescribed for home use are delivered not only by mouth but also via patches, injections, and intravenously. When the care recipient is seriously ill or severely impaired, the caregiver may also be managing technical procedures and equipment, such as feeding and drainage tubes, catheters, and tracheostomies, as well as managing symptoms and monitoring the care recipient's condition. During cancer treatment, for example, caregivers are called on for numerous health and medical care activities at home, including symptom and side effect management, nutrition, hands-on procedures (e.g., wound care and infusion pumps), management of acute conditions (e.g., fever, dehydration, or delirium), and management of complex medication regimens (e.g., oral chemotherapeutic agents, injections, and an array of symptom management medications) (Bond et al., 2012; Given et al., 2012; Krouse et al., 2004; Schumacher et al., 2000; Silver et al., 2004; Swore Fletcher et al., 2012; van Ryn et al., 2011). When older adults have other chronic medical conditions in addition to cancer, such as cardiovascular disease, diabetes, arthritis, or a mental health condition, the management of these co-morbidities may be greatly complicated by cancer treatment (Given et al., 2012; Glajchen, 2004).

Advocacy and Care Coordination

Family caregivers often serve as advocates and care coordinators. As advocates, their role is to identify and to help care recipients obtain needed community and health care resources. This may involve determining the care recipient's eligibility for specific services and the potential costs. More often than not, the older adult and the caregiver encounter bewildering and disconnected systems of care that involve an array of entities including health care providers, public- and private-sector community-based agencies, employers, and multiple potential payers (e.g., Medicare, Medicaid, and private Medigap plans) (Bookman and Kimbrel, 2011). Caregivers must navigate these multiple, evolving, and increasing complex systems, often without assistance.[3] The role of coordinator often falls to the family caregiver, who must patch together the services that an older adult needs and

[3] See Chapter 6 for a discussion of caregivers' interaction with the health care system.

also serve as the primary communication link among all the involved parties. Many people, such as some racial or ethnic groups, LGBT caregivers, and individuals with limited health literacy, face the additional challenge of finding culturally and linguistically tailored services appropriate to their care recipients' needs (Coon, 2007; Dilworth-Anderson, 2002; Fredriksen-Goldsen and Hooyman, 2007; Nápoles et al., 2010).

The role of family caregivers following discharge of their care recipient from a hospital or skilled nursing facility is important but currently understudied. The caregiver's specific role during this process may vary based on the care needs of the older adult, the caregiver's relationship to the older adult, and where the caregiver lives in relation to the older adult (Gitlin and Wolff, 2012). Given that current research shows the availability and preparedness of caregivers can affect the quality and course of care recipients' post-hospitalization care and that caregivers are often underequipped, outlining and defining these roles is important to designing possible interventions to help caregivers during the discharge process (Gitlin and Wolff, 2012). Chapter 6 discusses current interventions that seek to support caregivers during the discharge and care transition process.

More than three-quarters of caregivers (77 percent) reported helping with health systems interactions; many also assisted with making appointments (67 percent), speaking to doctors (60 percent), ordering medications (55 percent), adding or changing insurance (29 percent), or handling other insurance issues (39 percent) (see Figure 3-3).

Family caregivers continue to be involved with older adults who move into residential facilities (e.g., assisted living facilities and nursing homes). They perform tasks similar to those they carried out in the care recipient's home, providing emotional support and companionship, as well as feeding, grooming, managing money, shopping, and providing transportation. For example, in interviews with 438 such caregivers between 2002 and 2005, Williams and colleagues (2012) found that more than half of the caregivers had monitored care recipient health status, managed care, and assisted with meals; 40 percent assisted with self-care tasks. Caregivers may also take on new tasks when their care recipient moves into a residential facility, interacting with the facility's administration and staff, advocating for the resident, and serving as his or her surrogate decision maker (Friedemann et al., 1997; Ryan and Scullion, 2000).

Advocacy and care coordination in formal care settings can be especially challenging. A transition to a new care setting often requires the caregiver to coordinate a new array of services and providers, serve as a communication conduit between settings, and seek new information to ensure that the care recipient's needs are met.

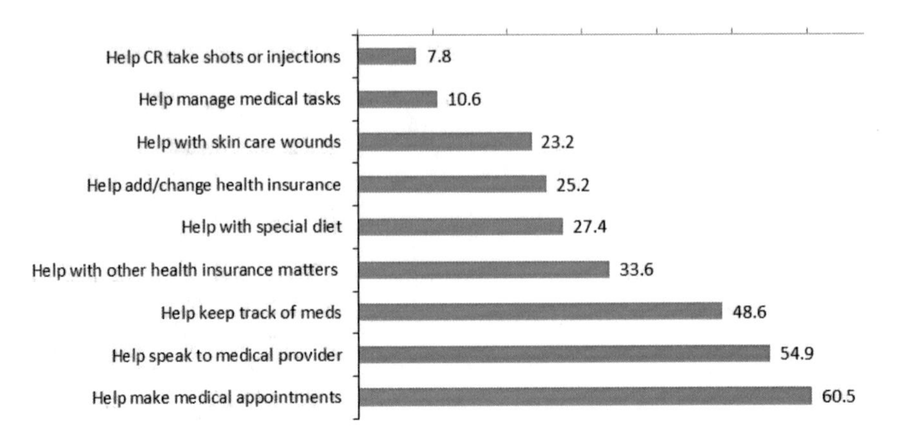

FIGURE 3-3 Percentage of caregivers coordinating care and providing medical tasks during the past month.
NOTES: Includes family caregivers of Medicare beneficiaries age 65 and older in the continental United States who resided in community or residential care settings (other than nursing homes) and received help with self-care, mobility, or household activities for health or functioning reasons. CR = care recipient.
SOURCES: Data from the 2011 NHATS and the companion NSOC.

Decision Making and Surrogacy

> In 2010, at my parents' request, I received both general and healthcare powers of attorney. The healthcare power of attorney contains both a living will and a HIPAA [Health Insurance Portability and Accountability Act] authorization, and gives me broad authority to get health information and make decisions. (I carry them with me at all times on a USB memory stick.) (Kenyon, 2015)

Caregivers are often involved in decision making with and, in some circumstances, for care recipients. However, the nature of caregivers' involvement varies. Types of decision-making roles include directive; participatory; supportive or guiding; advisory; advocacy; and trying to hold back and let the older adult decide (Garvelink et al., 2016). Care recipients with cognitive impairments may require surrogate decision making, as discussed below, although individuals with mild to moderate cognitive impairment often have the ability to express preferences and make choices (Feinberg and Whitlatch, 2001; Whitlatch, 2008). Frail older adults may be able to express their preferences, but lack executional autonomy or the ability to carry out their decisions without considerable assistance from a caregiver (Gillick,

2013). Caregivers and care recipients may confront many kinds of decisions, including decisions about treatment choices, location of care, and end-of-life care (Edwards et al., 2012; Garvelink et al., 2016; Gillick, 2013).

Decision making involves both older adult and caregiver values, preferences, needs, goals, abilities, and perceptions, which may or may not be congruent and in some instances may be in conflict (Garvelink et al., 2016; Kitko et al., 2015; Moon et al., 2016; Whitlatch and Feinberg, 2007). Decision making also involves religious considerations, family dynamics, finances, and feasibility (Garvelink et al., 2016). While respecting the rights of the care recipient and making sure his or her voice is primary, good communication and finding a balance between the care recipient's needs and preferences and the caregiver's ability to meet them contribute to the well-being of both parties (Whitlatch, 2008). Multiple legal tools such as health care and financial powers of attorney, living wills, and personal care agreements can help family caregivers and their families to better outline the preferences of the care recipient and the scope of his or her caregiver's decision making authority (Sabatino, 2015).

Although supported decision making attempts to give individuals the assistance they need to make decisions for themselves to the greatest extent possible, many individuals with advanced illnesses lack decision making capacity and therefore need to rely on surrogates. Studies show that family members are involved in decision making for nearly half (47 percent) of hospitalized older adults, including 23 percent needing all decisions made by a surrogate (Torke et al., 2009, 2014).

Most individuals prefer to involve family members in medical decisions and have family serve as surrogate decision makers when the individual loses decision-making capacity (Kelly et al., 2012). Some individuals step into the role of surrogate formally by being appointed under an advance directive or power of attorney or by a court in a guardianship proceeding. Others may fall into the role by default by virtue of being a close family member or friend. For health care decisions, the prevailing paradigm for default surrogate decision makers is a nuclear family hierarchy although some states also recognize close friends at the end of the hierarchy (ABA Commission on Law and Aging, 2014). This next-of-kin model lacks flexibility for accommodating diverse family structures and decision-making practices.

Family surrogates also face surrogate decision-making tasks far beyond health decisions. The management of the care recipient's affairs including financial, legal, and insurance issues is common. There is no counterpart to health care default surrogate decision-making laws for financial affairs. Family members must have some type of formal authority to make decisions for the care recipient by means of some form of co-ownership (e.g., joint bank accounts) or they must be appointed to manage financial affairs as a fiduciary typically by means of a durable power of attorney for finances or a trust. They are often unfamiliar with these legal options and unprepared to take on the fiduciary roles bestowed by these legal tools.

Preparedness for Caregiving

Given the multifaceted and complex nature of the caregiving role as described above, preparedness for caregiving is essential. Caregivers need specialized knowledge and skills relevant to their particular needs, as well as broadly defined competencies, such as problem-solving and communication skills (Gitlin and Wolff, 2012). Yet the available evidence indicates that many caregivers receive inadequate preparation for the tasks they are expected to assume. In the 2015 National Alliance for Caregiving and AARP Public Policy Institute survey, half (51 percent) of caregivers of older adults age 50 and older with Alzheimer's disease or dementia reported that they provide medical/nursing tasks without prior preparation. Thirty percent of Alzheimer's disease caregivers had informational needs about managing challenging behaviors and 21 percent wanted more help or information about incontinence. In the Home Alone study, more than 60 percent of the caregivers reported learning how to manage at least some medications on their own (Reinhard et al., 2012). Forty-seven percent reported never receiving training from any source. Caregivers described learning by trial and error and feared making a mistake.

In summary, the family caregiving role is broad in scope, and often requires a significant commitment of time. The complexity of the caregiving role has increased in recent years. Whereas families traditionally have provided emotional support and assisted their older members with household and self-care tasks, family caregivers now provide health and medical care at home, navigate complicated and fragmented health care and LTSS, and serve in a surrogacy role that has legal implications. Given the scope and complexity of the family caregiving role, ensuring that caregivers are well prepared is essential. Yet caregiver educational needs are not systematically addressed and training in the performance of caregiving tasks is inconsistent at best.

The scope, time commitment, and complexity of the family caregiving role make it unique in the care of older adults. No single health care or social service discipline is charged with providing assistance with self-care and household tasks, providing emotional support, and performing health and medical tasks around the clock, 7 days per week; advocating for an older adult's needs, values, and preferences in multiple health care and LTSS settings; and functioning in a legal capacity as a surrogate decision maker. Health and social service professionals and direct care workers "hand off" responsibility to others, whereas many family caregivers do not have the option of handing off their responsibilities. Given the essential role they play, involving family caregivers as key partners in health care and LTSS settings is vitally important, as discussed further in Chapter 6.

THE IMPACT OF CAREGIVING ON THE CAREGIVER

The effects of caregiving are both wide ranging and highly individualized. Caregivers are potentially at increased risk for adverse effects on their well-being in virtually every aspect of their lives, ranging from their health and quality of life to their relationships and economic security. However, the actual consequences for individual caregivers are variable, depending on a host of individual and contextual characteristics.

Data from NSOC provide an overview of both negative and positive impacts of caregiving. For example, more than 20 percent of caregivers report that caregiving is financially and physically difficult for them, and 44 percent report that it is emotionally difficult. High rates of difficulty are particularly prevalent among caregivers providing intensive levels of care. As one would expect, caring for persons with high care needs such as persons with dementia or self-care needs creates more difficulties for the caregiver than persons with lesser needs. These caregivers also report relatively high rates of exhaustion, being overwhelmed, and not having enough time for themselves (see Table 3-3).

Caregivers also find benefit in caregiving. As shown in Figure 3-4, helping the care recipients often instills confidence in the caregivers, teaches them how to deal with difficult situations, makes them feel closer to the care recipient, and assures them that the care recipient is well-cared for. It is important to note, however, that these positive effects can co-exist with the negative impact of caregiving. Caregivers can simultaneously feel highly distressed and report that they derive benefit from the caregiving experience (Beach et al., 2000).

Psychological Effects

As noted above, caregivers experience both positive and negative psychological effects from caregiving (Pinquart and Sörensen, 2003), but research has by far focused on negative effects. The effects of caregiving are variable, depending on characteristics intrinsic and extrinsic to the individual. Nevertheless, the body of evidence on negative effects is far larger than that on positive effects, as researchers have sought to assess the public health implications of caregiving and identify vulnerable at-risk caregivers. Documenting the adverse effects of family caregiving on both caregivers and care recipients is a requisite first step in developing interventions and public policy to address the needs of caregivers.

TABLE 3-3 Family Caregiver Reports of Emotional, Physical, and Other Difficulties, by Care Recipient's Dementia Status and Level of Impairment, by Percentage, 2011

	Care Recipient's Dementia Status and Level of Impairment			
Difficulties	Dementia Only	No Dementia; Has Two or More Self-Care Needs	Dementia; Has Two or More Self-Care Needs	No Dementia; Has Less Than Two Self-Care Needs
Percentage of caregivers reporting . . .				
Emotional difficulty	48.8	45.5	56.5	38.1
Physical difficulty	20.4	28.5	39.6	16.4
Percentage of caregivers responding "very much" . . .				
Exhausted at night	17.0	19.6	25.3	11.8
More things to do than they can handle	26.7	18.0	23.9	11.7
Don't have time for themselves	23.3	14.3	24.3	10.0
Population represented (in 1,000s)	2,931	2,745	2,828	9,190

NOTES: Includes family caregivers of Medicare beneficiaries age 65 and older in the continental United States who resided in community or residential care settings (other than nursing homes) and received help with self-care, mobility, or household activities for health or functioning reasons. Self-care activities include bathing, dressing, eating, toileting, or getting in and out of bed. Excludes caregivers of nursing home residents. "Dementia only" refers to care recipients with possible dementia and less than two self-care needs. "Probable dementia" includes individuals whose doctor said they had dementia or Alzheimer's disease and individuals classified as having probable dementia based on results from a proxy screening instrument and several cognitive tests.
SOURCES: Data from the 2011 NHATS and the companion NSOC.

Harms

Negative psychological effects of caregiving span a continuum ranging from the perception that caregiving is stressful or burdensome, to symptoms of depression and/or anxiety, to clinical depression diagnosed by a health professional, to impaired quality of life (Schulz and Sherwood, 2008; Zarit et al., 1980).

Assessment of psychological effects in research includes evaluation of individual psychological constructs (e.g., burden, depression, or anxiety) and the use of global inventories of mental health that encompass both depression and anxiety and instruments aimed at characterizing general

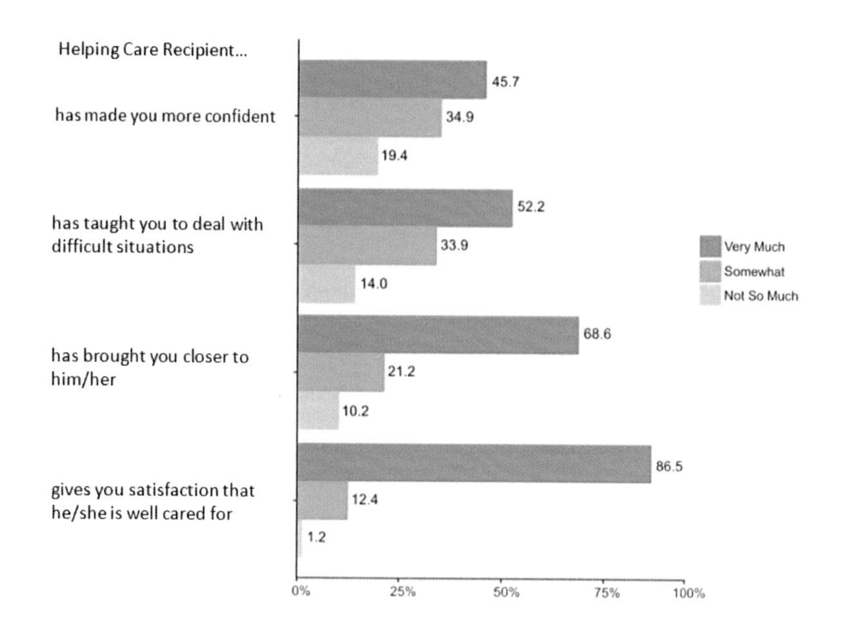

FIGURE 3-4 Percentage of caregivers responding very much, somewhat, not so much to positive aspects of caregiving.
NOTES: Includes family caregivers of Medicare beneficiaries age 65 and older in the continental United States who resided in community or residential care settings (other than nursing homes) and received help with self-care, mobility, or household activities for health or functioning reasons.
SOURCES: Data from the 2011 NHATS and the companion NSOC.

well-being and quality of life in the caregiver. Both caregiver self-report and clinical interviews with diagnostic criteria are used in research. Samples may be heterogeneous or more narrowly targeted to particular groups of caregivers (e.g., spouses or particular clinical populations).

A large and robust literature documents higher rates of psychological distress among caregivers compared with non-caregiver comparison groups. Evidence has been steadily accumulating during the 20 years that have elapsed since one of the earliest reviews by Schulz and colleagues (1995) and now includes a vast number of individual clinical studies, multiple systematic reviews (e.g., Cuijpers, 2005; Pinquart and Sörensen, 2003), and an increasing number of population-based epidemiological studies (Capistrant, 2016; Wolff et al., 2016). Much of this literature is based on cross-sectional studies in which caregivers are compared to comparable non-caregivers.

Since matching is always imperfect, these studies raise questions about the net effect of caregiving as opposed to selection biases that may be associated with caregiver outcomes. For example, shared life-style factors in married couples would predict that disability and psychological distress in one partner is associated with similar characteristics in the other. Thus, an outcome attributed to caregiving such as depression may be a reflection of underlying vulnerabilities shared by both partners (Roth et al., 2015). A more compelling case for the causal relationship between caregiving and psychological distress, for example, can be made from longitudinal studies in which individuals are followed into, throughout, and out of the caregiving role. These studies demonstrate significant declines in well-being as the person enters the caregiving role, further deterioration in well-being as care demands increase, and recovery after the care recipient dies (Beach et al., 2000; Dunkle et al., 2014; Hirst, 2005; Kurtz et al., 1995; Schulz et al., 2003). Intervention studies (see Chapter 5) showing improvement in caregiver health and well-being when caregiving needs are addressed also support causal connections between caregiving and well-being outcomes.

The prevalence of negative psychological effects among caregivers indicates that large segments of the caregiving population experience adverse effects. For example, 26 percent of all caregivers and 29 percent of those caring for the most disabled older adults reported substantial emotional difficulties in NSOC (Spillman et al., 2014). Thirteen percent of all caregivers and 15 percent of those caring for the most disabled older adults reported symptoms of anxiety and depression. In a study of caregivers of individuals who experienced a stroke, Haley and colleagues (2009) found that 14 percent of stroke caregivers reported clinically significant levels of depression. Even higher rates of depression are found in the dementia caregiving population. In a systematic review of 10 studies in this population, the prevalence rate for depressive disorders was 22.3 percent using standardized diagnostic criteria (Cuijpers, 2005). Among cancer caregivers, 25 percent reported clinically meaningful levels of depressive symptoms 2 years after the care recipient's diagnosis (Girgis et al., 2013; Kim et al., 2014).

In a meta-analysis of 84 studies, caregivers again were found to experience more depression and stress and less general subjective well-being than non-caregivers (Pinquart and Sörensen, 2003). Although differences in psychological well-being between whites and racial and ethnic subgroups are generally small, several systematic reviews report that African American caregivers tended to report lower levels of caregiver burden and depression than white, non-Hispanic caregivers while Hispanic and Asian American caregivers reported more depression than white caregivers (Nápoles et al., 2010; Pinquart and Sörensen, 2005). In a systematic review, Cuijpers (2005) found that the relative risk for clinical depression among dementia caregivers compared with non-caregivers in six studies ranged from 2.80

to 38.68. In an analysis of data from the prospective Nurses' Health Study, women who provided 36 or more hours of care per week to a disabled spouse were nearly 6 times more likely than non-caregivers to experience depressive or anxious symptoms (Cannuscio et al., 2002).

Family caregiver depressive symptoms and anxiety persist when the care recipient moves to a long-term care facility with similar severity as when they were providing in-home care, and antianxiety medication use has been found to increase before and after placement (Schulz et al., 2004). Indeed, the greater the hands-on care provided by the family caregivers, the higher their distress, and the lower their satisfaction with care provided by the nursing home staff (Tornatore and Grant, 2004). Causes of distress among caregivers include inadequate resident self-care, lack of communication with nursing home physicians, and challenges of surrogate decision making, including the need for education to support advance care planning and end-of-life decisions (Givens et al., 2012). Although the findings on the experience and impact of family caregiving in LTSS settings are consistent across studies (Gaugler, 2005), individual study samples are not necessarily representative of this population, making it difficult to generate population-level estimates for these indicators.

Longitudinal studies of psychological health effects among caregivers over time suggest that negative effects vary across the caregiving trajectory, although there may be critical periods when caregivers are most at risk for elevated psychological distress. In an analysis of longitudinal data from the British Household Panel Survey, Hirst (2005) found that negative psychological effects among heavily involved caregivers were most pronounced around the transitional periods of the start of caregiving and when caregiving ends. Longitudinal data from the Nurses' Health Study (Cannuscio et al., 2002) and the Health and Retirement Study (Dunkle et al., 2014) also indicate that the transition into the caregiving role is a time of elevated risk for increased depressive symptomatology.

However, caregiving over a long period of time may also have negative psychological effects. The American Cancer Society National Quality of Life Survey for Caregivers, which included follow-up assessments 2 and 5 years after cancer diagnosis, found that those who were still caregiving at 5 years had the largest increase in depressive symptoms and the poorest quality of life when compared to caregivers for a recipient now in remission or bereaved caregivers of recipients who had died (Kim et al., 2014). Among the group that was still caregiving, the level of clinically meaningful depressive symptoms rose from 28 percent at 2 years to 42 percent at 5 years (Kim et al., 2014).

A different longitudinal pattern was found in the stroke population, suggesting that the impact of caregiving over time may vary across clinical populations. In the Caring for Adults Recovering from the Effects of Stroke

(CARES) study, caregivers at 9 months after a stroke had significantly higher depressive symptoms than non-caregiving controls. However, this difference decreased over time, suggesting that caregivers are able to adapt to caregiving demands that remain relatively stable over time (Haley et al., 2015).

Positive Aspects

Although a substantial proportion of the caregiver population experiences negative psychological effects, many also find caregiving rewarding. Thus, a growing number of studies focus on the positive effects of caregiving in order to better understand the potential for personal growth and the mental health-promoting aspects of caregiving (Brown and Brown, 2014; Roth et al., 2015). However, as yet, fewer systematic reviews and population-based studies are available for positive effects compared with negative effects. Nevertheless, such research has introduced a more balanced treatment of psychological effects into the literature.

The positive psychological effects of caregiving have been defined in various ways. Most common are caregiving rewards or benefits, appreciation of life, personal growth, enhanced self-efficacy, competence or mastery, self-esteem, and closer relationships (Haley et al., 2009; J. H. Kim et al., 2007; Y. Kim et al., 2007). Prevalence rates for positive psychological effects are high across the caregiving population as a whole, with variation evident among demographic subgroups of caregivers. In NSOC, for example, 46 percent of caregivers reported feeling "very much" more confident about their abilities (see Figure 3-4). Percentages are substantially higher on this indicator for African American caregivers (68 percent), Hispanic caregivers (60 percent), caregivers with less than a high school education (67 percent), caregivers with income below $20,000 (67 percent), and caregivers who help more often with self-care tasks (58 percent). Similarly, in NSOC, 52 percent of caregivers reported feeling "very much" better able to deal with difficult situations. Again, percentages are higher for African American caregivers (67 percent), caregivers with less than a high school education (64 percent), and caregivers who help more often with self-care tasks (66 percent). These findings are consistent with literature reviews showing that racial and ethnic minority caregivers experienced higher levels of subjective well-being and perceived uplifts than white, non-Hispanic caregivers (Pinquart and Sörensen, 2005).

Positive psychological effects may mitigate some of the negative effects of caregiving, as several studies find that positive effects are associated with lower levels of burden and depression and better overall mental health. For example, van der Lee and colleagues (2014) found that a sense of competence or self-efficacy was associated with less caregiver burden and greater mental health, while Y. Kim and colleagues (2007) found that caregivers' esteem from caregiving was associated with lower psychological distress and better mental functioning.

In summary, a large body of literature, including population-based cross-sectional and longitudinal studies, provides strong evidence that a substantial proportion of the caregiving population experiences negative psychological effects, even though caregiving has some positive effects as well. Regardless of the mental health indicator used, levels of distress are high enough to constitute a public health concern.

Evidence about predictors of negative psychological health effects suggests that prevalence rates vary across subgroups of caregivers, placing some caregivers at higher risk for negative effects than others. Further evidence suggests that risk factors are multifactorial and may be cumulative. Women providing many hours of care weekly to a care recipient with challenging behavioral symptoms may be at particularly high risk. Thus, multidimensional assessment is needed to identify the specific array of risk factors present for any given caregiver. Likewise, interventions need to be tailored to specific subpopulations of caregivers.

Physical Health Effects

A variety of indicators have been used to assess the physical health of caregivers including global health status indicators, physiological measures, and health behaviors (see Table 3-4). Global health status indicators include standardized self-assessment tools such as health-related quality of life, chronic conditions, physical symptoms (e.g., Cornell Medical Index), mortality, and health service use, including clinic visits, physician or nurse practitioner visits, and days in the hospital (Schulz and Sherwood, 2008). For example, in a review of 176 studies of family caregivers of older adults assessing the physical health of caregivers, Pinquart and Sörenson (2007) found 66 percent of studies used a "single-item indicator" self-report measure, 21 percent incorporated measures related to physical impairment (activities of daily living or instrumental activities of daily living scales), 19 percent included measures based on a symptom checklist (e.g., SF-36[4]), 15 percent used the number of medical or chronic conditions, three studies assessed use of medications, and three measured usage of hospital or doctor visits. Saban and colleagues (2010) identified a similar list of health outcomes in their review of the literature and noted that overall studies focused on physical health are much rarer than studies assessing psychological outcomes such as stress and depression.

[4] The SF-36 is a 36-item patient-reported survey that is commonly used to assess physical and mental health and quality of life.

TABLE 3-4 Summary of Findings on the Physical Health Outcomes of Family Caregiving of Older Adults

Type of Measure/Health Indicator	Findings
Global Health Measures	
• Self-reported health (current health, health compared to others, changes in health status) • Chronic conditions (chronic illness checklists) • Physical symptoms (Cornell Medical Index) • Medications (number and types) • Health service usage (clinic visits, days in hospital, physician visits) • Mortality	Negative effects found for all indicators but effects are small to medium; self-report measures are most common and show largest negative effects High-stress caregiving associated with increased mortality in several studies
Physiological Measures	
• Antibodies and functional immune measures (immunoglobulin, Epstein-Barr virus, T-cell proliferation, responses to mitogens, response to cytokine stimulation, lymphocyte counts) • Stress hormones and neurotransmitters (ACTH, epinephrine, norepinephrine, cortisol, prolactin) • Cardiovascular measures (blood pressure, heart rate) • Metabolic measures (body mass, weight, cholesterol, insulin, glucose, transferrin) • Speed of wound healing • Telomere erosion	Negative effects for most indicators are generally small; larger negative effects found for stress hormones and antibodies than other indicators; some evidence for adverse metabolic effects and telomere erosion
Health Behaviors	
• Sleep, diet, exercise, smoking • Self-care, preventive care, medical compliance	Some evidence supporting impaired health behaviors in all domains; evidence is strongest for sleep problems in dementia caregivers

NOTE: ACTH = adrenocorticotropic hormone.
SOURCE: Adapted from Schulz and Sherwood, 2008.

The diversity of methods and instruments used to measure caregiver health makes cross-study comparisons and meta-analyses difficult (Grady and Rosenbaum, 2015). Methodological rigor of studies that assess impacts on the physical health of caregivers is often limited by study sample size, selection of comparison or control groups, timeline for data collection and longitudinal assessments as well as by the statistical methods used (Cameron and Elliott, 2015; Grady and Rosenbaum, 2015). Thus, caution is advised in overattributing negative health outcomes to the effects of caregiving. The physical health status and outcomes for caregivers may be relatively independent of the caregiving role or related to individual characteristics that existed prior to assuming the caregiving role, such as socioeconomic status, health habits, and prior illness (Brown and Brown, 2014; Robison et al., 2009; Roth et al., 2015; Schulz and Sherwood, 2008). Nevertheless, the data support the conclusion that at least some caregivers are at risk for adverse health outcomes (Capistrant, 2016). In the discussion below, we identify a broad range of individual and contextual factors that contribute to adverse health outcomes in caregivers.

Caregivers' Reports on their Health Status

Caregivers tend to rate their health as poorer than non-caregivers. Caregivers for older care recipients consistently report poorer subjective health status than non-caregivers (Berglund et al., 2015; Pinquart and Sörenson, 2003). Poorer caregiver physical health is closely associated with greater caregiver burden and depressive symptoms and is associated to a lesser degree with hours of care provided, the number of caregiving tasks, months in the caregiver role, as well as the physical, cognitive, and behavioral impairments and problems of the care recipient (Pinquart and Sörenson, 2007). Family caregivers in England responding to a national survey of users of primary care services also reported poorer health and a worse primary care individual experience compared with non-caregiver individuals with similar demographics, including age, gender, ethnicity, and level of social deprivation (Persson et al., 2015). In NSOC, 20 percent of all caregivers and 39 percent of caregivers of high-need older adults reported that they experienced a substantial level of physical difficulty.[5] Sleep problems affected more than 40 percent of caregivers and were highly correlated with reports of substantial negative effects of caregiving (Spillman et al, 2014).

Using the Health and Retirement Study (HRS), a large representative sample of U.S. adults, Capistrant and colleagues (2012) found that being a spousal caregiver independently predicted incident cardiovascular disease. Longer-term caregivers had twice the risk of short-term caregivers. However, this effect was observed only among whites, not among non-whites. Ji and colleagues (2012) reported similar results for spousal caregivers of persons with cancer. After cancer diagnosis in their spouse, the risk of coronary heart disease (CHD) and stroke were higher in both husband and wife caregivers when compared to husbands and wives without an affected

---

[5] Committee calculations.

spouse. These effects were more pronounced when the type of cancer had a high mortality rate, such as pancreatic and lung cancers. These findings suggest that psychological distress associated with the diagnosis may play a role in the risk of CHD and stroke.

Also based on data from the HRS collected from 1998 to 2010, Dassel and Carr (2014) showed that spousal caregivers of persons with dementia are significantly more likely to experience increased frailty (i.e., unintentional weight loss, self-reported exhaustion, weakness, slow walking speed, and low physical activity [as defined by Fried et al., 2001]) over time when compared to non-dementia spousal caregivers. Similarly, a systematic review of 192 articles focused on cancer caregiving (1990-2008) found that the most prevalent problems for caregivers included sleep disturbance, fatigue, pain, loss of physical strength, loss of appetite, and weight loss (Stenberg et al., 2010).

One of the consistent themes in the caregiver health effects literature concerns the role of caregiver strain in predicting negative health effects (Schulz et al., 1997), including mortality. Schulz and Beach (1999) found increased risk of mortality (63 percent) among older spousal caregivers, but only if they reported emotional strain in the caregiving role. Perkins and colleagues (2013) reported similar results showing that caregivers who reported high levels of caregiving strain had an excess 55 percent mortality risk when compared with those reporting no stress. Living with a person with Parkinson's disease 5 years after first Parkinson hospitalization was associated with higher risk of all-cause mortality for both husbands and wives in a study by Nielsen and colleagues (2014).

In contrast to these studies, several recent population-based studies suggest the opposite—that caregiving is associated with lower mortality risk (Brown et al., 2009). Fredman and colleagues (2015) found a 26 percent lower mortality risk among older adult caregivers when compared to non-caregivers, and several U.S. Census-based studies show lower mortality rates among caregivers (O'Reilly et al., 2008, O'Reilly et al., 2015; Ramsay et al., 2013). These opposing perspectives on caregiving and mortality may be reconcilable if we consider that negative impact studies are typically based on vulnerable, older, strained caregiving spouses providing intense levels of care while studies reporting positive effects focus on all caregivers regardless of age of caregiver, relationship to the care recipient, or type and amount of care provided.

Caregiving-Related Injuries

Providing care to an older adult is often physically demanding. In NSOC, 20 percent of all caregivers and 39 percent of high-need caregivers reported that providing care was physically difficult. Caregiving tasks such as transfers, lifts, bathing, dressing, and repositioning the care recipient place physical strain on the caregiver and may result in musculoskeletal injury such as back ache, muscle strain, and contusions (Brown and Mulley, 1997; Darragh et al., 2015; Hartke et al., 2006). These effects are likely to be exacerbated among older caregivers with impaired vestibular function, limited motion due to arthritis, and weakness due to age-related changes in muscle mass. The risk of injury is further compounded by the home environments of the care recipient, which may include small spaces, crowded and cluttered rooms, and steep stairways (NRC, 2011). Although reliable data on injury rates among caregivers are not available, the fact that paid home health aides as well as home care nursing and rehabilitation personnel sustain high rates of work-related musculoskeletal disorders suggests that this is likely to be a problem among family caregivers as well. Workplace injuries among direct-care workers that result in time away from work are four times the average rate of all occupations (BLS, 2007). Mitigating injuries related to caregiving requires a careful assessment of the home environment, an understanding of caregiving task demands, and the physical capabilities of the caregiver. This information can then be used to develop a treatment plan that may involve home alterations, caregiver training on how to safely perform required caregiving tasks, and the use of paid professionals to perform tasks that place the caregiver at risk of injury (Cornman-Levy et al., 2001).

Physiological Measures

Biological indicators include a broad array of measures aimed at assessing physiological markers that are thought to be responsive to chronic stress exposure and affect downstream illness and disease. These markers include measures of stress hormones and neurotransmitters such as cortisol, epinephrine, and norepinephrine; measures of immunologic function such as natural killer cell activity and healing response to a standardized skin puncture wound (wound healing); antibody markers such as vaccination response; cardiovascular markers such as blood pressure and heart rate; and metabolic markers such as insulin, transferrin, and plasma lipids (Vitaliano et al., 2003). These markers have been studied primarily in case control studies comparing stressed dementia caregivers with demographically similar non-caregiving controls. In a meta-analysis of the literature in this area, Vitaliano and colleagues (2003) found moderately sized statistically significant differences between dementia caregivers and controls, indicating more adverse effects among dementia caregivers. Subsequent studies have shown an increased risk of cardiometabolic changes and increased Framingham Coronary Heart Disease Risk Scores in dementia caregivers as well as proinflammatory changes and accelerated aging of the immune system (i.e., telomere erosion) (Damjanovic et al., 2007; Haley et al., 2010; Kiecolt-Glaser et al., 2003; Mausbach et al., 2007; von Känel et al., 2008). A recent study also examined kidney function in dementia caregivers over a study period of up to 3 years, but found no differences between caregivers and non-caregivers, possibly because the follow-up period was not long enough (von Känel et al., 2012). While the preponderance of evidence suggests an association between caregiving and physiological function, it is important to keep in mind that the caregivers selected for these studies are typically moderately to highly stressed dementia caregivers and therefore the generalizability of findings may be limited. In addition, some researchers have questioned the choice of control subjects in these case control studies, which may not adequately control for preexisting differences between caregivers and non-caregivers (O'Reilly et al., 2015).

Health Behaviors

For caregivers, neglect of their own health may worsen preexisting illnesses or increase vulnerability to stress-related problems (Son et al., 2007; Vitaliano et al., 2003; Yueh-Feng Lu and Austrom, 2005). Health-promoting self-care behaviors are designed to improve health, maintain optimal functioning, and increase general well-being. Health-promoting self-care for caregivers can include getting enough rest, maintaining a healthy diet, getting enough exercise, taking breaks, taking care of one's own health, seeking preventive health care, joining a support group, and locating respite care when needed (Acton, 2002; Collins and Swartz, 2011). Health risk behaviors for caregivers can include substance abuse, sleep problems, poor diets, sedentary behaviors (Vitaliano et al., 2003), smoking (Salgado-Garcia et al., 2015), and alcohol consumption (de Nooijer, et al., 2003).

Early work by researchers such as Gallant and Connell (1997), Pearlin and colleagues (1990), and Schulz and Beach (1999) suggested that health-promoting and self-care behaviors may be neglected by caregivers due to their caregiving duties, lack of time and energy to take care of themselves, or breakdown of social networks; health risk behaviors also may be triggered by care recipient behaviors or by coping mechanisms induced by the stress of caregiving. For example, in a study of dementia caregivers, nearly one-third frequently or occasionally missed medication doses and nearly a half did not keep their own health care appointments (Wang et al., 2015). In another dementia caregiving sample, 40 percent of caregivers reported smoking and 25 percent reported a recent increase in smoking (Salgado-Garcia et al., 2015).

Being female (Wang et al., 2015) and older (Rabinowitz et al., 2007) or younger (Salgado-Garcia et al., 2015) have all been associated with poorer caregiver health behavior. However, the relationship between caregiving and health behaviors/self-care is complex. In a review article of 23 studies, Vitaliano and colleagues (2003) found that dementia caregivers reported more risky health behaviors than non-caregivers. Although caregivers may have had poor health habits before caregiving (Vitaliano et al., 2003) or their health behaviors may be related to illness or other factors, these behaviors may also be triggered by the care recipient's behaviors or by distress.

This potential relationship between caregiving events and factors related to the caregiver can be seen clearly in the case of caregiver sleep disturbance. Caregivers of people with dementia have more sleep problems than non-caregiving adults, including waking up in the night or early morning, bathroom needs, sleep-onset difficulties, nighttime care recipient disruptions, and psychological distress (Wilcox and King, 1999). Behaviors of people with dementia may initially disrupt the caregiver's sleep patterns. However, subsequent caregiver sleep disturbances may be the result of factors related to risk factors for sleep difficulties (e.g., being an older woman, poor caregiver health), or subjective caregiver burden, depression, or anxiety (McCurry et al., 2007; Wilcox and King, 1999).

Evidence shows that burden, stress, and depression influence health behaviors. Caregivers who report high levels of stress are more likely to report risky health behaviors (Sisk, 2000; Zarit and Gaugler, 2000). Higher levels of objective (care recipient problem behaviors) and subjective (feeling of overload) burden are associated with negative health behaviors for dementia caregivers (Son et al., 2007), as is worse care recipient health (Rabinowitz et al., 2007). Increase in smoking for caregivers is associated with higher depression scores (Salgado-Garcia et al., 2015). Longer length of caregiving and more care recipient dependency in activities of daily living are associated with a decrease in the health-promoting behaviors of medication adherence and appointment keeping for caregivers (Wang et al., 2015). Conversely, caregivers who spend less time on duty for the care recipient use more health care services for themselves (Martindale-Adams et al., 2015). Caregivers perceiving lower subjective burden practice more health-promoting behaviors than those with higher subjective burden scores (Sisk, 2000).

Feeling capable of managing caregiving difficulties and positive caregiver health behaviors are associated. In a study of dementia caregivers, higher self-efficacy in controlling upsetting thoughts and obtaining respite is associated with fewer negative health risk behaviors and higher engagement in positive health behaviors (Rabinowitz et al., 2007). More caregiving skills are associated with less increase in smoking (Salgado-Garcia et al., 2015). Caregivers who practice health-promoting self-care behaviors are better protected from stress, and the effects of stress on well-being are reduced (Acton, 2002).

Social Effects

The social effects of caregiving range from changes in family relationships, including relationships with a spouse, children, and other close individuals, to changes in social activities with and social support from a wider network. Reduced time and energy for maintaining social relationships may occur, resulting in isolation and long-term constriction of social networks (George and Gwyther, 1986; Gwyther, 1998; Seltzer and Li, 2000; Skaff and Pearlin, 1992). In some instances, caregivers may experience extreme, life-changing social effects that irrevocably change relationships and even alter the life course, such as marital infidelity, spousal abuse, and/or divorce.

The time demands of caregiving often limit the opportunity to engage in other activities that caregivers enjoy (see Table 3-5). For example, 15.1 percent of caregivers responded "very much" and 26.2 percent responded "somewhat" when asked if they do not have time for themselves. Family caregivers who help with self-care tasks and/or care for persons with dementia report more limitations in their ability to spend time for themselves when compared to caregivers with less intense care responsibilities. As shown in Table 3-5, high-need caregivers who care for someone with probable dementia and with self-care needs report the highest level of restriction in their ability to visit with friends and family, to attend religious services, to go out for dinner or movies, or to do volunteer work.

Family Relationships

Family relationships and quality of life may also be impacted by caregiving demands, although this topic has received relatively little attention in the caregiving literature. In a large panel study of Health and Retirement Study participants, Amirkhanyan and Wolf (2006) found that adverse psychological effects of caregiving are dispersed throughout the family and not just the active caregivers. Bookwala (2009) found in a sample of adult caregiving daughters and sons that longer-term caregivers were significantly less happy in their marriages than those who recently assumed the caregiving role, suggesting that it takes time for negative impacts to manifest themselves.

The demands of caregiving may also generate familial conflict about care decisions. When caregivers were asked in NSOC how much family members disagreed over the details of the care recipient's care, 6.7 percent reported that family members disagreed "very much" and 13.9 percent disagreed "somewhat." These percentages were higher for Hispanic caregivers (11.0 percent and 17.5 percent), caregivers with less than a high school education (15.2 percent and 5.7 percent), and caregivers providing

TABLE 3-5 Family Caregiving's Social Impact, by Care Recipient's Dementia Status and Level of Impairment, by Percentage, 2011

	Care Recipient's Dementia Status and Level of Impairment			
Social Activities Identified by Caregivers as "Very" or "Somewhat" Important to Them	Dementia Only	No Dementia; Has Two or More Self-Care Needs	Dementia; Has Two or More Self-Care Needs	No Dementia; Has Fewer Than Two Self-Care Needs
Did caregiving keep you from . . .		Yes (Percentage)		
Visiting in person with friends or family	18.7	18	30.8	11.2
Attending religious services	5.7	10.7	16.4	4.1
Going out for enjoyment (e.g., dinner, movie, gamble)	14.7	13.5	23.7	6.1
Doing volunteer work	8.5	5.8	15.1	4.8
Population represented (in 1000s)	2,931	2,745	2,828	9,190

NOTES: Includes family caregivers of Medicare beneficiaries age 65 and older in the continental United States who resided in community or residential care settings (other than nursing homes) and received help with self-care, mobility, or household activities for health or functioning reasons. Self-care activities include bathing, dressing, eating, toileting, or getting in and out of bed. "Dementia only" refers to care recipients with possible dementia and less than two self-care needs. "Probable dementia" includes individuals whose doctor said they had dementia or Alzheimer's disease, and individuals classified as having probable dementia based on results from a proxy screening instrument and several cognitive tests.
SOURCES: Data from the 2011 NHATS and the companion NSOC.

high-intensity care defined as helping with two or more self-care needs (8.9 percent and 17.5 percent).

Sources of conflict include differing views about the appropriate boundaries for caregiving, disapproval of family members' actions or attitudes, disagreements about the nature and seriousness of the care recipient's condition, perceived failure to appreciate the demands on the primary caregiver and to provide adequate help or support, disapproval of the quality of care, and disagreements over financial matters pertaining to the care recipient (Aneshensel et al., 1995; Gwyther, 1995; Gwyther and Matchar, 2015; Strawbridge and Wallhagen, 1991). Aneshensel and colleagues (1995) found that although levels of conflict were low for most caregivers, one in four reported intense strife in at least one area of family conflict. In some instances, conflicts may be severe, resulting in severed relationships or legal action (Strawbridge and Wallhagen, 1991).

Anecdotal evidence in clinical and research contexts suggests that a small percentage of family caregivers experience severe conflict related to caregiving, resulting in abusive interactions with other family members and even divorce or other legal actions. Given the sensitive and potentially stigmatizing aspects of severe family conflict, it is surprising that this level of conflict has not been systematically examined in research. Thus, severe family conflict remains a hidden social effect of caregiving, recognized in clinical practice, but unexplored to date in research.

In sum, the time and energy demands of caregiving may compete with both work and leisure activities. The impact of caregiving on work is discussed in the following chapter. The brief review here highlights the consequences of caregiving for leisure activities, quality of married life, and family conflict. The small literature in this area emphasizes negative effects in all of these domains. Family systems approaches to caregiving in which family members are viewed as interacting elements that attempt to synchronize their efforts to deal with the challenges of providing care are relatively rare in the literature and deserve further attention. Because the caregiving literature has focused almost exclusively on the single primary caregiver, little is known about how care tasks are distributed within a family over time, how care responsibilities are negotiated, and how the physical and psychological effects of caregiving are shared among family members. A better understanding of these processes may help to identify new intervention opportunities for caregiving.

Elder Mistreatment and Neglect

A potential effect of caregiving stress is elder mistreatment and neglect. Mistreatment of older adults can take many forms including physical, emotional, and sexual abuse as well as financial exploitation, neglect, and abandonment (National Center on Elder Abuse, 2015). To qualify as mistreatment, a behavior has to intentionally cause harm or create a serious risk of harm to a vulnerable older adult. The term "domestic elder abuse" is used to refer to mistreatment committed by someone with whom the older adult has a special relationship such as a spouse, sibling, child, friend, or caregiver. Caregiver neglect is a specific type of mistreatment in which the caregiver intentionally fails to address the physical, social, or emotional needs of the older person. This neglect can include withholding food, water, clothing, medications, or assistance with activities of daily living such as help with personal hygiene.

Prevalence estimates of abuse have generally ranged from 7 to 10 percent of older adults annually, although physical abuse (less than 2 percent) and sexual abuse (less than 1 percent) prevalence are much lower (Acierno et al., 2010; Lachs and Berman, 2011; Laumann et al., 2008). Research suggests that family members commit most abuse, but it is not known if this abuse occurs primarily within a caregiving context. Rates of abuse are generally higher for older adults with dementia and/or adults who need physical assistance, suggesting that family caregivers are likely perpetrators of abuse (Beach et al., 2005).

Although the data suggest that family caregivers may play a significant role in committing elder mistreatment when it does occur, there is a lack of adequate data to address this issue. Based on responses from care recipients, studies of potentially harmful behaviors, defined as behaviors that are detrimental to the elder's physical and psychological well-being, show prevalence rates of nearly 25 percent among caregivers. By far the most prevalent potentially harmful caregiver behavior involved negative verbal interactions like screaming/yelling (22.2 percent) or using a harsh tone of voice/insulting/calling names/swearing (11.7 percent). Physical forms of abuse like hitting/slapping, shaking, and handling roughly in other ways were much less prevalent, reported by only about 1 percent of the care recipients (Beach et al., 2005). Level of care recipient impairment in cognitive and physical functioning was a strong predictor of potentially harmful behavior. Similar results with even higher prevalence rates were reported by Lafferty and colleagues (2016) in their survey of more than 2,000 caregivers in Ireland. The extent to which family caregivers experience abuse, by the older adults they care for, is not known. More research is needed on the prevalence of elder mistreatment among caregivers, the type of mistreatment they commit, the circumstances under which it occurs, and the factors that mitigate mistreatment or neglect. Of particular importance is gaining a better understanding of how and when a supportive caregiving relationship evolves into an abusive one.

Risk Factors for Adverse Outcomes

The above review clearly finds that a significant proportion of caregivers experience a broad range of adverse outcomes including impairment in psychological and physical health, disruptions in social relationships, and possible mistreatment of the care provider or recipient. These negative effects, however, are not universal. While nearly half of caregivers experience emotional distress associated with caregiving, a much smaller proportion exhibit adverse physical health effects. This begs the question, who is at risk for adverse outcomes as a result of caregiving?

All of the variables listed in Table 3-6 have been identified in one or more studies as risk factors for adverse caregiver outcomes. These risk factors fall into six categories:

1. Sociodemographic factors
2. Intensity and type of caregiving tasks
3. Caregivers' perceptions of care recipients' suffering
4. Caregivers' own health and functioning
5. Caregivers' social and professional supports
6. Care recipients' physical home environment (see Table 3-6)

Evidence for the strength of most of these predictors is mixed and considerable variability exists in study design, methods, and quality of the research. However, accumulating evidence suggests that caregiving intensity (i.e., hours of caregiving per week), gender, relationship to the care recipient (wives are more affected than adult daughters or others), living with the care recipient, and challenging behavioral symptoms in the care recipient are relatively robust predictors of negative psychological effects.

The intensity of caregiving has been found to be a consistent predictor of negative psychological effects in population-based studies. An analysis of the Nurses' Health Study, for example, found that the odds of increasing depressive or anxious symptoms rose with increasing caregiving time commitment (Cannuscio et al., 2002). Women providing care to an ill or disabled spouse 36 hours or more weekly were nearly six times more likely than non-caregivers to report depressive or anxious symptoms. Women who provided 36 hours of care weekly to a parent were two times more likely to report depressive or anxious symptoms than non-caregivers (Cannuscio et al., 2002). A longitudinal analysis of the British Household Panel Survey found that caregivers who provided long hours of care for extended periods of time had increased levels of psychological distress, and that this association was stronger for women than men (Hirst, 2005). The risk for onset of distress increased progressively with the amount of time spent in caregiving each week.

Caregivers who provide high-intensity care are also more likely to make treatment decisions for the care recipient, which the literature suggests may be a unique risk factor for adverse outcomes. In a meta-analysis of 2,854 surrogate decision makers, at least one-third experienced emotional burden as the result of making treatment decisions. Negative effects were often substantial and typically lasted months or, in some cases, years. The most common negative effects were stress, guilt over the decisions they made, and doubt regarding whether they had made the right decisions (Wendler and Rid, 2011).

Female caregivers have been found to experience more psychological distress than males in a meta-analysis (Pinquart and Sörensen, 2006), in an early literature review (Yee and Schulz, 2000), and in a recent systematic review (Schoenmakers et al., 2010). In their meta-analysis of 229 studies, Pinquart and Sörensen (2006) found that women had higher levels of

TABLE 3-6 Risk Factors for Adverse Outcomes Due to Family Caregiving

Sociodemographic factors

- Lower income
- Lower education (high school or less)
- Older age (50 or older)
- Spouse of care recipient
- Female
- Living with care recipient

Intensity/type of caregiving

- More than 100 hours of care per month
- High care recipient personal/mobility care needs
- Dementia care (including management of behavioral symptoms)
- Medical care (shots/injections, wound care)
- Coordinating care (appointments, interacting with providers, dealing with health insurance)

Caregiver's perceptions of the care recipient's physical, psychological, and existential suffering

- Lack of choice in taking on the caregiving role

Caregiver's health and physical functioning

- Poor/fair self-rated health
- Feeling stressed
- Having three or more medical conditions
- Sleep problems
- Difficulty breathing
- Pain
- Limited leg/arm strength
- Unwanted weight lost

Caregiver's social and professional supports

- No one to help with caregiving
- No one to talk to
- No time to socialize with others
- No access or use of professional support/care services

Care recipient's home physical environment

- Lacks appropriate home modifications
- Stairs, clutter

SOURCES: Adelman et al., 2014; Pinquart and Sörensen, 2003; Zarit et al., 2010.

burden and depression and lower levels of subjective well-being than men. Gender differences in depression were partially explained by differences in caregiver stressors, such as more hours of care given per week and a greater number of caregiving tasks performed by women.

Differences in psychological effects also exist across racial and ethnic groups. A meta-analyses of 116 studies showed that African American caregivers had lower levels of burden and depression than non-Hispanic white caregivers, but Hispanic and Asian American caregivers reported more depression than their white, non-Hispanic counterparts (Pinquart and Sörensen, 2005). Similar racial and ethnic differences were reported in a subsequent systematic review of dementia caregiving (Nápoles et al., 2010). Although some data are available on African American and Hispanic caregivers, the literature on racially and ethnically diverse populations has several limitations, including

1. Few large-scale comparative studies on a spectrum of outcome variables and their predictors with sufficient numbers and statistical power to report outcomes stratified by caregiver race and ethnicity (Apesoa-Varano et al., 2015; Aranda, 2001);
2. Few studies that directly compare caregiving in specific groups such as Asian Americans and Pacific Islanders, American Indians, black Caribbeans, and monolingual Spanish speakers, or the heterogeneity within such groups (Milne and Chryssanthopoulou, 2005; Weiner, 2008);
3. Lack of attention to clinically determined caregiver health indicators that go beyond self-report (e.g., clinically diagnosed depressive disorder, objective indicators of functional health status, etc.) (Hinton, 2002; Schulz and Sherwood, 2008); and
4. Minimal attention to racially and ethnically diverse caregivers in a variety of contexts that go beyond dementia-specific caregiving (e.g., frailty, diabetes, brain injury, end-of-life care, etc.) (Aranda and Knight, 1997).

Caregivers who live with the care recipient are at increased risk of adverse outcomes. Schulz and colleagues have shown that these effects are in part explained by the exposure to suffering of the care recipient (Monin and Schulz, 2009; Schulz et al., 2007, 2009). Living with an older adult who is physically or psychologically suffering takes its toll on the caregiver, above and beyond the pragmatic challenges of providing assistance.

Whether an individual has a choice in taking on the caregiving role may also make a difference. Nearly half of all caregivers report that they had no choice in taking on the caregiving role and lack of perceived choice is associated with increased levels of burden and depression (Reinhard et al., 2012; Schulz et al., 2012).

Care recipients' behavioral symptoms (e.g., agitation, irritability, combativeness) are also associated with negative effects for caregivers (Ballard et al. 2000; Gitlin et al. 2012; Pinquart and Sörensen, 2003; Schoenmakers et al., 2010; Schulz et al., 1995; Torti et al., 2004; van der Lee et al., 2014). In their examination of multivariate models predicting dementia caregiver burden, depression, and mental health, van der Lee and colleagues (2014) concluded that care recipient behavioral symptoms (e.g., waking up at night, rejecting needed care, agitation, and verbal and physical aggressiveness) were stronger predictors of caregiver burden and depression than the cognitive or functional status of the care recipient. Pinquart and Sörensen (2003) also found that care recipients' behavior problems had a greater impact on caregivers' burden and depression than care recipients' physical and cognitive impairments. Torti and colleagues (2004) reported that behavioral problems are associated with caregiver burden across geographic regions and cultures. Hinton and colleagues (2003) reported that behavioral problems are associated with depressive symptoms among family caregivers of cognitively impaired Latinos but that this association was most pronounced among non-spousal caregivers.

Definitive conclusions about the relative importance of different risk factors should be viewed cautiously, however, because many of these risk factors are correlated with each other, and no studies have examined all of these risk factors simultaneously in a single large population-based study. Nevertheless, existing findings on risk factors can help inform efforts to target caregivers in need of support and shape the type of support provided (Beach et al., 2005).

CONCLUSIONS

The committee's key findings and conclusions are described in detail in Box 3-1. In summary, this chapter raises profound concerns about our dependence on family caregivers to take on increasingly complex and demanding roles. As a society, we have always depended on families to provide emotional support and to assist their older members with household tasks and personal care. In today's health care and social service systems, providers expect family caregivers—with little or no training—to handle daunting technical procedures and equipment for seriously ill care recipients at home. Some family caregivers express concerns about making a life-threatening mistake.

The demands of caregiving appear to be taking a toll on family members on the front lines of supporting older adults. Substantial evidence indicates that family caregivers of older adults are at risk compared to non-caregivers; they have higher rates of depressive symptoms, anxiety, stress, and emotional difficulties. Evidence also suggests that caregivers have lower self-ratings of physical health, elevated levels of stress hormones, higher rates of chronic disease, and impaired health behaviors.

The effects of caregiving are not all negative. Numerous surveys suggest

BOX 3-1
Key Findings and Conclusions: Family Caregivers' Roles and the Impact on Their Mental and Physical Health

The family caregiver role is far more complex and demanding than in the past:

- Family caregivers have always provided the lion's share of long-term services and supports to older adults with impairments. Today, they are also tasked with managing difficult technical and medical procedures and equipment in older adults' homes, overseeing medications, and monitoring symptoms and side effects.
- As older adults' advocates and care coordinators, caregivers are often responsible for ensuring that care recipients obtain needed care from fragmented and complex health and social services systems.
- Family caregivers are often involved in older adults' decision making and may serve as surrogate decision makers when the care recipient loses the capacity to make important decisions.
- Many family caregivers help older adults without training, needed information, or supportive services.
- Physicians, hospitals, social service agencies, and other providers assume that family caregivers can carry out an older adult's care plan.

Family caregiving can negatively affect the caregiver's mental and physical health; it may also have positive effects:

- The impact of caregiving is highly individual and dependent on personal and family circumstances.
- Caregiving has positive effects for some individuals. It can instill confidence, provide meaning and purpose, enhance skills, and bring the caregiver closer to the older adult.
- However, compared to non-caregivers, family caregivers of older adults are more likely to experience emotional distress, depression, anxiety, or social isolation; report that they are in poor physical health; and have elevated levels of stress hormones and higher rates of chronic disease.
- The intensity and duration of caregiving and the older adult's level of impairment are consistent predictors of symptoms of depression or anxiety. Family members who spend long hours caring for older relatives with advanced dementia are especially vulnerable to adverse outcomes.
- Other factors associated with adverse outcomes for caregivers include low socioeconomic status, high levels of perceived suffering of the care recipient, living with the care recipient, lack of choice in taking on the caregiving role, poor physical health of the caregiver, lack of social support, and a physical home environment that makes care tasks difficult.

that, for some, caregiving instills confidence, provides lessons on dealing with difficult situations, brings them closer to the care recipient, and assures them that the care recipient is well-cared for. In fact, the caregiving experience and its impact are highly individual and dependent on a wide array of personal and family circumstances such as the caregiver's own health, the care recipient's level of impairment, financial resources, and competing demands from work and family. Gender, the caregiver–care recipient relationship, family dynamics, proximity to the care recipient, race and ethnicity, culture, personal values, and beliefs all play a part.

Few caregiving studies are designed to examine how race and ethnicity, rural residence, sexual orientation, or socioeconomic status affect caregivers. If providers and policy makers are to learn how best to support the nation's increasingly diverse aging population, future caregiving research should be sufficiently powered to enable meaningful subgroup analyses.

REFERENCES

ABA (American Bar Association) Commission on Law and Aging. 2014. *Default surrogate consent statutes chart as of June 2014*. Chicago, IL. http://www.americanbar.org/content/dam/aba/administrative/law_aging/2014_default_surrogate_consent_statutes.authcheckdam.pdf (accessed August 8, 2015).

Acierno, R., M. A. Hernandez, A. B. Amstadter, H. S. Resnick, K. Steve, W. Muzzy, and D. J. Kilpatrick. 2010. Prevalence and correlates of emotional, physical, sexual, and financial abuse and potential neglect in the United States: The National Elder Mistreatment Study. *American Journal of Public Health* 100(2):292-297.

Acton, G. J. 2002. Health-promoting self-care in family caregivers. *Western Journal of Nursing Research* 24(1):73-86.

Adelman, R. D., L. L. Timanova, D. Delgado, S. Dion, and M. S. Lachs. 2014. Caregiver burden: A clinical review. *Journal of the American Medical Association* 311(10):1052-1059.

Amirkhanyan, A. A., and D. A. Wolf. 2006. Parent care and the stress process: Findings from panel data. *Journal of Gerontology* 61(5):S248-S255.

Aneshensel, C. S., L. I. Pearlin, J. T. Mullan, S. H. Zarit, and C. J. Whitlatch. 1995. *Profiles in caregiving: The unexpected career.* San Diego, CA: Academic Press.

Apesoa-Varano, E. C., Y. Tang-Feldman, S. C. Reinhard, R. Choula, and H. M. Young. 2015. Multi-cultural caregiving and caregiver interventions: A look back and a call for future action. *Generations* 39(4):39-48.

Aranda, M. P. 2001. Racial and ethnic factors in dementia caregiving research in the U.S. *Aging and Mental Health* 5(S1):S116-S123.

Aranda, M. P., and B. Knight. 1997. The influence of ethnicity and culture on the caregiver stress and coping process: A sociocultural review and analysis. *The Gerontologist* 37(3):342-354.

Bakas, T., J. K. Austin, S. L. Jessup, L. S. Williams, and M. T. Oberst. 2004. Time and difficulty of tasks provided by family caregivers of stroke survivors. *Journal of Neuroscience Nursing* 36(2):95-106.

Ballard, C., K. Lowery, I. Powell, J. O'Brien, and I. James. 2000. Impact of behavioral and psychological symptoms of dementia on caregivers. *International Psychogeriatrics* 12(S1): 93-105.

Beach, S. R., R. Schulz, J. L. Yee, and S. Jackson. 2000. Negative and positive health effects of caring for a disabled spouse: Longitudinal findings from the Caregiver Health Effects Study. *Psychology and Aging* 15(2):259-271.

Beach, S. R., R. Schulz, G.M. Williamson, L. S. Miller, M. F. Weiner, and C. E. Lance. 2005. Risk factors for potentially harmful informal caregiver behavior. *Journal of the American Geriatrics Society* 53(2):255-261.

Berglund, E., P. Lytsy, and R. Westerling. 2015. Health and wellbeing in informal caregivers and non-caregivers: A comparative cross-sectional study of the Swedish general population. *Health and Quality of Life Outcomes* 13(1):1-11.

BLS (Bureau of Labor Statistics). 2007. *Nonfatal occupational injuries and illnesses requiring days away from work*. http://www.bls.gov/news.release/archives/osh2_11202008.pdf (accessed July 5, 2016).

Bond, S. M., M. S. Dietrich, J. L. Shuster, and B. A. Murphy. 2012. Delirium in patients with head and neck cancer in the outpatient treatment setting. *Supportive Care in Cancer* 20:1023-1030.

Bookman, A., and D. Kimbrel. 2011. Families and elder care in the twenty-first century. *The Future of Children* 21(2):117-140.

Bookwala, J. 2009. The impact of parent care on marital quality and well-being in adult daughters and sons. *The Journals of Gerontology Series B: Psychological Sciences and Social Sciences* 64B(3):339-347.

Brody, E.M. 1985. Parent care as a normative family stress. *The Gerontologist* 25(1):19-29.

Brown, A. R., and G. P. Mulley. 1997. Injuries sustained by caregivers of disabled elderly people. *Age and Ageing* 26(1):21-23.

Brown, R. M. and S. L. Brown. 2014. Informal caregiving: A reappraisal of effects on caregivers. *Social Issues and Policy Review* 8(1):74-102.

Brown, S. L., D. M. Smith, R. Schulz, M. U. Kabeto, P. A. Ubel, M. Poulin, J. Yi, C. Kim, and K. M. Langa. 2009. Caregiving behavior is associated with decreased mortality risk. *Psychological Science* 20(4):488-494.

Cagle, J. G. and J. C. Munn, 2012. Long-distance caregiving: A systematic review of the literature. *Journal of Gerontological Social Work* 55(8):682-707.

Cahill, E., L. M. Lewis, F. K. Barg, and H. R. Bogner. 2009. "You don't want to burden them": Older adults' views on family involvement in care. *Journal of Family Nursing* 15(3):295-317.

Cameron, J. I., and T. R. Elliott. 2015. Studying long-term caregiver health outcomes with methodologic rigor. *Neurology* 84(13):1292-1293.

Cannuscio, C. C., C. Jones, I. Kawachi, G. A. Colditz, L. Berkman, and E. Rimm. 2002. Reverberations of family illness: A longitudinal assessment of informal caregiving and mental health status in the Nurses' Health Study. *American Journal of Public Health* 92(8):1305-1311.

Capistrant, B. D. 2016. Caregiving for older adults and the caregivers' health: An epidemiologic review. *Current Epidemiology Reports* 3(1):72-80.

Capistrant, B. D., J. R. Moon, L. F. Berkman, and M. M. Glymour. 2012. Current and long-term spousal caregiving and onset of cardiovascular disease. *Journal of Epidemiology and Community Health* 66(10):951-956.

Carpentier, N., P. Bernard, A. Gernier, and N. Guberman. 2010. Using the life course perspective to study the entry into the illness trajectory: The perspective of caregivers of people with Alzheimer's disease. *Social Science and Medicine* 70(10):1501-1508.

Cavaye, J. E. 2008. *From dawn to dusk: A temporal model of caregiving: Adult carers of frail parents.* Paper presented at CRFR Conference, Understanding Families and Relationships over Time, Edinburgh, UK.

Collins, L. G., and K. Swartz. 2011. Caregiver care. *American Family Physician* 83(11): 1309-1317.
Coon, D. W. 2007. Exploring interventions for LGBT caregivers: Issues and examples. *Journal of Gay & Lesbian Social Services* 18(3-4):109-128.
Cornman-Levy, D., Gitlin, L.N., Corcoran, M.A. and Schinfeld, S., 2001. Caregiver aches and pains: The role of physical therapy in helping families provide daily care. *Alzheimer's Care Quarterly* 2(1):47-55.
Cuijpers, P. 2005. Depressive disorders in caregivers of dementia patients: A systematic review. *Aging & Mental Health* 9(4):325-330.
Damjanovic, A. K., Y. Yang, R. Glaser, J. K. Kiecolt-Glaser, H. Nguyen, B. Laskowski, Y. Zou, D. Q. Beversdorf, and N. P. Weng. 2007. Accelerated telomere erosion is associated with a declining immune function of caregivers of Alzheimer's disease patients. *The Journal of Immunology* 179(6):4249-4254.
Darragh, A. R., C. M. Sommerich, S. A. Lavender, K. J. Tanner, K. Vogel, and M. Campo. 2015. Musculoskeletal discomfort, physical demand, and caregiving activities in informal caregivers. *Journal of Applied Gerontology* 34(6):734-760.
Dassel, K. B., and D. C. Carr. 2014. Does dementia caregiving accelerate frailty? Findings from the Health and Retirement Study. *The Gerontologist* (Advance Access). https://gerontologist.oxfordjournals.org/content/early/2014/08/25/geront.gnu078.abstract (accessed April 7, 2016).
de Nooijer, J., L. Lechner, and H. de Vries. 2003. Social psychological correlates of paying attention to cancer symptoms and seeking medical help. *Social Science & Medicine* 56(5):915-920.
Dilworth-Anderson, P., I. C. Williams, and B. E. Gibson. 2002. Issues of race, ethnicity, and culture in caregiving research: A 20-year review (1980-2000). *The Gerontologist* 42(2):237-272.
Dunkle, R. E., S. Feld, A. J. Lehning, H. Kim, H. W. Shen, and M. H. Kim. 2014. Does becoming an ADL spousal caregiver increase the caregiver's depressive symptoms? *Research on Aging* 36(6):655-682.
Edwards, S. B., K. Olson, P. M. Koop, and H. C. Northcott. 2012. Patient and family caregiver decision making in the context of advanced cancer. *Cancer Nursing* 35(3):178-186.
Emanuel, E. J., D. L. Fairclough, J. Slutsman, and L. L. Emanuel. 2000. Understanding economic and other burdens of terminal illness: The experience of patients and their caregivers. *Annals of Internal Medicine* 132(6):451-459.
Feinberg, L. F. and C. J. Whitlatch, 2001. Are persons with cognitive impairment able to state consistent choices?. *The Gerontologist* 41(3):374-382.
Fredman, L., J. G. Lyons, J. A. Cauley, M. Hochberg, and K. M. Applebaum. 2015. The relationship between caregiving and mortality after accounting for time-varying caregiver status and addressing the healthy caregiver hypothesis. *The Journals of Gerontology Series A: Biological Sciences and Medical Sciences* 70(9):1163-1168.
Freedman, V. A., and B. C. Spillman. 2014. Disability and care needs among older Americans. *Milbank Quarterly* 92(3):509-541.
Fredriksen-Goldsen, K. I., and N. R. Hooyman. 2007. Caregiving research, services, and policies in historically marginalized communities. *Journal of Gay & Lesbian Social Services* 18(3-4):129-145.
Fredriksen-Goldsen, K., H. Kim, C. Emlet, A. Muraco, E. Erosheva, C. Hoy-Ellis, J. Goldsen, and H. Petry. 2011. *The aging and health report: Disparities and resilience among lesbian, gay, bisexual, and transgender older adults.* New York, NY: Services and Advocacy for GLBT Elders, LA Gay & Lesbian Center, New Leaf, LGBT Aging Project, SAGE at Center on Halsted, Senior Services, SAGE/Milwaukee, FORGE, Openhouse, GLBT Generations, and SAGE Metro St. Louis.

Fried, L. P., C. M. Tangen, J. Walston, A. B. Newman, C. Hirsch, J. Gottdiener, T. Seeman, R. Tracy, W. J. Kop, G. Burke, and M. A. McBurnie. 2001. Frailty in older adults: Evidence for a phenotype. *The Journals of Gerontology Series A: Biological Sciences and Medical Sciences* 56(3):M146-M157.

Friedemann, M. L., R. J. Montgomery, B. Maiberger, and A. A. Smith. 1997. Family involvement in the nursing home: Family-oriented practices and staff-family relationships. *Research in Nursing and Health* 20(6):527-537.

Gallant, M. P., and C. M. Connell. 1997. Predictors of decreased self-care among spouse caregivers of older adults with dementing illnesses. *Journal of Aging and Health* 9(3):373-395.

Garvelink, M. M., P. A. Ngangue, R. Adekpedjou, N. T. Diouf, L. Goh, L. Blair, and F. Légaré. 2016. A synthesis of knowledge about caregiver decision making finds gaps in support for those who care for aging loved ones. *Health Affairs* 35(4):619-626.

Gaugler, J. E. 2005. Family involvement in residential and long-term care: A synthesis and critical review. *Aging & Mental Health* 9(2):105-118.

George, L. K., and L. P. Gwyther. 1986. Caregiver well-being: A multidimensional examination of family caregivers of demented adults. *The Gerontologist* 26(3):253-259.

Gibbons, S. W., A. Ross, and M. Bevans. 2014. Liminality as a conceptual frame for understanding the family caregiving rite of passage: An integrative review. *Research in Nursing and Health* 37(5):423-436.

Gillick, M. R. 2013. The critical role of caregivers in achieving patient-centered care. *Journal of the American Medical Association* 310(6):575-576.

Girgis, A., S. D. Lambert, P. McElduff, B. Bonevski, C. Lecathelinais, A. Boyes, and F. Stacey. 2013. Some things change, some things stay the same: A longitudinal analysis of cancer caregivers' unmet supportive care needs. *Psycho-Oncology* 22(7):1557-1564.

Gitlin, L. N., and R. Schulz. 2012. Family caregiving of older adults. In *Public health for an aging society*, edited by T. R. Prohaska, L. A. Anderson, and R. H. Binstock. Baltimore, MD: The Johns Hopkins University Press. Pp. 181-205.

Gitlin, L. N., and J. Wolff. 2012. Family involvement in care transitions of older adults: What do we know and where do we go from here? *Annual Review of Gerontology and Geriatrics* 31(1):31-64.

Gitlin, L. N., H. C. Kales, and C. G. Lyketsos. 2012. Nonpharmacologic management of behavioral symptoms in dementia. *Journal of the American Medical Association* 308(19):2020-2029.

Given, B. A., C. E. Given, and P. R. Sherwood. 2012. Family and caregiver needs over the course of the cancer trajectory. *Journal of Supportive Oncology* 10(2):57-64.

Givens, J. L., R. P. Lopez, K. M. Mazor, and S. L. Mitchell. 2012. Sources of stress for family members of nursing home residents with advanced dementia. *Alzheimer Disease & Associated Disorders* 26(3):254-259.

Glajchen, M. 2004. The emerging role and needs of family caregivers in cancer care. *Journal of Supportive Oncology* 2(2):145-155.

Grady, P. A., and L. M. Rosenbaum. 2015. The science of caregiver health. *Journal of Nursing Scholarship* 47(3):197-199.

Gwyther, L. P. 1995. When "the family" is not one voice: Conflict in caregiving families. *Journal of Case Management* 4(4):150-155.

Gwyther, L. P. 1998. Social issues of the Alzheimer's patient and family. *American Journal of Medicine* 104(S1):17S-21S.

Gwyther, L. P., and B. G. Matchar. 2015. The Duke employee elder care consultation: Meeting employees where they are. *Generations* 39(4):105-108.

Haley, W. E., J. Y. Allen, J. S. Grant, O. J. Clay, M. Perkins, and D. L. Roth. 2009. Problems and benefits reported by stroke family caregivers: Results from a prospective epidemiological study. *Stroke* 40(6):2129-2133.

Haley, W. E., D. L. Roth, G. Howard, and M. M. Safford. 2010. Caregiving strain and estimated risk for stroke and coronary heart disease among spouse caregivers: Differential effects by race and sex. *Stroke* 41(2):331-336.

Haley, W. E., D. L. Roth, M. Hovater, and O. J. Clay. 2015. Long-term impact of stroke on family caregiver well-being: A population-based case-control study. *Neurology* 84(13): 1323-1329.

Hartke, R. J., R. B. King, A.W. Heinemann, P. Semik. 2006. Accidents in older caregivers of person surviving stroke and their relation to caregiver stress. *Rehabilitation Psychology* 51(2):150-156.

Hinton, L. 2002. Improving care for ethnic minority elderly and their family caregivers across the spectrum of dementia severity. *Alzheimer Disease & Associated Disorders* 16(2):S50-S55.

Hinton, L., M. Haan, S. Geller, and D. Mungas. 2003. Neuropsychiatric symptoms in Latino elders with dementia or cognitive impairment without dementia and factors that modify their association with caregiver depression. *The Gerontologist* 43(5):669-677.

Hirst, M. 2005. Carer distress: A prospective, population-based study. *Social Science & Medicine* 61(3):697-708.

Ji, J., B. Zoller, K. Sundquist, and J. Sundquist. 2012. Increased risks of coronary heart disease and stroke among spousal caregivers of cancer patients. *Circulation* 125(14):1742-1747.

Kasper, J. D., V. A. Freedman, B. C. Spillman. 2014. *Disability and care needs of older Americans by dementia status: An analysis of the 2011 National Health and Aging Trends Study*. Washington, DC: Office of the Assistant Secretary for Planning and Evaluation. http://aspe.hhs.gov/daltcp/reports/2014/NHATS-DS.pdf (accessed February 4, 2015).

Kelly, B., A. Rid, and D. Wendler. 2012. Systematic review: Individuals' goals for surrogate decision making. *Journal of American Geriatrics Society* 60(5):884-895.

Kenyon, K. 2015 January 16. *Insights from direct experience as a family caregiver. Testimony to the committee on family caregiving of older adults*. Testimony at IOM Workshop on Perspectives on Family Caregiving for Older Adults, Washington, DC.

Kiecolt-Glaser, J. K., K. J. Preacher, R. C. MacCallum, C. Atkinson, W. B. Malarkey, and R. Glaser. 2003. Chronic stress and age-related increases in the proinflammatory cytokine IL-6. *Proceedings of the National Academy of Sciences of the United States of America* 100(15):9090-9095.

Kim, J. H., B. G. Knight, and C. V. Longmire. 2007. The role of families in stress and coping processes among African American and white dementia caregivers: Effects on mental and physical health. *Health Psychology* 26(5):564-576.

Kim, Y., and R. Schulz. 2008. Family caregivers' strains: Comparative analysis of cancer caregiving with dementia, diabetes, and frail elderly caregiving. *Journal of Aging and Health* 20(5):483-503.

Kim, Y., F. Baker, and R. L. Spillers. 2007. Cancer caregivers' quality of life: Effects of gender, relationship, and appraisal. *Journal of Pain and Symptom Management* 34(3):294-304.

Kim, Y., K. M. Shaffer, C. S. Carver, and R. S. Cannady. 2014. Prevalence and predictors of depressive symptoms among cancer caregivers 5 years after the relative's cancer diagnosis. *Journal of Consulting and Clinical Psychology* 82(1):1-8.

King, R. B., C. R. Ainsworth, M. Ronen, and R. J. Hartke. 2010. Stroke caregivers: Pressing problems reported during the first months of caregiving. *Journal of Neuroscience Nursing* 42(6):302-311.

Kitko, L. A., J. E. Hupcey, C. Pinto, and M. Palese. 2015. Patient and caregiver incongruence in advanced heart failure. *Clinical Nursing Research* 24(4):388-400.

Krouse, H. J., S. F. Rudy, A. H. Vallerand, and E. M. Walizer. 2004. Impact of tracheostomy or laryngectomy on spousal and caregiver relationships. *ORL Head and Neck Nursing* 1(22):10-25.

Kurtz, M. E., J. C. Kurtz, C. W. Given, and B. Given. 1995. Relationship of caregiver reactions and depression to cancer patients' symptoms, functional states and depression—A longitudinal view. *Social Science & Medicine* 40(6):837-846.

Lachs, M., and J. Berman. 2011. *Under the radar: New York State Elder Abuse Prevalence Study*. Brighton, NY: Lifespan of Greater Rochester, Inc., Weill Cornell Medical Center of Cornell University, and New York City Department for the Aging.

Lafferty, A., G. Fealy, C. Downes, and J. Drennan. 2016. The prevalence of potentially abusive behaviours in family caregiving: Findings from a national survey of family carers of older people. *Age and Ageing* 45(5):703-707.

Laumann, E. O., S. A. Leitsch, and L. J. Waite. 2008. Elder mistreatment in the United States: Prevalence estimates from a nationally representative study. *The Journals of Gerontology Series B: Psychological Sciences and Social Sciences* 63(4):S248-S254.

Martindale-Adams, J., L. O. Nichols, J. Zuber, R. Burns, and M. J. Graney. 2015. Dementia caregivers' use of services for themselves. *The Gerontologist* (Advance Access). http://gerontologist.oxfordjournals.org/content/early/2015/09/08/geront.gnv121.abstract (accessed April 7, 2016).

Mausbach, B. T., T. L. Patterson, Y. G. Rabinowitz, I. Grant, and R. Schulz. 2007. Depression and distress predict time to cardiovascular disease in dementia caregivers. *Health Psychology* 26(5):539-544.

McCurry, S. M., R. G. Logsdon, L. Teri, and M. V. Vitiello. 2007. Sleep disturbances in caregivers of persons with dementia: Contributing factors and treatment implications. *Sleep Medicine Reviews* 11(2):143-153.

McLennon, S. M., T. Bakas, N. M. Jessup, B. Habermann, and M. T. Weaver. 2014. Task difficulty and life changes among stroke family caregivers relationship to depressive symptoms. *Archive of Physical Medicine and Rehabilitation* 95(12):2484-2490.

Milne, A., and C. Chryssanthopoulou. 2005. Dementia caregiving in Black and Asian populations: Reviewing and refining the research agenda. *Journal of Community and Applied Social Psychology* 15(5):319-337.

Monin, J. K., and R. Schulz. 2009. Interpersonal effects of suffering in older adult caregiving relationships. *Psychology and Aging* 24(3):681-695.

Moon, H., A. L. Townsend, C. J. Whitlatch, and P. Dilworth-Anderson. 2016. Quality of life for dementia caregiving dyads: Effects of incongruent perceptions of everyday care and values. *The Gerontologist* (Advanced Access).

NAC (National Alliance for Caregiving) and AARP Public Policy Institute. 2009. *Caregiving in the United States, 2009*. Washington, DC.

NAC and AARP Public Policy Institute. 2015. *Caregiving in the United States, 2015*. Washington, DC.

Nápoles, A. M., L. Chadiha, R. Eversley, and G. Moreno-John. 2010. Developing culturally sensitive dementia caregiver interventions: Are we there yet? *American Journal of Alzheimer's Disease and Other Dementias* 25(5):389-406.

National Center on Elder Abuse. 2015. *NCEA frequently asked questions*. http://www.ncea.aoa.gov/faq/index.aspx (accessed January 21, 2016).

Nielsen, M., J. Hansen, B. Ritz, H. Nordahl, E. Schernhammer, L. Wermuth, and N. H. Rod. 2014. Cause-specific mortality among spouses of Parkinson disease patients. *Epidemiology* 25(2):225-232.

NRC (National Research Council). 2010. Informal caregivers in the United States: Prevalence, caregiver characteristics, and ability to provide care. In *National Research Council, The role of human factors in home health care: Workshop summary*. Washington, DC: The National Academies Press. Pp. 117-143.

NRC. 2011. *Health care comes home: The human factors*. Washington, DC: The National Academies Press.

O'Reilly, D., S. Connolly, M. Rosato, and C. Patterson. 2008. Is caring associated with an increased risk of mortality? A longitudinal study. *Social Science & Medicine* 67(8): 1282-1290.

O'Reilly, D., M. Rosato, A. Maguire, and D. Wright. 2015. Caregiving reduces mortality risk for most caregivers: A census-based record linkage study. *International Journal of Epidemiology* 44(6):1959-1969.

Ory, M. G., R. R. Hoffman, J. L. Yee, S. Tennstedt, and R. Schulz. 1999. Prevalence and impact of caregiving: A detailed comparison between dementia and nondementia caregivers. *The Gerontologist* 39(2):177-185.

Peacock, S. C., K. Hammond-Collins, and D. A. Forbes. 2014. The journey with dementia from the perspective of bereaved family caregivers: A qualitative descriptive study. *BMC Nursing* 13(1):42-52.

Pearlin, L. I., J. T. Mullan, S. J. Semple, and M. M. Skaff. 1990. Caregiving and the stress process: An overview of concepts and their measures. *The Gerontologist* 30(5):583-594.

Penrod, J., J. E. Hupcey, B. L. Baney, and S. J. Loeb. 2011. End-of-life caregiving trajectories. *Clinical Nursing Research* 20(1):7-24.

Penrod, J., J. E. Hupcey, P. Z. Shipley, S. J. Loeb, and B. Baney. 2012. A model of caregiving through the end of life: Seeking normal. *Western Journal of Nursing Research* 34(2):174-193.

Perkins, M., V. J. Howard, V. G. Wadley, M. Crowe, M. M. Stafford, W. E. Haley, G. Howard, and D. L. Roth. 2013. Caregiving strain and all-cause mortality: Evidence from the REGARDS Study. *The Journals of Gerontology Series B: Psychological Sciences and Social Sciences* 68(4):504-512.

Persson, J., L. Holmegaard, I. Karlberg, P. Redfors, K. Jood, C. Jern, C. Blomstrand, and G. Forsberg-Warleby. 2015. Spouses of stroke survivors report reduced health-related quality of life even in long-term follow-up: Results from Sahlgrenska Academy Study on Ischemic Stroke. *Stroke* 46(9):2584-2590.

Pinquart, M., and S. Sörenson. 2003. Associations of stressors and uplifts of caregiving with caregiver burden and depressive mood: A meta-analysis. *The Journals of Gerontology Series B: Psychological Sciences and Social Sciences* 58(2):P112-P128.

Pinquart, M., and S. Sörenson. 2005. Ethnic differences in stressors, resources and psychological outcomes of family caregiving: A meta-analysis. *The Gerontologist* 45(1):90-106.

Pinquart, M., and S. Sörenson. 2006. Gender differences in caregiver stressors, social resources and health: Updated meta-analysis. *The Journals of Gerontology Series B: Psychological Sciences and Social Sciences* 61(1):P33-P45.

Pinquart, M., and S. Sörenson. 2007. Correlates of physical health of informal caregivers: A meta-analysis. *The Journals of Gerontology Series B: Psychological Sciences and Social Sciences* 62(2):P126-P137.

Rabinowitz, Y. G., B. T. Mausbach, L. W. Thompson, and D. Gallagher-Thompson. 2007. The relationship between self-efficacy and cumulative health risk associated with health behavior patterns in female caregivers of elderly relatives with Alzheimer's dementia. *Journal of Aging and Health* 19(6):946-964.

Ramsay, S., E. Grundy, and D. O'Reilly. 2013. The relationship between informal caregiving and mortality: An analysis using the ONS Longitudinal Study of England and Wales. *Journal of Epidemiology and Community Health* 67(8):655-660.

Reinhard, S., and L. Feinberg. 2015. The escalating complexity of family caregiving: Meeting the challenge. In *Family caregiving in the new normal*, edited by J. E. Gaugler and R. L. Kane. London, UK: Academic Press. Pp. 291-304.

Reinhard, S. C., C. Levine, and S. Samis. 2012. *Home alone: Family caregivers providing complex chronic care*. Washington, DC: United Hospital Fund and AARP Public Policy Institute.

Robison, J., R. Fortinsky, A. Kleppinger, N. Shugrue, and M. Porter. 2009. A broader view of family caregiving: Effects of caregiving and caregiver conditions on depressive symptoms, health, work, and social isolation. *The Journals of Gerontology Series B: Psychological Sciences and Social Sciences* 64(6):788-798.

Roth, D. L., L. Fredman, and W. E. Haley. 2015. Informal caregiving and its impact on health: A reappraisal from population-based studies. *The Gerontologist* 55(2):309-319.

Ryan, A. A., and H. F. Scullion. 2000. Family and staff perceptions of the role of families in nursing homes. *Journal of Advanced Nursing* 32(3):626-634.

Saban, K. L., P. R. Sherwood, H. A. DeVon, and D. M. Hynes. 2010. Measures of psychological stress and physical health in family caregivers of stroke survivors: A literature review. *Journal of Neuroscience Nursing* 42(3):128-138.

Sabatino, C. 2015. Into the matrix of law and caregiving. *Generations* 39(4):80-88.

Salgado-Garcia, F. I., J. K. Zuber, M. J. Graney, L. O. Nichols, J. L. Martindale-Adams, and F. Andrasik. 2015. Smoking and smoking increase in caregivers of Alzheimer's patients. *The Gerontologist* 55(5):780-792.

Schoenmakers, B., F. Buntinx, and J. Delepeleire. 2010. Factors determining the impact of care-giving on caregivers of elderly patients with dementia. A systematic literature review. *Maturitas* 66(2):191-200.

Schulz, R. 2013. Research priorities in geriatric palliative care: Informal caregiving. *Journal of Palliative Medicine* 16(9):1008-1112.

Schulz, R., and S. R. Beach. 1999. Caregiving as a risk factor for mortality—The Caregiver Health Effects Study. *Journal of the American Medical Association* 282(23):2215-2219.

Schulz, R., and P. R. Sherwood. 2008. Physical and mental health effects of family caregiving. *American Journal of Nursing* 108(9):23-27.

Schulz, R., A. T. O'Brien, J. Bookwala, and K. Fleissner. 1995. Psychiatric and physical morbidity effects of dementia caregiving—Prevalence, correlates, and causes. *The Gerontologist* 35(6):771-791.

Schulz, R., J. Newsom, M. Mittelmark, L. Burton, C. Hirsch, and S. Jackson. 1997. Health effects of caregiving: The Caregiver Health Effects Study: An ancillary study of the cardiovascular health study. *Annals of Behavioral Medicine* 19(2):110-116.

Schulz, R., A. B. Mendelsohn, W. E. Haley, D. Mahoney, R. S. Allen, S. Zhang, L. Thompson, and S. H. Belle. 2003. End of life care and the effects of bereavement on family caregivers of persons with dementia. *New England Journal of Medicine* 349(20):1936-1942.

Schulz, R., S. H. Belle., S. J. Czaja, K. A. McGinnis, A. Stevens, and S. Zhang. 2004. Long-term care placement of dementia patients and caregiver health and well-being. *Journal of the American Medical Association* 292(8):961-967.

Schulz, R., R. S. Hebert, M. A. Dew, S. L. Brown, M. F. Scheier, S. R. Beach, S. J. Czaja, L. M. Martire, D. Coon, K. M. Langa, L. N. Gitlin, A. B. Stevens, and L. Nichols. 2007. Patient suffering and caregiver compassion: New opportunities for research, practice, and policy. *The Gerontologist* 47(1):4-13.

Schulz, R., S. R. Beach, R. S. Hebert, L. M. Martire, J. K. Monin, C. A. Tompkins, and S. M. Albert. 2009. Spousal suffering and partner's depression and cardiovascular disease: The Cardiovascular Health Study. *The American Journal of Geriatric Psychiatry* 17(3):246-254.

Schulz, R., S. R. Beach, T. B. Cook, L. M. Martire, J. M. Tomlinson, and J. K. Monin. 2012. Predictors and consequences of perceived lack of choice in becoming an informal caregiver. *Aging & Mental Health* 16(6):712-721.

Schumacher, K. L., B. J. Stewart, P. G. Archbold, M. J. Dodd, and S. L. Dibble. 2000. Family caregiving skill: Development of the concept. *Research in Nursing & Health* 23(3):191-203.

Seltzer, M. M., and L. W. Li. 2000. The dynamics of caregiving: Transitions during a three-year prospective study. *The Gerontologist* 40(2):165-178.

Silver, H. J., N. S. Wellman, D. Galindo-Ciocon, and P. Johnson. 2004. Family caregivers of older adults on home enteral nutrition have multiple unmet task-related training needs and low overall preparedness for caregiving. *Journal of the American Dietetic Association* 104(1):43-50.

Sisk, R. J. 2000. Caregiver burden and health promotion. *International Journal of Nursing Studies* 37(1):37-43.

Skaff, M. M., and L. I. Pearlin. 1992. Caregiving-role engulfment and the loss of self. *The Gerontologist* 32(5):656-664.

Son, J., A. Erno, D. G. Shea, E. E. Femia, S. H. Zarit, and M. A. P. Stephens. 2007. The caregiver stress process and health outcomes. *Journal of Aging and Health* 19(6):871-887.

Spillman, B. C., J. Wolff, V. A. Freedman, and J. D. Kasper. 2014. *Informal caregiving for older Americans: An analysis of the 2011 National Study of Caregiving*. Washington, DC: Office of the Assistant Secretary for Planning and Evaluation. http://aspe.hhs.gov/report/informal-caregiving-older-americans-analysis-2011-national-health-and-aging-trends-study (accessed April 9, 2015).

Stenberg, U., C. M. Ruland, and C. Miaskowski. 2010. Review of the literature on the effects of caring for a patient with cancer. *Psycho-Oncology* 19(10):1013-1025.

Strawbridge, W. J., and M. I. Wallhagen. 1991. Impact of family conflict on adult child caregivers. *The Gerontologist* 31(6):770-777.

Swore Fletcher, B., C. Miaskowski, B. Given, and K. Schumacher. 2012. The cancer family caregiving experience: An updated and expanded conceptual model. *European Journal of Oncology Nursing* 16(4):387-398.

Torke, A. M., M. Siegler, A. Abalos, R. M. Moloney, and G. C. Alexander. 2009. Physicians' experience with surrogate decision making for hospitalized adults. *Journal of General Internal Medicine* 24(9):1023-1028.

Torke, A. M., G. A. Sachs, P. R. Helft, K. Montz, S. L. Hui, J. E. Slaven, and C. M. Callahan. 2014. Scope and outcomes of surrogate decision making among hospitalized older adults. *JAMA Internal Medicine* 174(3):370-377.

Tornatore, J. B., and L. A. Grant. 2004. Family caregiver satisfaction with the nursing home after placement of a relative with dementia. *The Journals of Gerontology Series B: Psychological Sciences and Social Sciences* 59(2):S80-S88.

Torti, F. M., L. P. Gwyther, S. D. Reed, J. Y. Friedman, and K. A. Schulman. 2004. A multinational review of recent trends and reports in dementia caregiver burden. *Alzheimer Disease & Associated Disorders* 18(2):99-109.

van der Lee, J., T. J. Bakker, H. J. Duivenvoordenc, and R. M. Droes. 2014. Multivariate models of subjective caregiver burden in dementia: A systematic review. *Ageing Research Reviews* 15:76-93.

van Ryn, M., S. Sanders, K. Kahn, C. van Houtven, J. M. Griffin, M. Martin, A. A. Atienza, S. Phelan, D. Finstad, and J. Rowland. 2011. Objective burden, resources, and other stressors among informal cancer caregivers: A hidden quality issue? *Psycho-Oncology* 20(1):44-52.

Vitaliano, P. P., J. P. Zhang, and J. M. Scanlan. 2003. Is caregiving hazardous to one's physical health? A meta-analysis. *Psychological Bulletin* 129(6):946-972.

von Känel, R., B. T. Mausbach, T. L. Patterson, J. E. Dimsdale, K. Aschbacher, P. J. Mills, M. G. Ziegler, S. Ancoli-Israel, and I. Grant. 2008. Increased Framingham Coronary Heart Disease Risk Score in dementia caregivers relative to non-caregiving controls. *Gerontology* 54(3):131-137.

von Känel, R., B. T. Mausbach, J. E. Dimsdale, P. J. Mills, T. L. Patterson, S. Ancoli-Israel, M. G. Ziegler, S. K. Roepke, E. A. Chattillion, M. Allison, and I. Grant. 2012. Effect of chronic dementia caregiving and major transitions in the caregiving situation on kidney function: A longitudinal study. *Psychosomatic Medicine* 74(2):214-220.

Wang, X., K. M. Robinson, and H. K. Hardin. 2015. The impact of caregiving on caregivers' medication adherence and appointment keeping. *Western Journal of Nursing Research* 37(12):1548-1562.

Weiner, M. F. 2008. Perspective on race and ethnicity in Alzheimer's disease research. *Alzheimer's Dementia* 4(4):233-238.

Wendler, D., and A. Rid. 2011. The effect on surrogates of making treatment decisions for others. *Annals of Internal Medicine* 154(5):336-346.

Whitlatch, C. J. and L. F. Feinberg. 2007. Family care and decision making. In *Dementia and social work practice: Research and interventions*, edited by C. Cox. New York: Springer. Pp. 129-148.

Whitlatch, D. 2008. Informal caregivers: Communication and decision making. *American Journal of Nursing* 103(9 Suppl):73-77.

Wilcox, S., and A. C. King. 1999. Sleep complaints in older women who are family caregivers. *The Journals of Gerontology Series B: Psychological Sciences and Social Sciences* 54(3):P189-P198.

Williams, S.W., S. Zimmerman, and C.S. Williams. 2012. Family caregiver involvement for long-term care residents at the end of life. *The Journals of Gerontology Series B: Psychological Sciences and Social Sciences* 67(5):595-604.

Wolff, J. L. 2007 (unpublished). *Supporting and sustaining the family caregiver workforce for older Americans: Paper commissioned by the IOM Committee on the Future Health Care Workforce for Older Americans.*

Wolff, J., S. Dy, K. Frick, and J. Kasper. 2007. End of life care: Findings from a national survey of family caregivers. *Archives of Internal Medicine* 167(1):40-46.

Wolff, J. L., B. C. Spillman, V. A. Freedman, and J. D. Kasper. 2016. A national profile of family and unpaid caregivers who assist older adults with health care activities. *JAMA Internal Medicine* 176(3):372-379.

Yee, J. L., and R. Schulz. 2000. Gender differences in psychiatric morbidity among family caregivers: A review and analysis. *The Gerontologist* 40(2):147-164.

Yueh-Feng Lu, Y., and M. G. Austrom. 2005. Distress responses and self-care behaviors in dementia family caregivers with high and low depressed mood. *Journal of the American Psychiatric Nurses Association* 11(4):231-240.

Zarit, S. H., K. E. Reever, and J. Bach Peterson. 1980. Relatives of the impaired elderly: Correlates of feelings of burden. *The Gerontologist* 20(6):649-655.

Zarit, S. H., and J. E. Gaugler. 2000. Caregivers and stress. In *Encyclopedia of stress Vol. 1*, edited by G. Fink. San Diego, CA: Academic Press. Pp. 404-407.

Zarit, S. H., E. E. Femia, K. Kim, and C. J. Whitlatch. 2010. The structure of risk factors and outcomes for family caregivers: Implications for assessment and treatment. *Aging & Mental Health* 14(2):220-231.

4

Economic Impact of Family Caregiving

ABSTRACT: This chapter examines the economic impact of unpaid caregiving on family caregivers of older adults who need help because of health or functional limitations and explores which caregivers are at greatest risk of severe financial consequences. Workplace and government policies and programs designed to support caregivers and/or mitigate these effects are also discussed. Caregivers of older adults can suffer significant financial consequences with respect to both direct out-of-pocket costs and long-term economic and retirement security. Spouses who are caregivers are especially at risk. More than half of today's caregivers are employed, yet current federal policy and most states' family leave is unpaid, making it difficult for many employed caregivers, particularly low-wage workers, to take time off for caregiving.

National surveys show that many family caregivers of older adults report financial strain associated with their roles as caregivers (NAC and AARP Public Policy Institute, 2015b; Spillman et al., 2014; Wolff et al., 2016), suggesting that there are important economic effects of taking on the caregiving role. This chapter examines the economic impact of unpaid family caregiving on family members and friends who care for older adults with functional or cognitive limitations, or a serious health condition, and identifies which caregivers are at greatest risk of severe financial consequences. It also explores the intersection of caregiving and work by examining the effects of caregiving on working caregivers and employers and describes workplace and government policies and programs designed to support working caregivers.

The economic effects of family caregiving can be examined at individual, family, and societal levels, including (1) reductions in available financial resources of the caregiver as a consequence of out-of-pocket expenses; (2) employment-related costs for the caregiver who must reduce work hours, exit the labor force, and forego income, benefits, and career opportunities in order to provide care; (3) employment-related costs to the employer who must replace workers who leave the labor force or reduce hours; and (4) societal benefits that include the potential cost savings to the formal health and long-term services and supports (LTSS) systems because of the care and support provided by family caregivers (Keating et al., 2014). The available research on these topics is limited and largely based on self-report data, studies that are too short in duration to capture long-term economic impact prospectively, and researchers disagree about assumptions made in economic impact analyses (e.g., replacement cost of a family caregiver) (Schulz and Martire, 2009).

BROAD IMPACTS

Feelings of "financial strain" are a frequently used global measure of the economic costs of caregiving. For example, a recent survey conducted by the National Alliance for Caregiving (NAC) and the AARP Public Policy Institute (2015b) asked caregivers about "financial strain" related to family caregiving. The survey found that 36 percent of the caregivers of adults older than the age of 50 reported moderate to high levels of financial strain. Those caregivers most likely to report high levels were caregivers who live at a distance from the older care recipient, those with high levels of caregiving burden, and those who report they are the "primary" caregiver. In a recent analysis of the 2011 National Health and Aging Trends Study (NHATS) and the National Study of Caregiving (NSOC)[1] for adults age 65 and older, caregivers who provided substantial assistance with health care activities (including care coordination and medication management) were more likely to report financial difficulty (23.0 percent) compared to their counterparts providing some assistance (12.0 percent) or no help (6.7 percent) (Wolff et al., 2016).

In 2011, nearly half (8.5 million of 17.7 million) of the nation's caregivers of older adults living at home or in residential care settings (other than

[1] The prevalence data presented in this report draw primarily from NHATS and NSOC, unless noted otherwise. See Chapter 2 and Appendix E for additional information about the surveys and the committee's methods in analyzing them.

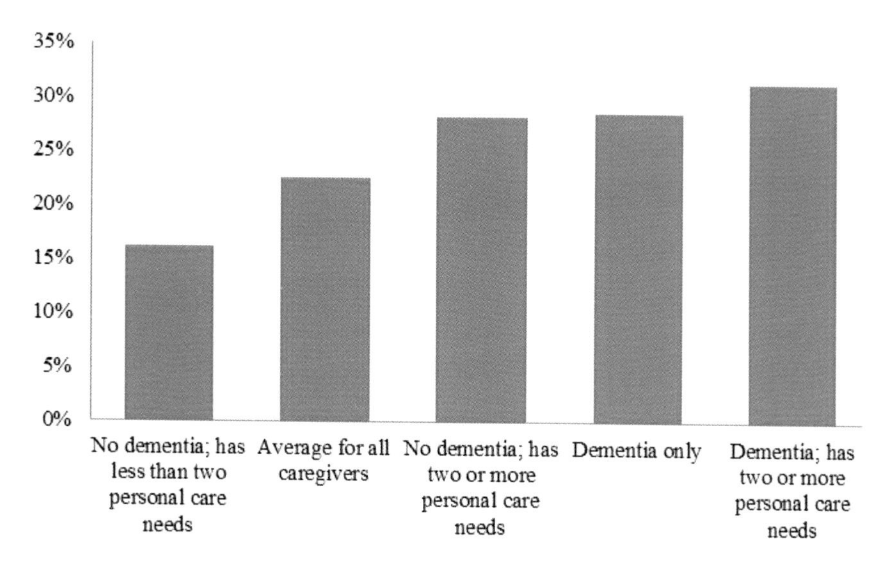

FIGURE 4-1 Percentage of caregivers reporting financial difficulties, by the care recipient's dementia status and level of impairment.
NOTES: Includes family caregivers of Medicare beneficiaries age 65 and older in the continental United States who resided in community or residential care settings (other than nursing homes) and received help with self-care, mobility, or household activities for health or functioning reasons. "Dementia only" refers to care recipients with possible dementia and fewer than two self-care needs. "Probable dementia" includes individuals whose doctor said they had dementia or Alzheimer's disease and individuals classified as having probable dementia based on results from a proxy screening instrument and several cognitive tests.
SOURCES: Data from the 2011 NHATS and the companion NSOC.

nursing homes)[2] provided care to high-need, older adults.[3] As Figure 4-1 illustrates, the caregivers who are helping older adults with the greatest needs are the most likely to report having financial problems. Nearly one-third (31.3 percent) of the caregivers (in NSOC) who helped significantly impaired persons—those with both dementia and the need for help with at least two personal care activities—reported having financial difficulties related to caregiving. In contrast, only 16.2 percent of the caregivers of indi-

[2] NSOC includes caregivers of older adults living in any type of residential care setting other than a nursing home. Residential care settings include assisted or independent living facilities, personal care and group home settings, continuing care retirement communities, and other settings (Kasper and Freedman, 2014).

[3] See Chapter 2 for additional statistics describing the caregiver population.

viduals who needed help with fewer than two personal care activities and do not have dementia reported financial difficulties (i.e., the care recipients).

The caregiving literature consistently shows that caregivers of significantly impaired older adults are the most likely to suffer economic effects (Butrica and Karamcheva, 2014; Jacobs et al., 2014; Langa et al., 2001; Lilly et al., 2007; NAC and AARP Public Policy Institute, 2015b; Van Houtven et al., 2013). The economic impact of intensive caregiving is likely related to the many hours of care and supervision that this population requires and the costs of hiring help. In a recent multivariate analysis of eight waves of the Health and Retirement Study (HRS), for example, Butrica and Karamcheva (2014) found that caregivers who helped with dressing, bathing, and eating provided nearly three times the number of caregiving hours than caregivers who provided only household help. They were also more likely than household helpers to provide at least 1,000 hours of help annually.

Other researchers, using longitudinal data, suggest that caregiving for an older adult places the caregiver at financial risk over time. For example, Wakabayashi and Donato (2006) found that caregiving increases the likelihood that women experience poverty and/or reliance on public assistance. Lee and Zurlo (2014) also found a positive association between caregiving and lower income later in life. In their examination of an eight-wave longitudinal study, Butrica and Karamcheva (2014) found that caregiving was associated with both reduced labor force participation and reduced net worth of family caregivers when compared with non-caregivers. These are examples of some of the broad economic impacts of caregiving. The discussion below examines in greater detail specific types of economic impact on the caregiver.

OUT-OF-POCKET SPENDING

Out-of-pocket spending generally refers to the purchase of goods and services on behalf of the person whom the caregiver is helping, including payment for medical/pharmaceutical co-pays, meals, transportation, and goods and services. Data on the dollar value of out-of-pocket costs are limited. The available estimates are based on self-reports that use rather broad and vague definitions of what constitutes an out-of-pocket caregiving expense. Little is known about the extent to which older adults and their family caregivers share the costs. One 2007 telephone survey asked caregivers about a wide range of spending including medical expenses, food and meals, household goods, travel costs, care recipient services (adult day services and home care), nursing home/assisted living costs, housing costs, caregiving services, home modifications, clothing, medical equipment/supplies, and legal fees. The caregivers reported an average annual amount of $5,531; long-distance caregivers had the highest average annual expenses ($8,728) (Evercare and NAC, 2007). One in five caregivers reported that older adults' out-of-pocket medical costs were their highest expense. The 2011 NSOC found that 8 percent of caregivers incurred more than $1,000 per year in out-of-pocket caregiving costs—defined as spending on medications or medical care, Medicare or other insurance premiums or copayments, mobility and other assistive devices, home modifications, and paid home health aides. For some caregivers these costs may mean drawing down assets, taking on debt, or foregoing treatment of their own health problems. Better data on economic effects of caregiving on the family caregiver are needed to provide an accurate picture of the magnitude and predictors of economic effects.

Out-of-pocket spending plays a significant part of financing for LTSS because insurance—public or private—is lacking for these services, including hiring direct care workers such as home health aides and personal care workers. In one national survey, one in four (25 percent) family caregivers said it was very difficult to get affordable services in the older adult's community that would help with their care (NAC and AARP Public Policy Institute, 2015b). Out-of-pocket expenses for older adults who are not Medicaid eligible or do not have long-term care insurance must be covered by the older adult or their family. Medicare does not cover LTSS and Medicaid is only available after people have become impoverished.

The wealthiest families may have funds to pay for supportive services but many middle-class families cannot afford the home- and community-based services that will enable their elders to remain at home and avoid even more expensive institutional care (Bookman and Kimbrel, 2011). In 2016 the cost of employing a home health aide full time for 1 year was nearly $46,480 and use of adult day services cost nearly $18,000. The median annual cost for an assisted living facility was $43,539 in 2016; the median annual cost for nursing home care was $92,378 in 2016 (Genworth, 2016).

EMPLOYMENT-RELATED COSTS TO CAREGIVERS

Today's caregivers of older adults are much more likely to be employed than in the past. The NSOC found that approximately half of all caregivers to older adults were employed either part- or full-time. Of those caregivers who worked, 69 percent were employed at least 35 hours weekly. In 2011, half of the estimated 17.7 million caregivers of older adults (8.7 million or 50.3 percent) in the United States worked (see Figure 4-2). Depending on the care needs and the intensity of the caregiving role, a caregiver may have to make accommodations in order to manage their caregiving responsibilities and their job. Researchers, advocates, and observers have raised

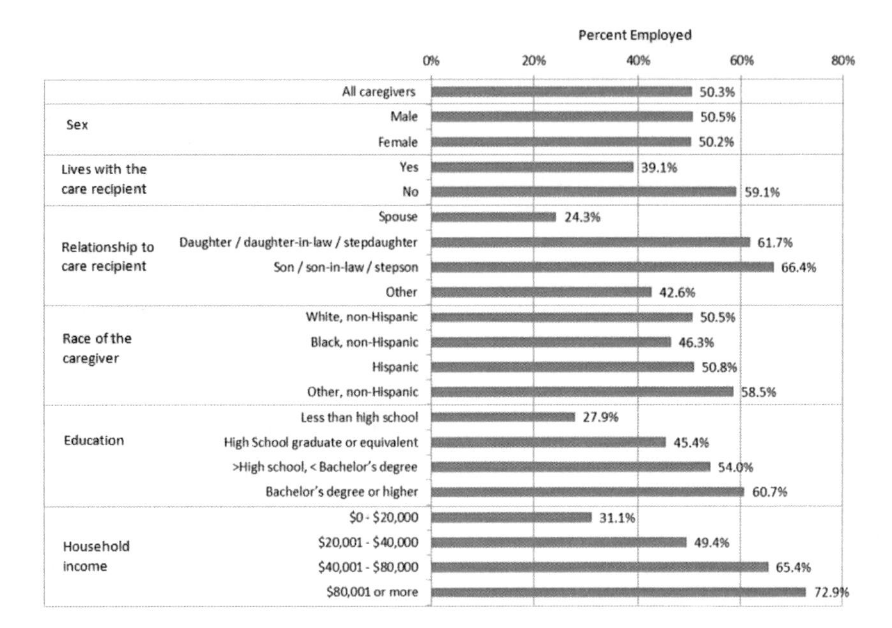

FIGURE 4-2 Employment status of family caregivers of older adults, by sex, co-residence, relationship, race, education, and household income.
NOTES: N = 8.7 million (employed caregivers). Includes family caregivers of Medicare beneficiaries age 65 and older in the continental United States who resided in community or residential care settings (other than nursing homes) and received help with self-care, mobility, or household activities for health or functioning reasons. Employment percentages are based on part- or full-time work.
SOURCES: Data from the 2011 NHATS and the companion NSOC.

concerns that the demands of caregiving can negatively impact caregivers' ability to stay in the workforce and thus jeopardize their income, job security, personal retirement savings, eventual Social Security and retirement benefits, career opportunities, and overall long-term financial well-being (Arno et al., 2011; Feinberg and Choula, 2012; Lilly et al., 2007; Munnell et al., 2015; Reinhard et al., 2015; Skira, 2015; Van Houtven et al., 2013; Wakabayashi and Donato, 2006).

Other survey data (NAC and AARP Public Policy Institute, 2015a) suggest that the majority (61 percent) of employed caregivers need to make some workplace accommodations such as coming in late to work or leaving early, taking time off to manage care situations, reducing work hours or level of responsibility, and/or taking a leave of absence. All of these accommodations have potential costs associated with them for both the caregiver and the employer. If an employee has exhausted his/her paid time off or has no paid time off to begin with, each hour of work lost due to caregiving activities bears a financial cost to the employee. Taking unpaid leave is expensive, as is cutting hours or taking a lower paying job with less responsibility. Not only does the caregiver have an immediate loss of income, his/her long-term economic status may be affected due to lower retirement savings or benefits.

As Chapter 2 describes, current trends point to higher rates of employment among caregivers in the future—especially for the wives and daughters of older adults (Stone, 2015). The U.S. Bureau of Labor Statistics projects that women's participation in the labor force will continue to increase during the same years they are most likely to be caregiving (Toossi, 2009). The percentage of women older than age 54 who work, for example, is expected to increase from 28.5 percent in 2012 to 35.1 percent in 2022. During the same period, the percentage of working women older than age 64—those most likely to be caring for a spouse—is expected to increase from 14.4 percent to 19.5 percent. As women work outside the home to make ends meet and grow the economy, the demands and pressures of working families to balance work, caregiving, and other family responsibilities have grown (Feinberg, 2013).

Caregivers' employment rates are highly variable across important subgroups (Bauer and Sousa-Poza, 2015; Jacobs et al., 2014; Lilly et al., 2007; Van Houtven et al., 2013). The 2011 NSOC found marked differences in employment between those caring for a spouse (24 percent) or a parent (more than 60 percent).

Although many people expect to work longer—primarily driven by financial considerations—family caregiving responsibilities can sometimes get in the way of continued employment (Feinberg, 2014). Surveys indicate a strong association between caregiving—especially high levels of caregiving—and reduced work for pay. One national survey found that one in five (19 percent) retirees left the workforce earlier than planned because of the need to care for an ill spouse or other family member (Helman et al., 2015). In the 2015 Caregiving in the U.S. survey (NAC and AARP Public Policy Institute, 2015a), working caregivers who quit their job or took early retirement reported doing so in order to have more time with the person they were helping (39 percent) or because their job did not provide flexible scheduling (34 percent). Caregivers with high care hours provided to the older person reported that they left the job because they could not afford to hire a paid caregiver. Co-resident caregivers were most likely to make income-related accommodations such as cutting back work hours, taking a leave of absence, quitting a job, or taking early retirement. A recent analysis of NHATS and NSOC data revealed that working caregivers who provide high levels of help with health care activities were three times more likely to experience work productivity loss[4] than caregivers who provided some or no help with health care (Wolff et al., 2016). Some research has also examined how family caregiving affects a woman's current and future employment situation and retirement security. One study, using data from HRS, found that women who leave work while caregiving may find it difficult to return to the labor force after they cease providing care to a parent (Skira, 2015). A study by Arno and colleagues (2011) based on HRS longitudinal data examined the long-term economic effects on workers who either reduced their hours at work or left the workplace before full retirement age. The analysis found that income-related losses sustained by family caregivers ages 50 and older who leave the workforce to care for a parent are $303,880, on average, in lost income and benefits over a caregiver's lifetime.[5] More research is needed to fully understand the factors influencing the working caregiver's productivity and decision to exit and later return to the workplace and whether there are strategies that could mitigate adverse economic effects.

Figure 4-2 illustrates the employment rates by selected characteristics. These rates suggest that factors that would predict the ability to continue working while providing care are related to higher education and income levels. Caregivers with a lower level of education or lower income are the least likely to be in the workforce and therefore are most at risk of the economic losses outlined earlier.

COSTS TO EMPLOYERS

Much less is known about caregiving-related costs to employers. Employer- or business-related costs may include the replacement costs for employees who quit due to their caregiving responsibilities, costs of absenteeism and workday interruptions, as well as management and administrative costs based on the time supervisors spend on issues of employed caregivers. Some estimates suggest that the cost to U.S. businesses due to caregiving may exceed $29 to $33 billion per year, but these estimates should be viewed cautiously as they are based on old data and the studies make debatable assumptions in carrying out their analysis (MetLife Mature Market Institute and NAC, 1997, 2006). Reliable data on the impact of eldercare on U.S. businesses are currently not available.

---

[4] "Work productivity loss" in this research was a composite variable based on measures of absenteeism (missed hours of work because of caregiving in relation to typical hours worked) and presenteeism (negative effect of caregiving on productivity when at work) (Wolff et al., 2016).

[5] In this study, the estimates range from a total of $283,716 for men to $324,044 for women, or $303,880 on average. The average figure breaks down as follows: $115,900 in lost wages, $137,980 in lost Social Security benefits, and conservatively $50,000 in lost pension benefits.

Some, primarily large, employers have invested resources in developing workplace programs for caregiving employees in an effort to support caregivers and retain workers. Anecdotal evidence suggests that these programs may be well received and helpful to employed caregivers. However, data do not exist to assess the effect of programs on employers or their return on investment. The few studies undertaken to explore these outcomes are largely dependent on self-reported data with the expected limitations (Gwyther and Matchar, 2015/2016; NAC and ReACT, 2012; Wagner et al., 2012). Only a few studies have been done to explore the small business environment (Matos and Galinsky, 2014; MetLife Mature Market Institute and NAC, 2006). Nonetheless, the topic of economic impact of family caregiving is an important one for both employers and caregivers who are employed. As new workplace policies emerge it will be important to assess employer acceptance, impact on business and industry, and benefit to the caregiver.

SOCIETAL BENEFITS

Family caregiving has the potential of substituting for formal health care services and the associated costs to Medicare and Medicaid in the form of reduced nursing home use and lower rates of home health care utilization (Charles and Sevak, 2005; Van Houtven and Norton, 2008). Both intervention and descriptive studies suggest that under some circumstances cost savings can be achieved in the form of delayed institutionalization, reduced rehospitalizations, and lower home health service use. These studies are described in subsequent chapters on interventions with caregivers (see Chapter 5) and health care and LTSS (see Chapter 6).

Some researchers estimate the societal benefit of family caregiving by calculating the replacement costs of the time spent by family caregivers on tasks that someone else could perform (and assuming an hourly wage that would be paid in lieu of caregiving). Estimates of the economic value of unpaid care depend on which data sources are used and how caregiving is defined. Most studies use survey data to estimate the number of family caregivers, the number of hours of care provided by caregivers, and the average wage of a home health aide (the replacement for the family caregiver). The Congressional Budget Office estimates that, in 2011, unpaid care provided by family caregivers to older adults was worth about $234 billion (CBO, 2013). However, estimating replacement costs is complex because not all caregivers are alike. For example, replacement costs for retired individuals would likely be different than replacement costs for younger caregivers in the workforce. In addition, as noted by Skira (2015), existing static estimates are likely to underestimate the true cost because they do not take into account dynamic wage and employment effects of elder parent care such as leaving the labor force permanently as a result of caregiving.

POLICIES AND PRACTICES THAT SUPPORT WORKING CAREGIVERS

Balancing work and caregiving responsibilities is a difficult task even under the best of circumstances. A *flexible workplace* can support employed caregivers with the time they need to handle emergencies and routine matters such as doctor's appointments. However, many family caregivers lack this flexibility and, for those who do not have the option of taking time off with pay, balancing work and family responsibilities can be nearly impossible. Employees may be absent from work for both planned and unplanned reasons. For example, taking a mother to a scheduled doctor's appointment is a *planned leave* from work. Going to the hospital to care for a father who has suffered a stroke is an example of *unplanned leave* that may happen due to an urgent and unexpected situation (Feinberg, 2013). The U.S. Department of Labor (DOL) (2015c) reports that 40 percent of the private-sector workforce lacks access to any paid sick leave, while 70 percent of workers who have earnings in the bottom 25 percent of the wage scale in the United States lacks any paid time off.

Flexible Workplaces

Flexible workplaces may include flexibility about where work occurs, when work takes place, and an option to modify work schedules according to competing responsibilities. In 2014, President Obama signed a Presidential Memorandum that gave federal workers a right to request flexible working arrangements. Flexible workplaces are not only good for the employees with caregiving responsibilities but benefit employers as well. Studies suggest that flexible work policies reduce turnover and absenteeism among employees and may improve productivity (Council of Economic Advisors, 2010). Flexible work schedules specifically with respect to eldercare have not been studied.

Family and Medical Leave Policies

The federal Family and Medical Leave Act (FMLA) has been in place in the United States since 1993. The Act allows workers to take unpaid, job-protected leave to care for a worker's own health needs, to bond with a new child, or to care for a seriously ill family member (child, parent, or spouse). FMLA only applies to governmental agencies and private employers with more than 50 employees. Eligibility for FMLA requires a worker to have been employed by the covered employer for at least 12 months and to have worked at least 1,250 hours. Up to 12 weeks of unpaid leave may be taken during any 12-month period and employees must be able to return to their job or equivalent with the same pay, benefits, and working conditions (Mayer, 2013). FMLA can be taken intermittently, over a 12-week period, or by working part time. In most states, the circumstances that define a worker's right to FMLA are limited to certain relationships: spouses, domestic partners, children, and parents. Many caregivers of older adults such as in-laws—daughters or sons—step-children, grandchildren, siblings, nieces and nephews, and other relatives are not eligible for the protection of FMLA. Overall 40 percent of U.S. workers do not qualify for FMLA due to their family relationship to the care recipient or because of the law's other restrictions (Klerman et al., 2014).

FMLA is also not a true option for low-income people who cannot afford to forego wages they would lose by taking it (Feinberg, 2013; Umberson and Montez, 2010). In a DOL-sponsored survey in 2011, 17 percent of caregivers did not take leave because they feared losing their job even though they were eligible for protected job leave, and 8 percent did not access unpaid leave benefits because they were not eligible due to the relationship with the care recipient (Klerman et al. , 2014).

Although DOL has sponsored a series of surveys to track the implementation of FMLA, the agency's data collection is not detailed enough to assess the law's specific impact on caregivers of older adults. The most recent DOL survey indicates that, in 2012, 18 percent of workers who took leave under FMLA did so to care for a child, parent, or spouse with a serious health condition (Klerman et al., 2014). The survey did not distinguish among the different caregiver categories, so data on leave taken specifically for eldercare are not available.

Fourteen states including the District of Columbia have enacted legislation to extend FMLA to other family relationships, most often to domestic partners and parents-in-law but also including grandparents, grandchildren, and siblings. Six states have also expanded eligibility to some workers in smaller firms. Table 4-1 lists the covered categories for each state.

Access to Paid Family Leave

The overwhelming majority of U.S. workers do not have access to paid family or medical leave (Glynn, 2015). According to the National Compensation Survey, only 12 percent of private-sector workers have access to paid family leave benefits through their employers (BLS, 2015a). In this survey, lower-wage workers were less likely than higher-wage workers to have access to paid family leave. Although paid family leave is not available to most workers, other forms of paid leave can support a working family

TABLE 4-1 States with Expansions in Unpaid Family and Medical Leave

State	Allows Leave for Family Members' Routine Medical Visits	Covers Employers with Fewer than 50 Employees	Broadens Definition of Family						
			Domestic Partner	Step-parent	Parent-in-Law	Grand-parent	Grand-parent in-Law	Sibling	All Relatives[a]
California			x	x	x	x		x	
Colorado									x
Connecticut			x	x	x				x
District of Columbia		x							x
Hawaii				x	x	x	x		
Maine		x	x					x[b]	
Massachusetts	x								
Minnesota		x				x		x	
New Jersey			x		x				
Oregon		x	x		x[c]	x			
Rhode Island		x	x		x				
Vermont	x	x	x		x[c]				
Washington		x	x		x	x			
Wisconsin			x		x[c]				

[a] Includes relatives by blood, legal custody, or marriage, and anyone with whom an employee lives and has a committed relationship.
[b] Limited to co-resident siblings.
[c] Includes parent of domestic partner or civil union partner.
SOURCES: A Better Balance, 2015b; Connecticut Department of Labor, 2015; District of Columbia Office of Human Rights, 2011; Employment Law HQ, 2012; GovDocs, 2013; Governor's Commission on Women, 2001; National Conference of State Legislatures, 2016; New Jersey Department of Children and Families, 2007; New Jersey Department of the Treasury, 2016; Oregon Bureau of Labor and Industries, 2015; U.S. Department of Labor, 2015a.

BOX 4-1
Paid Leave and Caregiving

Working caregivers who do not have paid family leave benefits may have one or more of the options below to take paid time off for caregiving. Access to paid leave and other employee benefits often depends on weekly work hours. Part-time workers are much less likely than full-time workers to be offered any form of paid leave.

Vacation time usually has to be scheduled in advance and is typically provided on an annual basis. The number of paid vacation days is typically linked with workers' length of employment.

Sick leave policies provide pay protection to sick or injured workers for a fixed number of paid sick days per year. In most cases, paid sick leave is voluntarily offered by employers. Some employers allow workers to use sick leave to care for an ill family member. In 2014, nearly half of covered workers could accumulate unused sick days from year to year (up to a specified maximum). Some states and localities require certain employers to provide paid sick days, including paid time off to accompany a family member to a medical appointment. In 2015, President Obama issued an executive order requiring federal contractors to offer paid sick days to their employees.

Personal leave is a general-purpose leave benefit usually limited to a fixed number of days per year. Some employers place restrictions on the purposes for which personal leave may be used.

Paid family leave plans cover employees' time spent attending to the needs of an ill family member or bonding with a new baby. Family leave allowances are separate from other pay protected days. In 2014, only 12 percent of private industry workers were covered by a family leave plan, paid in part or in full by their employer.

Consolidated leave packages provide a single bank of paid days off, sometimes referred to as Paid Time Off (PTO). An increasing proportion of employers offer PTO, which employees can use at their own discretion for vacation, illness, or other personal purposes. Although the leave may allow for unforeseeable events, such as illness or a family emergency, PTO is usually scheduled in advance.

SOURCES: Bishow, 2015; BLS, 2015a (Glossary); Matos, 2015; White House Office of the Press Secretary, 2015b; Wiatrowski, 2015.

TABLE 4-2 Workers Without Employer-Paid Leave, by Average Wage Category and Weekly Work Hours, 2015

Wage or Work Status	Percentage of Workers Without Paid Personal, Sick, Family, or Vacation Leave
Average wage	
Lowest 25 percent	44
Second 25 percent	12
Third 25 percent	7
Highest 25 percent	5
Weekly work hours	
Full-time	6
Part-time	56

NOTE: Includes private- and public-sector non-farm workers except private household and federal government employees.
SOURCE: BLS, 2015b (Table 46).

caregiver. When employers provide paid time off, it can be in the form of vacation days, sick leave, personal days, or as "PTO," paid time off for any reason (Bishow, 2015; BLS, 2015a). Box 4-1 outlines alternative paid leave options that may be available to employees. The form of leave benefits vary widely across occupations, type of worker, industries, establishment size, and geographic areas. Nearly all full-time federal, state, and local government employees are entitled to paid leave of some type (BLS, 2015a).

Table 4-2 shows the percentage of workers in wage categories without any paid leave. As can be seen, there is a clear association between low wages and part-time status and no paid leave options.

State and Local Efforts to Expand Access to Paid Leave for Family Caregivers

State governments provided the leadership in the development of the paid family and medical leave policies in place today. Connecticut was the first state to enact paid family leave for state employees in 1987. In 2004, California began the first paid family and medical leave program in the nation (Wagner, 2006). Today states are again leading in the development of paid family leave programs. Four states—California, New Jersey, New York, and Rhode Island—have enacted access to paid family and medical leave programs for new parents and caregivers of certain seriously ill family members. New York and Rhode Island incorporate job protection as a feature of their program. The four programs share the following design characteristics:

- Financed through an insurance model
- Fully funded by worker payroll deductions
- Provides partial pay replacement for a finite period of time
- Covers caregivers of spouses, parents, and domestic partners (California, New York, and Rhode Island also include parents-in-law and grandparents; siblings are eligible only in California)
- Uses an existing state infrastructure to finance and administer claims (i.e., Temporary Disability Insurance [TDI] agencies)

The annual payroll deductions are designed to fully cover the program costs (Fiscal Policy Institute, 2014). Some evidence indicates that costs are low because program utilization is low (Appelbaum and Milkman, 2011). Because New York's program was passed in 2016, data on the program will not be available until after the program starts in 2018 (A Better Balance, 2016).

Impact of Paid Family Leave Programs on Caregivers of Older Adults

Determining the direct impact of these programs on caregivers of older adults is difficult although the programs clearly offer some financial protection for those who can use them. The states collect some data on users but not in enough detail to identify the ages or conditions of the older adults who receive care. In every state, the programs are used primarily by new parents for bonding with infants (Andrew Chang & Company, 2015; Bartel et al., 2014; EDD, 2014a,b, 2015; Milkman and Appelbaum, 2014; National Partnership for Women and Families, 2015; New Jersey Department of Labor and Workforce Development, 2015) (see Table 4-3). People caring for spouses or adult children caring for parents constitute about 6 to 10 percent of claimants—presumably many of their care recipients are older adults. In New Jersey, 60 percent of family care claims in 2011 were made by employed caregivers aged 45 and older (Feinberg, 2013).

Public awareness of the programs is a problem particularly with respect to eligibility for paid leave to care for seriously ill family members. In California, the individuals who are most likely to benefit from paid family leave are among those groups least likely to know about it (Andrew Chang & Company, 2015; Field Research Corporation and California Center for Research on Women & Families, 2015). A survey conducted in late 2014, for example, found that only 36 percent of California registered voters knew about the program and its benefits; awareness was particularly low among ethnic minority groups (i.e., persons identifying as Latino, African American, or Asian American), individuals with no more than a high school education, low-income households, and women (Field Research Corporation and California Center for Research on Women & Families, 2015). A

TABLE 4-3 Characteristics of State Mandatory Paid Family and Medical Leave Programs

State (year implemented)	Eligible Caregivers of Older Adults	Affected Employers
California Paid Family Leave (2004, 2016)	Caregivers of seriously ill spouses, domestic partners, parents, parents-in-law, grandparents, or siblings	Private-sector employers; some government employers; self-employed individuals may elect to participate
New Jersey Family Leave Insurance (2009)	Caregivers of seriously ill spouses, domestic partners, parents, or grandparents	All private- and public-sector employers[d]
New York Paid Family Leave Program (2018)	Caregivers of seriously ill spouses, parents, parents-in-law, domestic partners, or grandparents	All private employers;[e] self-employed individuals may opt in
Rhode Island Temporary Caregiver Insurance (2014)	Caregivers of seriously ill spouses, domestic partners, parents, parents-in-law, or grandparents	Private-sector employers with 50+ employees; public agencies with 30+ employees

[a] In California, the maximum weekly pay is updated annually to equal the state's average weekly wage.
[b] Some adult caregiving recipients may be younger than age 65.
[c] Bonding with newborns includes adoptions.
[d] New Jersey employers may opt to use a private insurance plan in lieu of the state TDI program.
[e] New York public-sector unions may opt their members into the program.

Financing and Administration	Coverage	Utilization by Family Caregivers
Payroll tax fully paid by employees (0.9% of first $32,000 in earnings); $45/year per worker in 2015[a] Administered by the state's existing Temporary Disability Insurance (TDI) program	Currently 6 weeks with 55% of usual pay (up to $1,104). In 2018, low-wage employees will get 70% of usual pay and higher-wage employees, 60%	Since start of program: spouses caring for spouses or adult children caring for parents: 8%[b] newborn bonding: 88%[c] parents caring for children: 4%
Payroll tax fully paid by employees (0.12% of taxable wages); $31.50/year per worker in 2015 Administered by the state's existing TDI program or private insurer[d]	Six weeks with 66% of usual pay (up to $604 per week)	Since start of program: spouses caring for spouses or adult children caring for parents: 9%[b] newborn bonding: 82%[c] parents caring for children: 9%
Payroll tax fully paid by employees (amount will be set upon implementation) Will be administered by the state's existing TDI program	Twelve weeks with 67% of usual weekly wage, up 67% of statewide average weekly wage (when fully implemented)	The program will be phased in starting in 2018
Payroll tax fully paid by employees (1.2% of first $64,000 in earnings) Administered by the state's existing TDI program	Four weeks with 55% of usual pay (up to $795 per week)	In October 2015: adult children caring for parents: 5.7% spouses: 10.4%[b] newborn bonding: 79%[c]

SOURCES: A Better Balance, 2016; Andrew Chang & Company, 2015; Arsen, 2016; Bartel et al., 2014; EDD, 2014a,b, 2015; National Partnership for Women and Families, 2015; New Jersey Department of Labor and Workforce Development, 2014; New Jersey Department of the Treasury, 2016; New York State Legislature, 2016; Rhode Island Department of Labor and Training, 2015; Stoler and Lewis, 2010; White et al., 2013.

New Jersey poll found that 60 percent of the public did not know about the family caregiving benefit (White et al., 2013). Some workers may not use available paid family leave because the benefit does not guarantee job security, or because they cannot afford to take the time off because the paid leave benefit covers only partial wage replacement.

In 2014, the California legislature funded a public education and outreach campaign that including focused market research on the linguistic and cultural issues that may affect awareness and use of family leave benefits. Focus group discussions—structured to examine the perspectives of eligible Armenian, Chinese, Filipino, Latino, LGBTQ Californians, Punjabi, and Vietnamese—revealed significant challenges in communicating information about paid family leave (Andrew Chang & Company, 2015).

Impact of Paid Family Leave Programs on Employers

Most of the published reports on employers' response to their state's mandated paid leave program draw from small surveys and structured, in-depth interviews with selected employers. Most employers appear to have adapted to the mandates although some report additional costs. A 2010 survey of California employers found that nearly 90 percent of employers reported either a positive or no noticeable effect on productivity, profitability, or employee turnover (Appelbaum and Milkman, 2011). In-depth interviews with 18 New Jersey employers 4 years after the start of the program found largely positive responses (Lerner and Appelbaum, 2014). The surveyed employers represented businesses with as few as 26 employees and as many as 36,000 employees. All respondents had at least one employee who submitted a claim for paid family leave. Some employers said it improved morale and led to only small to moderate increases in paperwork. However, 2 of the 18 employers said the mandate led to lower profitability.

Prospects for New State and Local Paid Family Leave Programs

California, New Jersey, New York, and Rhode Island have been able to limit the cost of implementing paid family leave by using existing TDI state agencies. These states have extended TDI programs to provide a partial wage replacement benefit to employees caring for a relative with an illness (Feinberg, 2013; New York State Legislature, 2016). In April 2016, California expanded its paid family leave law to include more low-income workers and to provide higher pay to workers while on leave (effective in 2018). Only one other state—Hawaii—has the same TDI infrastructure but it does not have a paid family leave program (National Partnership for Women and Families, 2015).[6] Washington State—which does not have a TDI program—enacted paid family leave in 2007 but has yet to implement it due to lack of start-up funds (Glynn, 2015). Table 4-3 displays the characteristics of state mandatory paid family and medical leave programs.

Additional insights into other approaches for the design and implementation of paid family medical leave programs may be forthcoming from DOL. Since 2014, DOL has awarded more than $2 million in grants to 12 states and localities to either evaluate their existing programs or to conduct feasibility studies to encourage their development. The grantees are California; the District of Columbia; Massachusetts; Montana; Montgomery County, Maryland; New Hampshire; New York City; Rhode Island; Tennessee; Vermont; and Washington state (DOL, 2015b). Recently DOL announced the third round of $1 million in grants. Importantly, in this round of paid leave analysis grants, DOL is encouraging states/localities to study issues related to eldercare. DOL will award up to three points to applications that touch on paid family leave for workers with eldercare responsibilities (DOL, 2016).

Access to Mandatory Paid Sick Leave

Five states—California, Connecticut, Massachusetts, Oregon, and Vermont—have recently enacted paid sick leave laws affecting the employees of all or a large portion of the respective state's employers. The policies, described in Table 4-4, have important implications for employed caregivers because they stipulate that workers have access to paid sick time when caring for certain ill family members. Earned sick day policies differ from paid family and medical leave policies. Public policies covering sick days at work generally cover a limited number of paid days off per year (typically between 3 and 9 days, depending on state or locality) with full wage replacement (Reinhard and Feinberg, 2015). California has the most expansive definition of eligible family members; it includes spouses, domestic partners, parents, parents-in-law, grandparents, and siblings. Connecticut covers spouses only. The Massachusetts statute—a result of a 2014 ballot initiative—allows time off for workers taking family members to a medical appointment.

Employers in a growing number of major metropolitan areas are also subject to local paid sick leave mandates (National Partnership for Women and Families, 2015; Reyes, 2016). These include Eugene and Portland, Oregon; New York City; the San Francisco Bay Area; Los Angeles;

[6] Puerto Rico also has a TDI program.

TABLE 4-4 Characteristics of State Mandatory Paid Sick Leave Laws

State (effective date)	Eligible Caregivers of Older Adults	Affected Employers	Financing	Coverage
Connecticut[a] (2012)	Caregivers of spouses; adult children are not eligible if caring for their parents	Most employers with 50+ employees	Employer-paid	Up to 5 paid sick days per year for own illness or child or spouse's illness; includes an anti-discrimination provision prohibiting employers from asking workers about their familial responsibilities
California[b] (2015)	Caregivers of spouses, domestic partners, parents, parents-in-law, grandparents, or siblings	All employers	Employer-paid	3 days per year for own illness or to care for an ill family member
Massachusetts[c] (2015)	Caregivers of spouses, parents, or parents-in-law	All private and public employers with 11+ employees	Employer-paid	One hour of paid sick time for every 30 hours worked (up to 40 hours per year) Allows time off for medical appointments for family members

Oregon[d] (2016)	Caregivers of spouses, parents, parents-in-law, or grandparents	All private and public employers with 10+ employees Other employers must provide unpaid leave	Employer-paid	Up to 5 paid sick days per year for own illness or to care for an ill family member
Vermont[e] (2016)	Caregivers of spouses, parents, grandparents, siblings, or parents-in-law	All employers	Employer-paid	One hour per every 52 hours worked (up to 40 hours per year when fully implemented)

[a] Connecticut General Statute 31-57r through 31-57w – Paid Sick Leave.
[b] California Labor Code § 245-§249.
[c] Massachusetts General Laws Chapter 149 § 148C.
[d] 2015 Oregon Laws Ch. 537 (S.B. 454).
[e] Vermont H. 187 (Act 69).
SOURCES: A Better Balance, 2015a; Appelbaum and Milkman, 2011; Caterine and Theberge, 2016; National Partnership for Women and Families, 2015.

Montgomery County, Maryland; Philadelphia and Pittsburgh; Seattle and Tacoma; Washington, DC; and nine New Jersey cities.[7]

Federal workers and contractors also have access to sick leave. In January 2015, the White House issued a Presidential Memorandum directing federal agencies to advance up to 6 weeks of paid sick leave for federal employees to care for ill family members, including spouses and parents (White House Office of the Press Secretary, 2015a). In September 2015, the President signed an Executive Order requiring federal contractors to offer their employees up to 7 days of paid sick leave annually, including paid leave allowing employees to care for ill family members (White House Office of the Press Secretary, 2015b).

Caregiving and Social Security Benefits

Because Social Security benefits are based on one's earnings history, caregivers who cut their work hours or withdraw from the workforce will ultimately receive lower Social Security payments. Social Security caregiving credits have been proposed as one way to reduce the impact of foregone wages on future benefits (Estes et al., 2012; Morris, 2007; White-Means and Rubin, 2009). In its simplest form, a Social Security credit program would prospectively credit eligible caregivers with a defined level of deemed wages up to a specified time period. White-Means and Rubin (2009), for example, have proposed that full-time caregivers receive up to 4 years of Social Security work credits equal to the individual's average wage or self-employment income during the previous 3 years. The caregiver's eligibility would require certification by a physician as to the care recipient's level of need. Using 2008 estimates, the analysts projected that married caregivers who used the credit for the full 4 years would see a lifetime increase in Social Security benefits of $8,448 and single caregivers would receive $13,632 more.

The costs of developing and administering a Social Security caregiver credit program have not been fully explored. The direct cost of the credits would depend on several variables such as eligibility criteria (e.g., spouses, adult children, or others), the maximum number of creditable years, and the method used to calculate individual payments (Jankowski, 2011). The development and management of an infrastructure to administer the program would also have costs.

---

[7] The New Jersey cities are Bloomfield, East Orange, Irvington, Jersey City, Montclair, Newark, Passaic, Paterson, and Trenton.

Job Discrimination

Some employed caregivers of older adults may be subject to workplace discrimination because of their caregiving responsibilities (Bornstein, 2012; Calvert, 2010; Calvert et al., 2014; EEOC, 2007, 2009; Williams et al., 2012). Family responsibility discrimination (FRD), also called caregiver discrimination, is employment discrimination against someone based on his or her family caregiving responsibilities and the assumption that workers with family obligations are not dependable or less productive than their peers (Calvert, 2015). The outcome can be emotionally draining and costly to the working caregiver. Appendix G includes the stories of two workers who reported experiencing job discrimination as a consequence of their family caregiving responsibilities.

FRD usually results from unexamined assumptions about how an employee will or should act. For example, a supervisor may assume that a woman will not be as attentive or committed an employee after she advises her supervisor of her need to take periodic time off to care for her ill husband. FRD occurs when caregivers—regardless of their work performance—are rejected for hire, denied a promotion, demoted, harassed, terminated, or subjected to schedule changes that force the employee to quit (Calvert, 2010). One recent national study found that 5 percent of working caregivers age 65 or older had ever received a warning about their performance or attendance as a result of caregiving (NAC and AARP Public Policy Institute, 2015b).

Responses to evidence of FRD have been varied. No federal statutes or regulations specifically prohibit FRD. Some states and localities have enacted laws that protect workers with family responsibilities as a specific group or class from discrimination—but the protections are sometimes limited to childcare responsibilities (Reinhard et al., 2014; Williams et al., 2012). In January 2016, the Mayor of New York City signed legislation expanding the protections of the city's Human Rights law against employment discrimination to include caregivers of a minor child or an individual with a disability. The law adds "caregiver status" as an additional protected category for which employment discrimination is prohibited (McHone, 2016).

In 2007, the Equal Employment Opportunity Commission (EEOC) issued a report on FRD, *Enforcement Guidance: Unlawful Disparate Treatment of Workers with Caregiving Responsibilities* (EEOC, 2007). While the report acknowledges that federal equal employment opportunity laws do not prohibit discrimination against caregivers, it articulates the circumstances in which employment decisions affecting a caregiver might unlawfully discriminate on the basis of Title VII of the Civil Rights Act[8]

[8] Public Law 88-352.

or the Americans with Disabilities Act.[9] Further guidance is provided in an EEOC best practices guide for employers (EEOC, 2009). Although the EEOC efforts are valuable, the agency's advice does not carry the weight of regulation nor does it have authority over FMLA and other statutes outside of the agency's jurisdiction.

The magnitude of the impact of FRD on family caregivers of older adults is not known; most reported cases relate to pregnancy and parenthood. The Center for WorkLife Law, which tracks litigated cases of FRD cases decided by courts, agencies, and arbitrators, has compiled a dataset of more than 4,400 cases dating from 1996 to 2015 (Calvert, 2016). Overall, 11 percent of the cases were related to caregiving for aging relatives. The report author suggests that because FRD cases are identified primarily through publicly available court rulings, they may be a small fraction of the total number of actual cases.

PRIVATE EMPLOYER INITIATIVES

More than 30 years ago, employee surveys began to raise concerns among large employers and organized labor about the challenges faced by workers with caregiving responsibilities (Labor Project for Working Families, 1999; Travelers Insurance Companies, 1985). An often cited *Fortune* magazine survey found that even some CEOs reported they did not believe they could manage their own jobs if they had to care for a parent (Fortune Magazine and John Hancock Financial Services, 1989). In response, large employers began to provide workplace programs to support workers and mitigate the impact of caregiving on employees' temporary or permanent departures, lower productivity, absenteeism, coming to work late or leaving early, accidents or mistakes, and health problems (Galinsky and Stein, 1990; GAO, 1994; Wagner et al., 2012). The 2014 Society for Human Resource Management (SHRM) survey of employers estimates that 5 percent of employers provide eldercare referral services, 1 percent geriatric counseling and 1 percent eldercare in-home assessments (Matos and Galinsky, 2014). There is little empirical evidence about outcomes of the workplace programs and the extent to which they either assist the employee with caregiving responsibilities or mitigate work–family conflicts. Early research supports the idea that many employees do not feel comfortable bringing a family issue into the workplace and may, as a result, not use available programs (Wagner and Hunt, 1994). However, there is evidence as discussed earlier, that workplace flexibility supports those employees with eldercare responsibilities. The three eldercare workplace programs shown in Box 4-2 were selected as examples because of their successes over

[9] Public Law 101-336.

BOX 4-2
Three Noteworthy Eldercare Workplace Programs

- *Fannie Mae*, one of the nation's leading providers of residential home mortgages, has provided geriatric case manager (GCM) services to its more than 3,000 employees in the Washington, DC, area for more than a decade. The service is offered with the assurance that the GCM's advice and counsel is totally independent of the employer's interest—a critical factor for employees who are concerned about bringing family issues to the workplace. Although the service is provided onsite, the GCM is an employee of a local aging service provider—not Fannie Mae. Twelve percent of Fannie Mae employees have used the services—an unusually high utilization rate that speaks to its value to employees.
- *Emory University*, which employs more than 29,000 people in the Atlanta, Georgia, area, is in the midst of a transformational shift for its workforce. Employee surveys had found that 15 percent had eldercare responsibilities and nearly 60 percent of the caregivers were concerned about balancing their work and eldercare responsibilities. The university spent 2 years developing a plan for a family-friendly workplace. It conducted external and internal audits and engaged employees in the planning effort with the goal of increasing employee engagement, reducing absenteeism, and minimizing caregivers' need to miss work or drop out of the workforce. The Emory initiative is likely to yield important insights into the possibilities of workplace supports for elder caregivers.
- In 2000, *Duke University*, an employer of about 34,000 people in Durham, North Carolina, launched its Employee Elder Care Consultation Services in response to employee surveys indicating increasing need for eldercare assistance. All Duke employees and their family members are eligible for a free, confidential eldercare consultation. The individual 60- to 90-minute consultations are provided in face-to-face meetings or by phone or e-mail. Follow-up information or telephone consultations are available as are ongoing support groups, presentations to employee groups, and "lunch and learn" events. The services are provided by staff experts in geriatric social work, family caregiving, and Alzheimer's disease. Although new employees are told about the service during orientation, most referrals come from supervisors or colleagues who have used the service. Approximately 169 Duke families use the service each year.

SOURCES: Gwyther and Matchar, 2015/2016; NAC and ReACT, 2012; Wagner et al., 2012.

time (Fannie Mae and Duke University) and the thoughtfulness and careful planning that went in to the newly developed Emory University program. The university used consultants and studied both the campus needs and the resources in the community in their planning.

CONCLUSIONS

The committee's key findings and conclusions are described in detail in Box 4-3. In summary, the committee concludes that family caregiving of older adults poses substantial financial risks for some caregivers. Although the relevant evidence is based primarily on caregivers' self-reports, research consistently shows that family caregivers of older adults with significant physical and cognitive impairments (and associated behavioral symptoms)

BOX 4-3
Key Findings and Conclusions: Economic Impact of Family Caregiving

Although the dynamics of the economic consequences of family caregiving are not well understood, surveys of caregivers suggest that the following factors are associated with financial harm:

- The older adult's level of physical and cognitive impairment, including behavioral symptoms;
- Co-residence with the older adult needing help;
- The older adult's, caregiver's, and family's existing financial resources;
- Limited or no access to paid leave or a flexible workplace, if employed;
- Limited or no availability of other family members to share responsibilities and out-of-pocket costs; and
- Residing a long distance from the older adult needing help.

Research consistently shows that family caregivers of significantly impaired older adults are at the greatest risk of economic harm, in part because of the many hours of care and supervision that these older adults need.

Economic impacts on family caregivers may include:

- Loss of income and career opportunities if the caregiver cuts back on his/her paid work hours or leaves the workforce in order to meet caregiving responsibilities;
- Reduced Social Security and other retirement benefits (because of fewer hours in paid employment); and
- Significant out-of-pocket expenses for the older adult's care, which may draw from the family caregiver's own savings and undermine the caregiver's future financial security.

Family caregiving of older adults has significant workplace implications for employees:

are at the greatest risk of economic harm. This risk is especially true for low-income caregivers (and families) with limited financial resources, caregivers who reside with or live far from the older adult who needs care, and caregivers with limited or no access to paid leave benefits (if they are employed).

Some caregivers cut back on paid work hours or leave the workforce altogether to care for an older adult. As a result, they lose income and may

- More than half of today's family caregivers of older adults are employed, and the proportion is expected to grow with women's increasing participation in the workforce;
- Low-wage and part-time workers are the most vulnerable to financial harm because they are the least likely to have any paid personal, sick, family, or vacation leave. If they have access to *unpaid leave*, they may not be able to afford the time off without pay; and
- Family caregivers are at risk of job discrimination because of eldercare responsibilities.

Federal, state, and municipal laws provide some protections for employed family caregivers, but little is known about their impact on caregivers of older adults or employers:

- Daughters- and sons-in-law, stepchildren, grandchildren, and siblings of older adults are not eligible for the Family and Medical Leave Act (FMLA) protections nor are employees of small firms (although 14 states and the District of Columbia have expanded eligibility). FMLA enables eligible workers to take *unpaid* family leave with job protection.
- Four states have expanded their Temporary Disability Insurance programs to administer *paid* family and medical leave programs. The programs offer partial wage replacement and are fully financed by worker-paid payroll taxes, however:
- In states where paid family leave is available, the programs are used primarily by new parents, and the public is largely unaware of the benefits for caregivers of older adults.
- Five states and a growing number of major metropolitan areas have enacted paid sick leave mandates.

Little is known about the practical and economic consequences of potential caregiver-related workplace reforms on employers:

- Reliable data on the economic impact of family caregiving on employers are not available. The impact is likely to vary by type, size, and other characteristics of employers.

receive reduced Social Security and other retirement benefits. They may also incur significant out-of-pocket expenses to pay for help and other caregiving expenses. There is also some evidence of increasing job-related discrimination against workers with eldercare responsibilities.

Caregiving of older adults has substantial implications for the workplace. Today's family caregivers of older adults are more likely to be in the workforce than ever before—more than half are employed either part- or full-time. Moreover, the cohort of Americans most likely to care for older adults—women age 55 and older—are expected to participate in the workforce at increasing rates.

Federal policies provide little protection to many employed caregivers in these circumstances. For example, daughters- and sons-in-law, stepchildren, grandchildren, nieces and nephews, and siblings of older adults are not eligible for FMLA's unpaid leave or job protections for family leave. Low-wage and part-time workers are particularly vulnerable because they cannot afford to take unpaid leave and their employers are less likely to offer paid time off. A handful of states and local governments have taken action to assure access to some form of paid family or sick leave. However, much remains to be learned about how these efforts have specifically affected caregivers of older adults or their employers.

The impact of family caregiving on employers has not been well studied. Some large employers have established programs to support workers with eldercare responsibilities. Unfortunately, there is little empirical evidence about the costs and outcomes of workplace programs or the extent to which they help working caregivers juggle their caregiving and job responsibilities. Data and research are clearly needed to learn how to effectively support working caregivers of older adults through workplace leave benefits, protections from job discrimination, or other approaches.

REFERENCES

A Better Balance. 2015a. *Overview of paid sick time laws in the United States*. New York. http://www.abetterbalance.org/web/images/stories/Documents/sickdays/factsheet/PSDchart.pdf (accessed December 9, 2015).

A Better Balance. 2015b. *The Family and Medical Leave Act: What should LGBT families know?* New York. http://abetterbalance.org/web/images/stories/Documents/FMLA-LGBT.pdf (accessed August 24, 2016).

A Better Balance. 2016. *Overview of the New York Paid Family Leave program*. New York. http://www.abetterbalance.org/web/images/stories/Documents/PFLNY.pdf (accessed April 8, 2016).

Andrew Chang & Company. 2015. *Paid family leave market research*. Sacramento, CA: California Employment Development Department. http://www.edd.ca.gov/disability/pdf/Paid_Family_Leave_Market_Research_Report_2015.pdf (accessed April 8, 2016).

Appelbaum, E., and R. Milkman. 2011. *Leaves that pay: Employer and worker experiences with paid family leave in California*. Washington, DC: Center for Economic and Policy Research. http://www.cepr.net/publications/reports/leaves-that-pay (accessed November 22, 2015).

Arno, P., D. Viola, and Q. Shi. 2011. *The MetLife Study of Caregiving Costs to Working Caregivers: Double jeopardy for baby boomers caring for their parents*. Westport, CT: MetLife Mature Market Institute; Center for Long-Term Care Research and Policy, New York Medical College; and National Alliance for Caregiving. http://www.caregiving.org/wp-content/uploads/2011/06/mmi-caregiving-costs-working-caregivers.pdf (accessed February 12, 2016).

Arsen, H. S. 2016. *California governor signs paid family leave expansion into law*. https://www.shrm.org/legalissues/stateandlocalresources/pages/california-paid-family-leave-expansion.aspx (accessed May 3, 2016).

Bartel, A., C. Baum, M. Rossin-Slater, C. Ruhm, and J. Waldfogel. 2014. *California's paid family leave law: Lessons from the first decade*. Washington, DC: U.S. Department of Labor. http://www.dol.gov/asp/evaluation/reports/PaidLeaveDeliverable.pdf (accessed March 13, 2015).

Bauer, J. M., and A. Sousa-Poza. 2015. Impacts of informal caregiving on caregiver employment, health, and family. *Journal of Population Ageing* 8(3):113-145.

Bishow, J. L. 2015. *Monthly Labor Review. The relationship between access to benefits and weekly work hours*. Washington, DC: Bureau of Labor Statistics. http://www.bls.gov/opub/mlr/2015/article/pdf/the-relationship-between-access-to-benefits-and-weekly-work-hours.pdf (accessed December 22, 2015).

BLS (Bureau of Labor Statistics). 2015a. *National Compensation Survey: Glossary of employee benefit terms*. Washington, DC. http://www.bls.gov/ncs/ebs/glossary20142015.pdf (accessed December 22, 2015).

BLS. 2015b. *Table 46. Paid leave combinations: Access, civilian workers, National Compensation Survey, March 2015*. Washington, DC. http://www.bls.gov/ncs/ebs/benefits/2015/ownership/civilian/table46a.pdf (accessed December 23, 2015).

Bookman, A., and D. Kimbrel. 2011. Families and elder care in the twenty-first century. *The Future of Children* 21(2):117-140.

Bornstein, S. 2012. Work, family, and discrimination at the bottom of the ladder. *Georgetown Journal on Poverty Law Policy* 19(1):1-42.

Butrica, B., and N. Karamcheva. 2014. *The impact of informal caregiving on older adults' labor supply and economic resources*. Washington, DC: U.S. Department of Labor http://www.dol.gov/ebsa/pdf/impactofinformalcaregivingonolderadults.pdf (accessed April 8, 2015).

Calvert, C. T. 2010. *Family responsibilities discrimination: Litigation update 2010*. San Francisco, CA: The Center for WorkLife Law.

Calvert, C. T. 2015. *Family responsibilities discrimination. Presentation to the Committee on Family Caregiving for Older Adults*, January 16, 2015, Washington, DC.

Calvert, C. T. 2016. *Caregivers in the workplace: Family responsibilities discrimination litigation update 2016*. San Francisco, CA: The Center for Worklife Law. http://www.worklifelaw.org/pubs/FRDupdate2016.pdf (accessed May 19, 2016).

Calvert, C. T., J.C. Williams, and G. Phelan. 2014. *Family responsibilities discrimination*. Arlington, VA: Bloomberg BNA.

Caterine, M., and S. Theberge. 2016. *Vermont becomes the fifth state to pass paid sick leave legislation*. https://www.littler.com/publication-press/publication/vermont-becomes-fifth-state-pass-paid-sick-leave-legislation (accessed May 3, 2016).

CBO (Congressional Budget Office). 2013. *Rising demand for long-term services and supports for elderly people*. Washington, DC: Congressional Budget Office.

Charles, K. K., and P. Sevak. 2005. Can family caregiving substitute for nursing home care? *Journal of Health Economics* 24(6):1174-1190.

Connecticut Department of Labor. 2014. *Guidance from the Connecticut Department of Labor regarding Connecticut General Statutes §§ 31-57r – 31-57w – paid sick leave*. https://www.ctdol.state.ct.us/wgwkstnd/SickLeaveGuidance.pdf (accessed December 22, 2015).

Connecticut Department of Labor. 2015. *Family and Medical Leave Act (FMLA)*. https://www.ctdol.state.ct.us/wgwkstnd/fmla.htm (accessed December 22, 2015).

Council of Economic Advisors. 2010. *Work-life balance and the economics of workplace flexibility*. https://www.whitehouse.gov/files/documents/100331-cea-economics-workplace-flexibility.pdf (accessed December 10, 2015).

District of Columbia Office of Human Rights. 2011. *District of Columbia Family & Medical Leave Act frequently asked questions*. http://ohr.dc.gov/sites/default/files/dc/sites/ohr/release_content/attachments/20373/DCFMLA-Website_Facts_Questions_Answers.pdf (accessed July 29, 2016).

DOL (U.S. Department of Labor). 2015a. *Federal vs. Vermont Family and Medical Leave laws*. http://www.dol.gov/whd/state/fmla/vt.htm (accessed February 12, 2016).

DOL. 2015b. *Department awards $1.55 m to study paid family, medical leave implementation*. http://www.dol.gov/opa/media/press/wb/WB20151927.html (accessed February 12, 2016).

DOL. 2015c. *Get the facts on paid sick time*. http://www.dol.gov/featured/paidleave/get-the-facts-sicktime.pdf (accessed February 12, 2016).

DOL. 2016. *Paid leave analysis grants*. https://www.dol.gov/wb/media/paidleavegrants.htm (accessed August 1, 2016).

EDD (State of California Employment Development Department). 2014a. *Paid family leave. Ten years of assisting Californians in need*. http://www.edd.ca.gov/disability/pdf/Paid_Family_Leave_10_Year_Anniversary_Report.pdf (accessed December 27, 2015).

EDD. 2014b. *State Disability Insurance (SDI) statistical information*. http://www.edd.ca.gov/Disability/pdf/qspfl_PFL_Program_Statistics.pdf (accessed December 27, 2015).

EDD. 2015. *October 2015 Disability Insurance (DI) fund forecast*. http://www.edd.ca.gov/About_EDD/pdf/edddiforecastoct15.pdf (accessed December 10, 2015).

EEOC (Equal Employment Opportunity Commission). 2007. *Enforcement guidance: Unlawful disparate treatment of workers with caregiving responsibilities*. Washington, DC. http://www.eeoc.gov/policy/docs/caregiving.html (accessed July 2, 2015).

EEOC (Equal Employment Opportunity Commission). 2009. *Employer best practices for workers with caregiving responsibilities*. Washington, DC. http://www.eeoc.gov/policy/docs/caregiver-best-practices.html (accessed July 2, 2015).

Employment Law HQ. 2012. *FMLA laws by state*. http://www.employmentlawhq.com/state-by-state-map.html (accessed December 10, 2015).

Estes, C., T. O'Neill, and H. Hartmann. 2012. *Breaking the social security glass ceiling: A proposal to modernize women's benefits*. Washington, DC: Institute for Women's Policy Research, National Committee to Preserve Social Security & Medicare Foundation, and National Organization for Women. http://www.iwpr.org/publications/pubs/breaking-the-social-security-glass-ceiling-a-proposal-to-modernize-womens-benefits (accessed December 10, 2015).

Evercare, and National Alliance for Caregiving (NAC). 2007. *Family caregivers: What they spend, what they sacrifice*. Minnetonka, MN. http://www.caregiving.org/data/Evercare_NAC_CaregiverCostStudyFINAL20111907.pdf (accessed July 2, 2015).

Feinberg, L. F. 2013. *Keeping up with the times: Supporting family caregivers with workplace leave policies*. Washington, DC: AARP Public Policy Institute.

Feinberg, L. F. 2014. Recognizing and supporting family caregivers: The time has come. *Public Policy & Aging Report* 24(2):65-69.

Feinberg, L., and R. Choula. 2012. *Understanding the impact of family caregiving on work.* Washington, DC: AARP Public Policy Institute.

Field Research Corporation, and California Center for Research on Women & Families. 2015. *A survey of California registered voters about the state's paid family leave program.* San Francisco, CA. http://www.field.com/fieldpollonline/subscribers/Rls2494.pdf (accessed December 29, 2015).

Fiscal Policy Institute. 2014. *Reform of New York's Temporary Disability Insurance program and provision of family leave: Estimated costs of proposed legislation.* Albany, NY: Fiscal Policy Institute.

Fortune Magazine and John Hancock Financial Services. 1989. *Corporate and employee response to caring for the elderly: A national survey of U.S. companies and the workforce.* New York: *Fortune* Magazine and John Hancock Financial Services.

Galinsky, E., and P. J. Stein. 1990. The impact of human resource policies on employees: Balancing work/family life. *Journal of Family Issues* 11(4):368-383.

GAO (Government Accountability Office). 1994. *Long term care: Private sector elder care could yield multiple benefits.* Washington, DC: Government Accountability Office.

Genworth. 2016. *Genworth 2016 cost of care survey.* https://www.genworth.com/about-us/industry-expertise/cost-of-care.html (accessed June 9, 2016).

Glynn, S. J. 2015. *Administering paid family and medical leave: Learning from international and domestic examples.* Washington, DC: Center for American Progress. https://cdn.americanprogress.org/wp-content/uploads/2015/11/19060022/PaidLeaveProposal-report-11.19.15.pdf (accessed November 24, 2015).

GovDocs. 2013. *Colorado extends FMLA coverage for family members.* http://www.govdocs.com/colorado-fmla-revised (accessed August 24, 2016).

Governor's Commission on Women. 2001. *Vermont guide to parental and family leave.* http://women.vermont.gov/sites/women/files/pdf/Parental_Family_Leave_Guide.pdf (accessed August 1, 2016).

Gwyther, L. P., and B. G. Matchar. 2015/2016. The Duke employee elder care consultation: Meeting employees where they are. *Journal of the American Society on Aging* 39(4):105-108.

Helman, R., C. Copeland, J. VanDerhei. 2015. *The 2015 Retirement Confidence Survey: Having a retirement savings plan a key factor in Americans' retirement confidence.* Employee Benefit Research Institute Issue Brief 413. https://www.ebri.org/pdf/briefspdf/EBRI_IB_413_Apr15_RCS-2015.pdf (accessed December 15, 2015).

Jacobs, J., C. Van Houtven, A. Laporte, and P. Coyte. 2014. *The impact of informal caregiving intensity on women's retirement in the United States.* Toronto, CA: Canadian Centre for Health Economics. http://www.canadiancentreforhealtheconomics.ca/wp-content/uploads/2014/04/Jacobs-et-al.pdf (accessed October 13, 2015).

Jankowski, J. 2011. Caregiver credits in France, Germany, and Sweden: Lessons for the United States. *Social Security Bulletin* 71:61-77.

Kasper, J. D., and V. A. Freedman. 2014. Findings from the 1st round of the National Health and Aging Trends Study (NHATS): Introduction to a special issue. *Journals of Gerontology, Series B: Psychological Sciences and Social Sciences* 69(7):S1-S7.

Keating, N. C, J. E. Fast, D. S. Lero, S. J. Lucas, J. Eales. 2014. A taxonomy of the economic costs of family care to adults. *The Journal of the Economics of Ageing* 3:11-20.

Klerman, J. A., K. Daley, and A. Pozniak. 2014. *Family and medical leave in 2012: Technical report (2014 revision).* Cambridge, MA: Abt Associates.

Labor Project for Working Families. 1999. *Bargaining for elder care.* Berkeley, CA: Labor Project for Working Families.

Langa, K. M., M. E. Chernew, M. U. Kabeto, A. Regula Herzog, M. B. Ofstedal, R. J. Willis, R. B. Wallace, L. M. Mucha, W. L. Straus, and A. M. Fendrick. 2001. National estimates of the quantity and cost of informal caregiving for the elderly with dementia. *Journal of General Internal Medicine* 16(11):770-778.

Lee, Y., and K. A. Zurlo. 2014. Spousal caregiving and financial strain among middle-aged and older adults. *International Journal of Human Development* 79(4):302-321.

Lerner, S., and E. Appelbaum. 2014. *Business as usual: New Jersey employers' experiences with family leave insurance*. Washington, DC: Center for Economic and Policy Research. http://cepr.net/publications/reports/business-as-usual-new-jersey-employers-experiences-with-family-leave-insurance (accessed August 4, 2015).

Lilly, M. B., A. Laporte, and P. C. Coyte. 2007. Labor market work and home care's unpaid caregivers: A systematic review of labor force participation rates, predictors of labor market withdrawal, and hours of work. *Milbank Quarterly* 85(4):641-690.

Matos, K. 2015. *Paid time off, vacations, sick days and short-term caregiving in the United States: 2014 National Study of Employers*. New York: Families and Work Institute, Society for Human Resource Management, and When Work Works. http://familiesandwork.org/downloads/paid-leave-nse.pdf (accessed March 16, 2015).

Matos, K., and E. Galinsky. 2014. *2014 National Study of Employers*. http://familiesandwork.org/downloads/2014NationalStudyOfEmployers.pdf (accessed November 22, 2015).

Mayer, G. 2013. *The Family and Medical Leave Act (FMLA): Policy issues*. Washington, DC: Congressional Research Service.

McHone, K. 2016. *New York City protects caregivers under expanded law*. Western Springs, IL: The National Law Review. http://www.natlawreview.com/article/new-york-city-protects-caregivers-under-expanded-law (accessed February 16, 2016).

MetLife Mature Market Institute and NAC (National Alliance for Caregiving). 1997. *The MetLife Study of Employer Costs for Working Caregivers. Based on data from Family Caregiving in the U.S.: Findings from a national survey*. http://www.geckosystems.com/downloads/empcosts.pdf (accessed December 4, 2015).

MetLife Mature Market Institute and NAC. 2006. *The MetLife Caregiving Cost Study: Productivity losses to U.S. business*. Westport, CT: MetLife Mature Market Institute and NAC.

Milkman, R., and E. Appelbaum. 2014. Low-wage workers and paid family leave: The California experience. In *What works for workers: Public policies and innovative strategies for low-wage workers*, edited by S. Luce, J. Luff, J. A. McCartin, and R. Milkman. New York: Russell Sage Foundation. Pp. 305-328.

Morris, J. L. 2007. Explaining the elderly feminization of poverty: An analysis of retirement benefits, health care benefits, and elder care-giving. *Notre Dame Journal of Law, Ethics & Public Policy* 21(2):571-607.

Munnell, A. H., G. T. Sanzenbacher, and M. S. Rutledge. 2015. *What causes workers to retire before they plan? Center for Retirement Research, Boston College*. http://crr.bc.edu/wp-content/uploads/2015/09/wp_2015-22.pdf (accessed June 9, 2016).

NAC (National Alliance for Caregiving) and AARP Public Policy Institute. 2015a. *Caregiving in the U.S.* Washington, DC: NAC and AARP Public Policy Institute.

NAC and AARP Public Policy Institute. 2015b. *Caregivers of older adults: A focused look at those caring for someone age 50+*. Washington, DC: NAC and AARP Public Policy Institute.

NAC and ReACT (Respect a Caregiver's Time). 2012. *Best practices in workplace eldercare*. Washington, DC. http://www.caregiving.org/pdf/research/BestPracticesEldercareFINAL.pdf (accessed March 16, 2015).

National Conference of State Legislatures. 2016. *State family and medical leave laws*. http://www.ncsl.org/research/labor-and-employment/state-family-and-medical-leave-laws.aspx (accessed August 24, 2016).

National Partnership for Women and Families. 2015. *First impressions: Comparing state paid family leave programs in their first years. Rhode Island's first year of paid leave in perspective.* Washington, DC. http://www.nationalpartnership.org/research-library/work-family/paid-leave/first-impressions-comparing-state-paid-family-leave-programs-in-their-first-years.pdf (accessed February 15, 2016).

New Jersey Department of Children and Families. 2007. *Federal Family and Medical Leave Act (FMLA) and the New Jersey Family Leave Act (FLA).* http://www.state.nj.us/dcf/policy_manuals/DCF-III-A-1-005.2007_issuance.shtml (accessed August 1, 2016).

New Jersey Department of Labor and Workforce Development. 2014. *Family leave program statistics.* http://lwd.dol.state.nj.us/labor/fli/content/fli_program_stats.html (accessed December 27, 2015).

New Jersey Department of Labor and Workforce Development. 2015. *Family leave insurance.* http://lwd.dol.state.nj.us/labor/fli/fliindex.html (accessed December 27, 2015).

New Jersey Department of the Treasury. 2016. *New Jersey Family Leave Act and Family and Medical Leave Act of 1993: Frequently Asked Questions and Answers.* Employers' Pensions and Benefits Administration Manual (EPBAM). http://www.state.nj.us/treasury/pensions/epbam/additional/fmla-qa.htm (accessed August 16, 2016).

New York State Legislature. 2016. *Budget Article VII (Internal # 7 - 2016).* http://public.leginfo.state.ny.us/navigate.cgi (accessed April 8, 2016).

Oregon Bureau of Labor and Industries. 2015. *Oregon Family Leave Act (OFLA).* http://www.oregon.gov/boli/TA/pages/t_faq_oregon_family_leave_act_01-2011.aspx (accessed December 27, 2015).

Reinhard, S., and L. F. Feinberg. 2015. The escalating complexity of family caregiving: Meeting the challenge. In *Family caregiving in the new normal*, edited by J. E. Gaugler and R. L. Kane. London, UK: Academic Press. Pp. 291-304.

Reinhard, S. C., E. Kassner, A. Houser, K. Ujvari, R. Mollica, and L. Hendrickson. 2014. *Raising expectations: A state scorecard on long-term services and supports for older adults, people with physical disabilities, and family caregivers.* Washington, DC: AARP, The Commonwealth Fund, and The SCAN Foundation. http://www.aarp.org/content/dam/aarp/research/public_policy_institute/ltc/2014/raising-expectations-2014-AARP-ppi-ltc.pdf (accessed April 8, 2015).

Reinhard, S. C., L. F. Feinberg, R. Choula, and A. Houser. 2015. *Valuing the invaluable: 2015 update.* Washington, DC: AARP Public Policy Institute.

Reyes, E. 2016. *6 paid sick days for workers in L.A.? City council says yes.* The Los Angeles Times, April 19. http://www.latimes.com/local/lanow/la-me-ln-los-angeles-sick-days-20160419-story.html (accessed May 3, 2016).

Rhode Island Department of Labor and Training. 2015. *Launching the Rhode Island Temporary Caregiver Insurance program (TCI): Employee experiences one year later.* Providence, RI.

Schulz, R., and L. M. Martire. 2009. Caregiving and employment. In *Aging and work: Issues and implications in a changing landscape.* Baltimore, MD: Johns Hopkins University Press. Pp. 35-50.

Skira, M. M. 2015. Dynamic wage and employment effects of elder parent care. *International Economic Review* 56(1):63-93.

Spillman, B. C., J. Wolff, V. A. Freedman, and J. D. Kasper. 2014. *Informal caregiving for older Americans: An analysis of the 2011 National Study of Caregiving.* Washington, DC: Office of the Assistant Secretary for Planning and Evaluation. https://aspe.hhs.gov/report/informal-caregiving-older-americans-analysis-2011-national-study-caregiving (accessed April 9, 2015).

Stoler, J., and L. M. Lewis. 2010. *New hurdles for N.J. employers seeking to comply with paid leave law*. New York: Sheppard, Mullin, Richter & Hampton LLC. https://www.sheppardmullin.com/media/article/814_SHRM%20-%20New%20Hurdles%20for%20NJ%20Employers%20-%20Stoler%20Lewis.pdf (accessed November 22, 2015).

Stone, R. I. 2015. Factors affecting the future of family caregiving in the United States. In *Family caregiving in the new normal*, edited by J. E. Gaugler and R. L. Kane. London, UK: Academies Press. Pp. 57-78.

Toossi, M. 2009. *Labor force projections to 2018: Older workers staying more active*. Washington, DC: Bureau of Labor Statistics.

Travelers Insurance Companies. 1985. *The Travelers Employee Caregiver Survey: A survey on caregiving responsibilities of Travelers employees for older Americans*. Hartford, CT: The Travelers.

Umberson, D., and J. K. Montez. 2010. Social relationships and health a flashpoint for health policy. *Journal of Health and Social Behavior* 51(1 Suppl):S54-S66.

Van Houtven, C. H., and E. C. Norton. 2008. Informal care and Medicare expenditures: Testing for heterogeneous treatment effects. *Journal of Health Economics* 27(1):134-156.

Van Houtven, C. H., N. B. Coe, and M. M. Skira. 2013. The effect of informal care on work and wages. *Journal of Health Economics* 32(1):240-252.

Wagner, D. L. 2006. Families, work, and an aging population: Developing a formula that works for the workers. *Journal of Aging and Social Policy* 18(3):115-125.

Wagner, D. L., and G. Hunt. 1994. The use of workplace eldercare programs by employed caregivers. *Research on Aging* 16(1):69-84.

Wagner, D. L., A. Lindemer, K. N. Yokum, and M. DeFreest. 2012. *Best practices in workplace eldercare*. Washington, DC: National Alliance for Caregiving, Respect a Caregiver's Time, and Alzheimer's Immunotherapy Program. http://www.caregiving.org/wp-content/uploads/2010/01/BestPracticesEldercareFinal1.pdf (accessed December 8, 2014).

Wakabayashi, C., and K. M. Donato. 2006. Does caregiving increase poverty among women in later life? Evidence from the Health and Retirement Survey. *Journal of Health and Social Behavior* 47(3):258-274.

White, K., L. Houser, and E. Nisbet. 2013. *Policy in action: New Jersey's Family Leave Insurance program at age three*. New Brunswick, NJ: Rutgers Center for Women and Work. http://smlr.rutgers.edu/CWW-report-FLI-at-age-three (accessed December 29, 2015).

White House Office of the Press Secretary. 2015a. *Presidential Memorandum—modernizing federal leave policies for childbirth, adoption and foster care to recruit and retain talent and improve productivity*. https://www.whitehouse.gov/the-press-office/2015/01/15/presidential-memorandum-modernizing-federal-leave-policies-childbirth-ad (accessed May 3, 2016).

White House Office of the Press Secretary. 2015b. *Executive Order—establishing paid sick leave for federal contractors*. https://www.whitehouse.gov/the-press-office/2015/09/08/executive-order-establishing-paid-sick-leave-federal-contractors (accessed May 3, 2016).

White-Means, S. I., and R. M. Rubin. 2009. *Retirement security for family elder caregivers with labor force employment*. Washington, DC: National Academy of Social Insurance. https://www.nasi.org/sites/default/files/research/White-Means_and_Rubin_January_2009_Rockefeller.pdf (accessed December 23, 2015).

Wiatrowski, W. J. 2015. *Monthly Labor Review: Pay protection during temporary absences from work: What we know and what we don't know*. Washington, DC: Bureau of Labor Statistics. http://www.bls.gov/opub/mlr/2015/article/pdf/pay-protection-during-temporary-absences-from-work.pdf (accessed December 23, 2015).

Williams, J. C., R. Devaux, P. Petrac, and L. Feinberg. 2012. *Protecting family caregivers from employment discrimination*. Washington, DC: AARP Public Policy Institute. http://www.aarp.org/home-family/caregiving/info-08-2012/insight-protecting-family-caregivers-from-employment-discrimination-AARP-ppi-health.html (accessed August 5, 2015).

Wolff, J., B. Spillman, V. Freedman, and J. Kasper. 2016. A national profile of family and unpaid caregivers who assist older adults with health care activities. *JAMA Internal Medicine* 176(3):372-379.

5

Programs and Supports for Family Caregivers of Older Adults

ABSTRACT: This chapter reviews what is known about the effectiveness of interventions designed to support family caregivers of older adults, including education and skills training, environmental modifications, care management, counseling, and multicomponent models. Well-designed randomized clinical trials show that effective caregiver interventions tend to share several characteristics including, for example, assessments of caregiver risks and needs, tailored interventions that address multiple areas of risk or caregiver need and preferences, and active involvement of caregivers in skills training (rather than a didactic, prescriptive approach). Trials also suggest the potential that some caregiver interventions reduce the resource use of care recipients by delaying nursing home placement, reducing re-hospitalizations, and shortening hospital stays. Despite demonstrated effectiveness, however, promising interventions have not been disseminated and adopted in everyday settings. A variety of barriers, outlined in the chapter, have to be overcome if family caregivers are to benefit from this research.

Family members form the backbone of our health care and long-term services and supports (LTSS) systems, representing the largest single source of care for older adults. Although family caregivers assume a wide array of roles and responsibilities, as Chapter 3 described, they typically do so without sufficient education, training, or support. Caregiving can result in positive outcomes for the caregiver such as personal growth due to longstanding expectations of mutual support (e.g., a spouse caring for a partner) or a sense of giving back to someone who has cared or provided support for them at some other time (e.g., an adult child caring for a parent). Caregiving can also result in a myriad of negative consequences for caregivers including financial strain, emotional distress, social isolation, disruption in work and other family roles, and even physical morbidities for those who are most distressed.

With the number of potential family caregivers projected to decline in the next few decades, the United States faces a looming care gap just as the population rapidly ages and many older adults have longer periods of care needs (Redfoot et al., 2013). Finding ways to support families has been and will continue to be a pressing public health focus. The past three decades have generated considerable research on the identification of interventions and supportive approaches for family caregivers and the need for advancing supportive policies will only continue. Research to date on developing, evaluating, and implementing programs for family caregivers provides invaluable insight on the challenges and consequences of caregiving and approaches for providing caregivers with needed skills for care provision, alleviating caregiver distress, and improving the quality of life for the caregiver and the older adult receiving care.

This chapter reviews the evidence on interventions directed at supporting family caregivers of older adults. Given the vast literature in this area, the committee used a framework to facilitate organization of the literature and to illustrate that, although the caregiver is the ultimate target of intervention programs, programs vary in focus, scope, funding, and the service settings and environments in which they are delivered. It also illustrates the complexity of the caregiving experience and the interactions that occur among the caregiver, the care recipient, the community, and the larger social/political environment. Because most interventions include a protocol for assessing both the caregiver (e.g., problems, needs, strengths, and resources) and the older adult, this review also includes a brief review of protocols used for caregiver assessment. A summary of the evidence for interventions is presented according to the various levels of the framework (recognizing that there are interactions among them): the individual/social level (older adult and caregiver, family, friends) organized by the specific health conditions of the older adult care recipient; the organizational level (e.g., workplace or formal health care organization); and the broader societal level.

Approach Used in the Review of the Literature

The committee defined intervention broadly to represent therapeutic strategies, care delivery models, programs, and services intended to support family caregivers of older adults. As noted, interventions may target the family caregiver or older adult (or both), organizations or the broader social context (or some combination) with the intent of modifying a particular risk factor (e.g., depression, social isolation, poor physical health, economic strain), behavioral process (e.g., communication strategies, self-care behaviors), or set of relationships (e.g., family caregiver and health and service providers; caregiver and care recipient). An intervention may include a set of social-behavioral strategies (e.g., education, skills training), psychosocial therapies (e.g., cognitive behavioral therapy), programmatic organizational strategies (e.g., workplace provisions for caregivers) or broad policy initiatives (e.g., the Family and Medical Leave Act, or FMLA). The review excluded pharmacological interventions and other interventions targeting the older adult unless caregiver outcomes were also reported.

The committee's approach overall was to summarize the available evidence regarding intervention strategies for family caregivers of older adults with varying conditions and to draw conclusions as to what types of interventions are effective. This chapter does not present a formal systematic review of the available literature as that is beyond the scope of this report. Rather, it summarizes the characteristics of interventions, their impact on the caregiver and care recipient, and general findings regarding the extent to which diversity and issues of cost were considered. For health conditions of older adults for which the caregiver intervention literature is extensive (e.g., dementia, cancer) and recent meta-analyses or systematic reviews have been conducted, the committee summarized the results of these analyses/reviews and then examined individual articles that were not included in or published after the review was completed. For conditions such as spinal cord injury and mental health disorders in which the literature is not as extensive, the key existing intervention studies were summarized. In summary, the committee examined several important factors:

- Interventions directed at families caring for older adults with a very wide range of conditions including dementia, stroke, cancer, spinal cord injuries, and mental illnesses, were included.
- Five categories of outcomes and their measurements were considered. These included outcomes related to the psychological, physical, social/support service use, economic, and positive effects on caregiving. Encompassed in these broad outcomes is utilization of available resources by the caregiver and placement of the older adult. For example, in the National Institutes of Health (NIH)-supported Resources for Enhancing Alzheimer's Caregiver Health II (REACH II) trial, changes in use of formal care and services by the caregiver were evaluated as the intervention included information on strategies to enhance existing use of resources.

- Consideration was given to the heterogeneity of the caregiving experience and the longitudinal trajectory of providing care, thus recognizing that different intervention approaches may be warranted for different caregivers, older adult populations, and stages in the caregiving career and stages in the life course of caregivers (e.g., young adult caregivers may require different types and levels of support than older spouses).
- Special attention was given to how interventions do (or do not) address issues of diversity given that caregivers and older adults are very heterogeneous. Diversity was defined using a broad lens to include variations in race, ethnicity/culture, geography, socioeconomic status, caregiver–older adult relationship, care arrangements, and care contexts.
- Special consideration was given to the role of technology in delivering supportive services to families. Technology can be used to provide support for the caregiver (e.g., information websites, social media); to serve as an interface with the health care system; or to foster support through the development of caregiver networks. It is also playing an increasingly important role in health care delivery, and thus caregivers often need to interact with sophisticated technologies in the delivery of care.
- In evaluating the evidence for intervention studies, deliberation was given to intervention implementation considerations such as factors that may influence access to evidence-based interventions, approaches to the design of interventions (e.g., person centeredness, tailoring to caregiver needs, training needs of health and human service providers to provide evidence-based interventions), and factors that may impede the implementation of evidence-based interventions in real-world settings, including home care, primary care, hospitals, or the aging service network.

Organizational Framework for the Interventions

To organize the available literature and understand the evidence and gaps in knowledge regarding caregiver interventions, as noted, the committee adopted a framework that recognizes that caregiving occurs within a multifaceted context that encompasses the care setting (e.g., the home or residential setting of the older adult who is impaired), the social/community networks (e.g., family members), organizations such as the workplace and health care organizations, and societal/policy environments.

Using this framework, interventions were categorized as targeting and/or delivered in various levels of the caregiver's experience and his or her life space: the individual (older adult or caregiver), organizations (workplace,

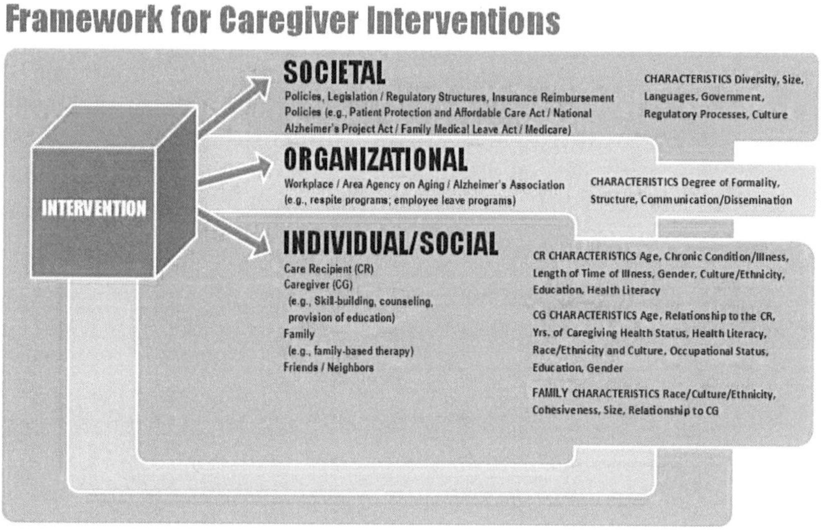

FIGURE 5-1 Organizational framework for reviewing family caregiving interventions.

health systems, community-based agencies), or society (policy initiatives), or their combination. Each of these levels has a unique set of characteristics that influence the caregiving experience. There is also a dynamic interplay among the various levels (see Figure 5-1).

Individual Level

Interventions at this level directly target the caregiver (the relative, partner, friend, or neighbor who assists the older adult who needs help due to physical, mental, cognitive, or functional limitations), and caregiver outcomes such as their physical and emotional health, knowledge and skills, social support, coping strategies, well-being, and quality of life. Interventions at this level also include interventions that target or are delivered to entities that are proximal to a caregiver such as the family, or the immediate community in which the caregiver interacts such as the neighborhood or neighborhood organizations. Interventions targeting this level include family-based interventions (e.g., family meetings) that attempt to increase the cohesiveness or support of other family members or a support group at a neighborhood senior center, naturally occurring retirement communities, or faith-based organizations. The interventions encompass a broad range of strategies including but not limited to: education, skill building, social support groups, cognitive behavioral therapy, environmental modifications, mindfulness training, information provision, stress management, and education. Many interventions are multicomponent and target several areas of caregiver risk. Interventions at this level may also target the dyad (both the caregiver and the older adult) or the older adult. Studies, which evaluate interventions directed at the older adult care recipient (e.g., cognitive training programs, prescription drugs) and for which caregiver outcomes are reported, are briefly summarized.

Organizational Level

The organizational level includes formal organizational structures such as health care and social service providers, the workplace, formal care settings, or community agencies (e.g., hospitals, Area Agencies on Aging). Examples of interventions that target this level include workplace benefits for caregivers, employee education and referral programs, adult day services, and in-home and outside-of-the-home respite programs.

Societal/Policy

This level includes interventions targeted at a societal and policy level, and includes insurance reimbursement policies, the National Family Caregiver Support Program (NFCSP), the National Alzheimer's Project Act (NAPA), the Patient Protection and Affordable Care Act, FMLA, or requirements for electronic health record (EHR) technology for caregiver access to the care recipient's health information. This chapter discusses interventions at this level briefly; more detail about them can be found in Chapters 1 and 6.

ASSESSMENT STRATEGIES

Interventions at the individual level and sometimes at the organizational level typically include an assessment of the family caregiving situation. In this report, caregiver assessment generally refers to a systematic process of gathering information about a caregiving situation, from the caregiver's perspective, about (1) specific problems, needs, strengths, and resources; (2) the emotional and physical functioning of the caregiver and care recipient; (3) the caregiver's ability to help meet the needs of the older adult; and (4) caregiver interactions or relationships with health care teams and/or LTSS systems. However, it may also include an assessment of the environment (e.g., clutter, safety hazards) or of the interaction between the caregiver and older adult. The specific topics of assessments vary according to the health condition of the older adults (e.g., dementia versus cancer). An assumption of caregiver assessment is that direct contact has occurred between the person performing the assessment and the family caregiver. In other words, family caregiver assessment involves asking questions of the family caregiver about themselves, not asking the caregiver questions about the care recipient (Kelly et al., 2013). However, it frequently also involves some assessment of the care recipient such as the assessment of cognitive status. Many measures may be used to assess family caregivers and domains of assessment vary (see Box 5-1). In this regard, a comprehensive inventory of caregiver assessment measures was recently compiled and is available at the website of the Family Caregiver Alliance (2012).

In intervention research and clinical settings, a caregiver assessment is generally conducted for three purposes. First, a caregiver assessment may be motivated for the purpose of identifying caregiver eligibility for an inter-

BOX 5-1
Domains of Caregiver Assessment

1. ***Context:*** describes situational information regarding the relationship between the caregiver and the older adult such as the living arrangement, environmental characteristics, duration of caregiving, caregiver's interactions with health care teams and long-term services and supports systems, financial status, and employment status, among other factors.
2. ***Caregiver's perception of health and functional status of care recipient:*** describes activities of daily living, instrumental activities of daily living, psychosocial needs, cognitive impairment, behavioral problems, and medical tests and procedures. This is sometimes supplemented with the assessment of the care recipient's cognitive status.
3. ***Caregiver values and preferences:*** measures the caregiver and care recipient's willingness to assume or accept care, perceived obligation to provide care, cultural norms that influence the care preferred or provided, as well as preferences for scheduling and delivering care and services.
4. ***Well-being of the caregiver:*** encompasses self-rated health, health conditions and symptoms, depression or emotional distress, and life satisfaction or quality of life.
5. ***Consequences of caregiving:*** describes the perceived challenges and perceived benefits of providing care.
6. ***Skills/abilities/knowledge to provide care recipient with needed care:*** reflects caregiving confidence and competencies as well as appropriate knowledge of the care recipient's health conditions and medical care tasks.
7. ***Potential resources that caregiver could choose to use:*** describes services, education, and training provided by formal and informal networks to assist in supporting the care recipient, caregiver, or both.

SOURCE: Family Caregiver Alliance, 2006.

vention trial. Second, a caregiver assessment may be incorporated in the intervention process to determine how to appropriately tailor services and skill-building strategies to best benefit family caregivers and persons receiving care (Belle et al., 2006; Fortinsky et al., 2009; Judge et al., 2011). This might involve, for example, culturally tailoring an intervention to accommodate differences in cultural values and preferences. Data from assessments may also be used in the interpretation of intervention study findings to understand how family caregiver factors relate to study outcomes.

One example of an assessment instrument that was used in a research study to tailor the intervention and that is becoming widely used in other research and clinical settings is the REACH II Risk Appraisal Measure (RAM). The RAM is a 16-item measure based on psychometric analysis of the responses of 642 caregiver dyads to the REACH II 59-item baseline assessment. It was developed as a brief, face-valid method to identify and prioritize specific areas of risk for caregivers of individuals with dementia that were amenable to intervention and relevant across diverse cultural and ethnic groups. The six RAM domains include depressive symptomatology (one item), burden (three items), self-care (two items), social support (two items), care recipient problem behaviors (two items), and safety (four items) (Czaja et al., 2009). Assessment for caregivers of individuals with other conditions such as cancer might have a strong focus on a caregiver's ability to manage the cancer symptomatology, medication regime, and other medically oriented procedures (e.g., infusion of fluids, cleaning of feeding tubes) of the care recipient. Irrespective of the assessment instrument, the rationale for conducting a family caregiver assessment is based on the recognition that family caregivers are highly diverse and that services and supports need to be tailored to address the unique and varying needs of caregivers (Brodaty et al., 2003).

Caregiver assessment is not commonly integrated in health delivery settings. At the system level, with rare exception, health care or LTSS providers have not adopted caregiver assessment into everyday practice (Feinberg and Levine, 2015). Less than one-third of states include family caregiver assessments in their Medicaid home- and community-based services (HCBS) waiver programs, with considerable variability in the scope of the assessment used (Kelly et al., 2013). The challenges of implementing caregiver assessment in practice are multifaceted. Problems not only span organizational and provider pushback but caregivers themselves may not understand the purpose of the assessment or want to be assessed (Levine et al., 2013). Importantly, caregiver assessments should also include an assessment of family structures, dynamics, and resources. In many cases, marshaling family resources can provide needed support to family members (e.g., Eisdorfer et al., 2003). Understanding the characteristics and resources of the family can also help service providers work effectively with multiple caregiver families (or groups) and suggest strategies for sharing caregiving responsibilities. Similarly, the social/community context of the caregiver should be considered and would help to gain an understanding of interventions that are acceptable to and effective for caregivers that are population-specific and accommodate language or cultural caregiving norms.

INDIVIDUAL-LEVEL INTERVENTIONS

Interventions at the individual level employ a variety of therapeutic strategies including problem solving, skills training, information provision, support groups, counseling, and family therapy; and target various aspects of caregiver risk (e.g., symptom management, behavioral problems, lack of support and resources). They may vary in dose, intensity, and mode of delivery (e.g., face-to-face, Internet). Research evaluating individual-level interventions employs a variety of study designs such as randomized controlled trials (RCTs), case control, and pre-test/post-test designs, and includes varying outcomes related to the psychological (positive and negative), physical, social, and economic effects of caregiving. The following section summarizes the evidence regarding individual-level interventions organized according to the health condition of the older adult.

Alzheimer's Disease/Dementia Caregiving

Alzheimer's disease and related disorders (ADRD) are progressive, neurodegenerative conditions that result in cognitive, social, and physical functional decline, as well as behavioral and psychological symptoms. Most of the 3.6 to 5.2 million individuals with dementia in the United States live at home and are cared for by family members. In fact, families provide more than 80 percent of the LTSS that people with ADRD receive (Friedman et al., 2015; Kasper et al., 2015). As the disease progresses, the caregiving responsibilities of families increase and include advocacy, hands-on assistance with personal care and mobility tasks, emotional and social support, medical care, and surrogacy, as well as ensuring safety and quality of life and preventing and managing behavioral symptoms (Black et al., 2013; Callahan et al., 2012; Hodgson et al., 2014).

As noted in Chapter 3, compared to caregivers of older adults without cognitive impairment, caregivers of individuals with ADRD spend more time in caregiving, have more care responsibilities, and report greater objective (e.g., financial burdens, time spent in daily care routines) and subjective negative consequences (e.g., poor physical health, emotional upset and distress) (Alzheimer's Association, 2014; Bertrand et al., 2006; Friedman et al., 2015; Kasper et al., 2015; Moon et al., 2014; Ory et al., 1999). Many interventions have been developed for this population and tested in RCTs.

Overall, an estimated 200 interventions have been tested using randomized designs (Gitlin et al., 2015; Maslow, 2012). Seven meta-analyses and 17 systematic reviews of research conducted between 1966 and 2013 have been published.

Unfortunately, there is no agreed-on categorization system for classifying caregiver interventions by their content. However, for heuristic purposes, interventions for families of persons with dementia can be categorized as follows: professional support for depression (e.g., psychotherapy); psychoeducation (e.g., education about the disease, stress reduction and support, providing information about resources); behavior management/skills training (e.g., instruction in particular approaches such as using activities, adaptive equipment, or the use of cueing to prevent and manage behaviors); situational counseling (e.g., family counseling, instruction in cognitive reframing or other positive coping techniques, mindfulness training); self-care/relaxation training (e.g., meditation, yoga); and multicomponent interventions (Gitlin and Hodgson, 2015). Multicomponent interventions tend to target caregivers of individuals at the moderate disease stage and include combinations of approaches such as dementia education, care management, environmental modification, counseling, skills training, and/or referral to community resources, all tailored to the identified unmet needs of caregivers identified via a systematic assessment.

Programs targeting family caregivers of persons with dementia have been delivered through various modalities including face-to-face (Belle et al., 2006; Gitlin et al., 2010b), group (Gallagher-Thompson et al., 2003), telephone (Bass et al., 2003; Kwok et al., 2013; Martindale-Adams et al., 2013; Tremont et al., 2015), videophone (Czaja et al., 2013), or Web-based platforms (Kajiyama et al., 2013). They range in level of dose and intensity from a brief number of sessions (e.g., four sessions delivered over 2 to 3 months) (Nichols et al., 2016) to 1 or more years of contact (Mittelman et al., 2006) and are delivered by different health and social service professionals including nurses, occupational therapists, community health workers, social workers, and care managers. Some interventions are offered in a variety of modalities. For example, the Savvy Caregiver, a psychoeducation intervention, which provides basic disease education, coping skills, and behavioral management strategies, is available in a variety of modalities (telephone, classroom, online) making it more accessible and responsive to family preferences (Hepburn et al., 2003, 2007). A few interventions have targeted both the family caregiver and the person with dementia (e.g., Whitlatch et al., 2006).

Outcome measures for dementia caregiver interventions are wide ranging and have primarily included caregiver knowledge, burden, self-efficacy, psychological morbidity (anxiety/depression), upset, confidence, skills, and desire or time to caregiver placement of the person with dementia in assisted living or nursing homes. Many interventions, using rigorous trial designs, demonstrate effectiveness for one or more outcomes that are targeted in the trial such as reducing caregiver burden and for some interventions, reducing institutionalization and other care recipient-related outcomes such as symptomatology (Brodaty and Arasaratnam, 2012; Gitlin et al., 2006, 2008; Mittelman et al., 2006). However, the outcomes that are positively or not positively impacted vary vastly among studies (e.g., one study may report benefits for depression whereas another will focus on efficacy). An example is the Mittelman and colleagues (2006) New York University Caregiver Intervention (NYUCI), which showed reduced nursing home placement rates and increased caregiver feelings of efficacy and social support. In addition, while the intervention does not appear to change the frequency of care recipient problem behaviors overall, it does appear to help caregivers feel less distressed by these behaviors. In contrast, the REACH II intervention (see Box 5-2) resulted in improvements in a multivariate quality of life indicator that assessed caregiver burden, depressive symptoms, self-care, social support, and care recipient problem behaviors for the intervention group compared to the control group (Belle et al., 2006). For the most part, multicomponent interventions show the largest effects for most outcomes. Most changes from program participation are examined for only short duration (e.g., 3, 4, or 6 months), with few studies examining long-term benefits (i.e., more than 9 months) (Gitlin et al., 2010b; Mittelman et al., 2006). Also, most studies report positive effects on outcomes such as increased confidence in dealing with challenging situations, with very few showing no benefits at all, and no studies reporting worsening or adverse effects.

Only a few studies directly target people with dementia and also evaluate the potential benefits of the intervention for family caregivers. Of these, there are inconsistent outcomes, with some studies showing benefits for caregivers and others not. For example, Stanley and colleagues' (2013) cognitive behavioral therapy intervention targeting anxiety in persons with dementia (Peaceful Mind) reduced caregiver distress associated with the anxiety of the person with dementia. A meta-analysis of 17 studies examining the effects on caregivers of antidementia clinical drugs administered to individuals with dementia found a small beneficial effect for caregivers including reductions in burden and time spent caregiving (Lingler et al., 2005). Gitlin and colleagues' (2010a) activity intervention study to reduce behavioral symptoms in persons with dementia resulted in significant reductions in objective burden (e.g., time spent in providing direct care), confidence in engaging in activities (e.g., preparing light meals, grooming, and exercise), and improved mastery among caregivers, with other aspects of well-being (e.g., depressive symptoms, burden) not affected. Similarly, Tappen and colleagues' (2014) cognitive training intervention for persons

BOX 5-2
A Successful Intervention for Dementia Caregivers: Resources for Enhancing Alzheimer's Caregiver Health II (REACH II)

REACH II was a randomized controlled trial (RCT), funded by the National Institute on Aging and the National Institute of Nursing Research, to assess the impact of a multicomponent intervention on dementia caregivers' quality of life and depression. The trial was conducted in five U.S. cities in 2004. It was unique in that it included roughly equal numbers of white, African American, and Hispanic caregivers and thus had the potential to measure racial or ethnic differences in the effectiveness of the intervention. The success of the trial has led to its adaptation in a shorter form by the U.S. Department of Veterans Affairs, the U.S. Department of Health and Human Services, including the Administration for Community Living, hospital systems such as Baylor Scott & White Health, several state agencies, and social service programs in Hong Kong. These organizations have found similar results despite using an intervention with fewer sessions.

The REACH II Intervention: Caregivers participate in nine in-home and three telephone sessions and five structured telephone support group sessions over a 6-month period. During the sessions, trained interventionists with at least a bachelor's degree provide the following:

- Educational materials on dementia, caregiving, caregiving stress, and information on local resources;
- Role playing exercises to practice management of problem core recipient (CR) behaviors;
- Problem solving to identify and address problem CR behaviors
- Skills training for managing burden of caregiving, emotional well-being, and social support; and
- Stress management techniques such as breathing exercises, listening to music, and stretching exercises.

The Control Group: Caregivers in the control group received basic educational materials on dementia and Alzheimer's disease, caregiving, safety, and community resources but only two brief "check-in" calls at 3 and 5 months during the study period.

Results: Hispanic and white caregivers in the intervention group had a significantly larger improvement in quality of life compared to the control group. For African American caregivers, only spousal caregivers showed a significant improvement when compared to the control group. Prevalence of clinical depression in all racial groups was lower in the intervention group than in the control group at the end of the trial.

SOURCES: Belle et al., 2006; Cheung et al., 2015; HHS, 2014; Nichols et al., 2011; Rosalynn Carter Institute, 2012; Stevens et al., 2012.

with dementia did not result in reductions in depression or upset with behavioral symptoms for caregivers.

Although the literature is limited, interventions may also target the family or social networks of the caregiver, neighbors, neighborhoods, churches, or community-level groups such as senior centers. Family group interventions providing psychoeducation and/or counseling show positive benefits for families including reductions of caregiver negative reactions to behavioral symptoms in persons with dementia and caregiver depression (Eisdorfer et al., 2003; Ostwald et al., 1999). Home-Based Supportive Services programs that provide stipends to families to offset care expenses of individuals with disability of all ages demonstrate a wider range of benefits to family caregivers, including fewer out-of-pocket care expenses, better mental health and access to health care, and improved self-efficacy, than caregivers on a waitlist for this service (Caldwell, 2006; Heller and Caldwell, 2006; Heller et al., 1999).

The community represents a largely untapped resource for supporting families for which there are no tested interventions (see Box 5-3 for an example). Communities have a wide range of naturally occurring resources such as churches or religious places of worship, libraries, community or senior centers, or schools. Each of these could provide a range of emotional and logistical supportive services for families, including support groups, friendly visitors, chore services, and education, and serve as a supportive network for families. For example, the Naturally Occurring Retirement Communities (NORCs) and villages, which have been developing primarily in urban areas throughout the United States to provide supportive services for and to neighbors, could more purposely support family caregivers (Greenfield et al., 2013). However, the benefit of these resources for family caregivers has not been evaluated. This is a critical gap in the literature. Future research needs to be conducted concerning models for supporting family caregivers using these naturally occurring resources and other models of livable communities. There is also a lack of community-engaged interventions targeting ethnic/racial groups through outreach to ethnic media, churches, and community-based organizations that serve ethnic communities. The community can also play an important role in terms of providing support and services to "hard to reach" caregivers, such as those who live in rural locations, ethnic/racial minorities, or those who have no other source of support for the care recipient and are often unaware of or have difficulty accessing available resources and sources of caregiver support. Specifically, community programs or workers may help identify and "recruit" caregivers into educational or support programs by marketing these programs in newsletters, through service providers, or other forms of community engagement using targeted, culturally appropriate messaging. Engagement of caregivers in these programs might be facilitated by pro-

BOX 5-3
An Example from a Community-Based Intervention

Tom is 88 and was diagnosed with Alzheimer's disease 5 years ago. His wife Betsy, also his primary caregiver, is 85. Betsy's initial REACH assessment found her to be at high risk for safety issues, depression, and anxiety due to the burden of caregiving for her very difficult husband. She reported that he was a kind and gentle man to her and to their children who always put family first. After he was diagnosed, he became self-centered, demanding, and violent, threatening his wife with a hunting knife and a loaded gun and hitting her. He also spent their entire savings by investing online with a fraudulent broker; Betsy was too embarrassed to report it until her son intervened several months later.

Betsy's dementia care specialist worked closely with her to develop a safety plan and called on her adult children to be included in her plan. Betsy and her children removed all guns, knives, and ammunition from the home, cut up his credit cards, and disabled his computer. Two of their daughters moved into the house to protect their mother and continue to live with her in order to help keep their father home for as long as possible. At the end of her REACH participation, Betsy was empowered to find time for herself, to delegate some of the caregiving to her daughters and sons, to open her own bank account and control the finances, and most importantly, to develop ways of de-escalating her husband's aggression. She has now joined a support group, has returned to church, and has rekindled old, forgotten friendships. In her exit assessment, she commented, "My REACH specialist was the first beacon of light I have seen in a lot of years. I had forgotten how to laugh, to sleep through the night, and to feel strong. Thank you so much for this help."

SOURCE: Stevens et al., 2016.

viding transportation or respite services, offering home-based programs, implementing more flexible programs with respect to scheduling, integrating them within other services, or having satellite programs in rural locations (Navaie, 2011).

Overall, although interventions vary widely in purpose, dose, intensity, and mode of delivery, effective interventions tend to share several common characteristics: adjusting dose, intensity, and specific focus of an intervention based on a caregiver's risk or need profile (Belle et al., 2006; Czaja et al., 2009; Richards et al., 2007); active involvement of caregivers in learning a particular skill such as managing a problem behavior rather than a didactic, prescriptive approach in which information or instructions are provided (Belle et al., 2006; Chee et al., 2007; Czaja, 2009); addressing multiple areas of identified need or risk (Belle et al., 2006; Kansagara et al., 2010; Zarit and Femia, 2008); and longer interventions or episodic

BOX 5-4
Case Example of the COPE Intervention

Background: Robert, an 85-year-old African American man with moderate dementia, lives with his 80-year-old wife Beverly. He exhibits difficult behaviors (resistance to care, pacing, and repetitive vocalizations) and is dependent in dressing and grooming. He sits in front of the television most days disengaged and bored. Beverly is worried about his and her own quality of life and questions how long she can keep Robert home. Prescribed medications have not decreased Robert's behaviors and he also suffered side effects. Beverly initially wanted to work on his bathing difficulties and lack of activity in the COPE intervention.

COPE Intervention: In general, COPE participants received up to 10 sessions with occupational therapists (OTs) over 4 months and 1 face-to-face session and 1 telephone session with an advance practice nurse. Based on assessments in sessions 1 and 2, the OT identified that Robert is able to follow simple verbal cues, respond to visual cues, has good upper body strength and endurance, and can participate in activity for up to 30 minutes. The OT observes that Beverly's communications are too complex, the home is cluttered, and the tub is slippery. The OT also discerns that Robert was previously an accountant who enjoyed fishing and physical activity. The next visit is made by an advanced practice nurse who found no underlying medical infections but expressed concern about polypharmacy and the possibility of pain when Robert ambulated. The nurse (sessions 3 and 4) showed Beverly how to detect pain and reviewed questions to ask Robert's physician. The OT (sessions 5-12) next provided Beverly with education about dementia, how Robert's behaviors and functional changes are a consequence of disease (versus intention), and techniques to reduce her own stress. Different activities reflecting Robert's interests and abilities were developed and Beverly was taught how to help Robert initiate and participate in them. The OT helped Beverly remove unnecessary objects from the bathroom and helped her to secure bathroom equipment (grab bar, tub bench, and hand-held shower). The OT modeled verbal and tactile cueing with Robert and trained Beverly how to bring him to the shower and sit him on the tub bench.

Outcomes: At post-test, Beverly reported more time to herself, less distress, and Robert's increased pleasure and engagement in activities. His agitated behaviors were minimal and he was less resistant to bathing. Beverly used better communication and simplification strategies resulting in Robert's greater independence in other activities of living. She also met with Robert's doctor to review medications and evaluate his ambulation. Beverly felt more hopeful about continuing to care for Robert and keeping him at home awhile longer.

SOURCE: Gitlin et al., 2010b.

(i.e., booster) support over time for the duration of caregiving (Mittelman et al., 2006).

Overall, interventions directed at the individual level (i.e., target the older adult with dementia and/or the family caregiver) appear to be feasible to implement (they can be delivered and received) and are acceptable (well received) to families. These interventions regardless of dose and intensity or place of delivery also appear to make a real and important difference in the lives of family caregivers. Box 5-4 briefly describes one such intervention—In it Together: Learning to COPE with Dementia—designed to improve the well-being of both the person with dementia and the family caregiver.

The few cost studies that have been conducted suggest that interventions directed at the individual level can be low cost and result in cost savings to the caregiver in terms of reductions in time spent in caregiving, a highly valuable resource for caregivers (Gitlin et al., 2010a; Jutkowitz et al., 2010; Nichols et al., 2008). However, few studies have examined the cost effectiveness of an intervention.

Implementation of Interventions for Caregivers of Persons with Dementia

Generally a strong body of research evidence, some cost analyses, intervention feasibility, and caregiver acceptability of an intervention are factors necessary for moving forward with the widespread translation, dissemination, and implementation of these proven interventions for delivery in service and practice settings (Gearing et al., 2011; Gitlin et al., 2015). Despite the generally positive benefit of interventions for caregivers of older adults with dementia, few studies have been translated for implementation in systems of care (see Table 5-1). One exemplar exception is the National Institutes of Health (NIH)-supported REACH II initiative. The original trial was found to improve quality of life in Hispanic and white caregivers and spousal African American caregivers (Belle et al., 2006). It has since been adapted for delivery and implemented throughout the U.S. Department of Veterans Affairs (VA) and other organizations (see Box 5-2). Initially, its 12-session structure served as a barrier to full implementation in social service settings; however, a modified four-session adaptation has shown similar outcomes as the original trial (Burgio et al., 2009; Nichols et al., 2011, 2016). Although REACH II and other evidence-based programs are currently being tested in various care settings such as Medicaid waiver programs, social services, the aging network, and home care, few caregivers of persons with dementia currently have access to such programs unless they are located in the specific regions in which the demonstration programs are being evaluated through grant-supported funds (Gitlin et al., 2015) or through VA-supported programs.

A major challenge to implementation of interventions to support caregivers of older adults by the health care delivery system is the paucity of

TABLE 5-1 Outcomes and Implementation of Selected Family Caregiver Interventions

Intervention	Description	Caregiver and Care Recipient Outcomes	Implementation Sites
BRI Care Consultation	Consumer-driven coaching program focused on finding solutions for family caregivers (CGs) and their care recipients (CRs).	Improved psychosocial outcomes for CGs and CRs (e.g., reductions in burden); reduced hospital readmissions and return emergency department visits.	21 organizations are licensed to deliver BRI Care Consultation. Licensees have diverse missions, locations, and target populations.
Collaborative Care Model for Alzheimer's Disease and Related Dementias	For CGs of persons with dementia. Primary care management by an interdisciplinary team led by an advanced practice nurse. Uses standard protocols to initiate treatment and to identify, monitor, and treat behavioral and psychological symptoms of dementia. Emphasizes non-pharmacological management.	Improved CG distress and depression; CRs had fewer behavioral and psychological symptoms of dementia.	Has been evaluated in primary care practices in two university-affiliated health care systems.
New York University Caregiver Intervention (NYUCI)	For CGs of persons with dementia. Task-oriented counseling and support groups to provide emotional and instrumental support to CGs and to promote communication among family members and to teach techniques for problem solving and management of difficult CR behaviors.	Improved CG competence, self-confidence, social supports, and coping with problem behaviors. Reduced CR depression and nursing home placements.	Multiple Alzheimer's Associations and four project sites selected by the Minnesota Board on Aging and the Area Agency on Aging (AAA).

TABLE 5-1 Continued

Intervention	Description	Caregiver and Care Recipient Outcomes	Implementation Sites
REACH II	For CGs of persons with dementia. Education, support, and skills training to improve CG's health, safety, social support, handling of problem behaviors, and depression.	Improved CG quality of life as measured by decreased burden and depression, enhanced self-care and social support, and fewer CR fewer behavior problems.	Numerous VA sites; state aging services programs, AAAs; implemented in South Korea, Hong Kong, and Germany.
Savvy Caregiver	For CGs of persons with dementia. Education and skills training for CGs to help them manage stress and carry out the caregiving role effectively.	Improved CG competence, personal gain, management, positive experiences, depression, and ability to keep the CR occupied.	4 AAA Caregiver Programs and 25 communities (including rural areas).
$Skills_2Care$	For CGs of persons with dementia. Home-based intervention designed to develop a more supportive environment through modifications to the home environment and CG education and skill building.	Improved CG knowledge and skills, ability to engage persons with dementia in activities, confidence in managing behaviors, functional dependence, and care of themselves.	20 home care agencies; AAAs and by occupational therapists in private practice; covered by Medicare.

New Ways Better Days: Tailored Activity Program (TAP)	Home-based occupational therapy intervention for individuals with dementia. Focuses on identifying the CR's abilities, previous roles, habits, and interests; developing activities customized to the individual; and training their CGs in activity use and stress management.	Well-received by CGs and CRs; reduced CR behavioral symptoms; CGs gained more personal time.	Being implemented in several states through the Administration for Community Living's Dementia-Friendly Community initiative; has been adapted in hospital settings; is undergoing testing in Baltimore and Florida; and is used in Australia, Brazil, England, and Scotland. An online adaptation is under development.
Care of Older Persons in the Home Environment (COPE)	For CGs of persons with dementia. Designed to support CR's abilities by reducing environmental stressors and improving CG skills, problem-solving, and stress.	Improved CGs sense of well-being and confidence; improved CRs dependence and increased their engagement.	Being tested in Medicaid home and community-based programs.

SOURCES: Belle et al., 2006; Callahan et al., 2006; Clark et al., 2004; Gitlin et al., 2001, 2003, 2010a, 2010b, 2010c; Hepburn et al., 2001; Jutkowitz et al., 2010; Mittelman, 2008; Mittelman et al., 1993, 1995, 1996, 2006; Nichols et al., 2011; Ostwald et al., 1999.

Current Procedural Terminology (CPT) or Healthcare Common Procedure Coding System (HCPCS) codes to recognize the services rendered. One exception to this model is the REACH I $Skills_2Care$ intervention, which was structured for implementation in home care delivery by occupational therapists and is reimbursed through Medicare Part A and B as long as the caregiver training is linked to the health and functional goals of the care recipient with dementia (Gitlin et al., 2015).

Table 5-2 describes the barriers to moving evidence-based interventions from the research phase to implementation in real-world, health, and social service settings. The challenges include limitations of existing evidence; funding; lack of knowledge of providers, health and social service organizations, and administrators of available evidence-based programs; and various contextual barriers. Table 5-3 outlines several strategies for addressing these barriers and facilitating the translation of evidenced-based intervention programs into clinical and community settings.

There are also notable limitations of intervention studies that point to the need for additional and new research. For example, samples are poorly characterized in terms of the disease etiology and disease stage of the person with dementia. Most interventions target the needs of families who care for persons at the moderate disease stage with a primary diagnosis of Alzheimer's disease, with few studies targeting families caring for persons with mild cognitive impairment, early-stage dementia, severe stages of the disease, or for specific dementias such as Frontotemporal Dementia or Lewy bodies that impose unique care challenges for caregivers. Also, caregivers of older adults with dementia may also have to handle other disease challenges such as diabetes or sensory impairments such as difficulty seeing or hearing (Feil et al., 2011; Maslow, 2011). This makes it challenging for clinicians or service providers to know which families would benefit from which interventions. Also, as noted earlier, few intervention studies report long-term outcomes (i.e., more than 12 months) (Gitlin et al., 2006; Mittelman et al., 2006; Samus et al., 2014), evaluate adherence (Chee et al., 2007), or identify mechanisms by which an intervention works or why desired benefits are achieved (Roth et al., 2005). Further, interventions are, for the most part, tested outside of clinical and practice settings requiring yet additional translation and then implementation test phases (Gitlin et al., 2015; Nichols et al., 2016).

Furthermore, a psychosocial stress-process model guides most interventions and thus their focus has been on reducing stressors and caregiver burden. Consequently, the practical issues that many caregivers confront have been largely ignored such as financial and physical strain, balancing caregiving with employment responsibilities or their need for specific skills for overseeing complex medical conditions (e.g., wound care, diabetes care, vision impairments, or fall risk), or managing frustrating encounters with

TABLE 5-2 Challenges in Moving Family Caregiver Interventions from Research to Large-Scale Implementation

Challenge	Examples
Limitations of the existing evidence	• Not evaluated in real-world delivery settings subject to Medicare, Medicaid, or other payment rules • Too complex • Staff require training to implement the intervention • Limited to caregivers' needs at one time point (not addressing changing needs over time) • Limited outcome data on cost, health care usage, financial distress, and physical health • Limited evidence for subgroups of caregivers (e.g., men, minority populations, rural, long-distance caregivers, multiple caregivers)
Funding	• Existing funding sources have limited resources for translation efforts • Administration for Community Living Alzheimer's Disease Supportive Services Program • NIA/AoA research grant program (Translational Research to Help Older Adults Maintain Health and Independence in the Community) • U.S. Department of Veterans Affairs • Rosalynn Carter Institute for Caregiving
Provider knowledge	• Do not know that effective interventions can be implemented • Do not know how to obtain or pay for the intervention or how to train staff to provide it • Do not know how to identify and reach caregivers who might benefit • Do not know how to assess the feasibility of implementing the intervention in specific settings
Contextual barriers	• Limited reimbursement or payment mechanisms to support provision of evidence-based interventions • Lack of workforce preparation in working with caregivers and knowing about and how to adopt interventions • Lack of time and funding of health and social agencies and organizations for training in evidence-based interventions • Lack of guidelines when to use which intervention • Needs of families are complex and may require using more than one program • Lack of understanding as to how to identify families, referral mechanisms

NOTES: NIA = National Institute on Aging; AoA = Administration on Aging.
SOURCES: Gitlin et al., 2015, 2016; Nichols et al., 2016; Reinhard et al., 2008.

TABLE 5-3 Selected Strategies for Addressing Barriers to Intervention Implementation

- Development of a Web-based classification system for categorizing interventions by who they target, their delivery characteristics, and outcomes and how to access training in programs for health and human service organizations and families to access.
- Development and testing of dissemination and implementation strategies to enable reach and scaling up of proven programs and integration in existing systems of care.
- Development of bundled or reimbursement payment mechanisms for providers to use proven caregiver interventions.
- Expansion of funding for purposeful adoption of existing evidence-based programs for delivery to diverse family caregivers.
- Identification of core competencies by professional organizations required for engaging with families and using caregiver interventions in existing educational programs.
- Linking health organizations with aging network of services to implement proven caregiver interventions.

SOURCES: Gitlin et al., 2015; Nichols et al., 2016; Reinhard et al., 2008.

health care providers. Another limitation is that interventions target single individual caregivers even though evidence suggests that families often share care responsibilities. Finally, most interventions have been tested with white caregivers. Only a few studies have involved African Americans (Belle et al., 2006; Martindale-Adams et al., 2013), Latino (Belle et al., 2006; Gallagher-Thompson et al., 2003), and Asian (Heller and Caldwell, 2006; Reuben et al., 2013) caregivers. Other groups such as lesbian, gay, bisexual, and transgender (LGBT) caregivers, long-distance caregivers, and rural caregivers have largely been ignored. Further studies have not systematically examined caregiver health care utilization as a possible outcome of caregiving even though existing research suggests that caregiver self-care may be compromised, which has the potential of causing downsteam adverse health effects. Spouses of individuals with dementia have significantly higher monthly Medicare use than spouses of non-demented individuals, suggesting interdependence between the health and health care costs of the dyad (Dassel et al., 2015).

Impact of Pharmacological Treatments for Alzheimer's Disease and Related Dementias on the Caregiver

The most commonly prescribed medications for older adults with ADRD are cholinesterase inhibitors (ChEIs). The majority of the research examining positive benefits of ChEIs are focused on care recipient outcomes and based on clinical trial data that support clinical effectiveness of these medications at small to modest levels for some individuals. In some cases other benefits of ChEIs have been examined such as improvements in caregiver burden, care recipient and caregiver quality of life, and time to nursing home placement. Given the critical role that caregivers play in providing support to individuals with ADRD caregiver-specific outcome measures are gaining attention while specifying endpoints in clinical trials. Lingler and colleagues (2005) conducted a systematic review of ChEI trials that also examined indirect treatment effects, including caregiver-specific outcomes. The authors identified 17 studies involving 4,744 subjects; four trials met the inclusion for the burden analysis and six trials met the inclusion criteria for the time-use analysis. Overall the analysis revealed that providing ChEIs to care recipients had a small beneficial effect on caregiver burden and active time use among caregivers of persons with ADRD. Another systematic review by Knowles (2006) summarized major findings of effectiveness studies focusing on treatment effects of donepezil. The major findings of this review include significant improvement in cognitive function for the care recipients, delays in nursing home placement, as well as modest evidence for improvements in caregiving burden and time use. Generally, given the critical role of caregivers in providing support to older adults with ADRD, caregiver outcomes such as burden, quality of life, and time spent on caregiving should be included in any evaluation examining the effectiveness of ChEIs.

Caregivers of People Who Have Had a Stroke

Although the literature is less extensive than for persons with ADRD, interventions have also been developed for family caregivers of older adults who have had a stroke. These caregivers are typically thrust into the caregiver role with little or no warning. They typically need skills in the physical aspects of caring for the individual who had a stroke, play a large role in the person's care coordination, and also provide emotional support to the individual, which is especially challenging if the person is confronted with long-term disabilities. They may also live with the fear that a stroke may happen again.

Overall, the evidence suggests the available programs are beneficial for both survivors of stroke and their family caregivers. The American Heart Association and American Stroke Association (AHA/ASA) (Bakas et al., 2014) recently reviewed the evidence for the efficacy of family caregiving interventions in stroke. The review examined the stroke intervention literature to determine the impact of interventions on outcomes for both stroke survivors and their family caregivers. The review included 32 interventions; 22 interventions were evaluated in RCTs. Survivor outcomes included physical functioning, anxiety, depression, social functioning, service use, and knowledge. Family caregiver outcomes included preparedness to care for survivor, burden, stress and strain, anxiety, depression, quality of life, social functioning, coping, health care utilization, and knowledge. Intervention strategies are similar to those employed in interventions for other types of family caregiving. Psychoeducation elements in stroke interventions commonly include the presentation of information and warning signs of the survivor's health. Skills training techniques include problem solving and stress management for managing the care, medication, and personal needs of the survivor, and managing emotions and behaviors. The caregiver's emotions and health care needs are also the target of skills training techniques. Specific techniques used include problem solving, goal setting, and communication with health care professionals; hands-on training in skills such as lifting and mobility techniques and assistance with activities of daily living; and communication skills tailored to the needs of the care recipient.

Caregiver- and dyad-focused interventions have been tested. Of the 32 studies identified, 17 were caregiver focused and 15 were dyad focused. Overall, Kalra and colleagues (2004) provide strong evidence for the dyadic approach, which resulted in positive outcomes for both survivors and caregivers. However, there is also an absence of studies that target diverse groups of caregivers.

Caregivers of Older Adults with Cancer

Family members also serve as caregivers and provide critical support for older adults with cancer. For example, family caregivers can play an essential role in the delivery of medications directed at the cancer; monitoring and managing symptoms; and providing emotional support that is important to treatment and survival of the care recipient. Family caregivers of care recipients with cancer are often introduced into situations that require a working knowledge of complex medical procedures and medication regimens in the context of a life-threatening diagnosis to a member of the family. When the individual is in remission, the possibility of cancer recurrence is a concern. Interventions for family caregivers of persons with cancer have been designed to address these medical and emotional demands.

In 2010, Northouse and colleagues reported a meta-analysis of 29 RCTs of interventions for family caregivers of individuals with cancer that included an analysis of the types of interventions and their effects on various caregiver outcomes. The intervention RCTs were carried out from 1983 to 2009 and met the following criteria: (1) they had to involve family caregivers, either alone, or with the person with cancer; (2) they were psychosocially, cognitively, or behaviorally oriented; (3) the participants were randomly assigned to the intervention or control arm of the study; and (4) they were published in a peer-reviewed journal. The majority of interventions was psychoeducational and provided information regarding symptom management and other physical aspects of the individual's care.

Attention was also directed to the emotional and psychosocial needs of care recipients, caregivers, and/or marital or family relationships. Skills training interventions that focused primarily on the development of coping, communication, and problem-solving skills with a focus on behavioral change were also included. The least frequent intervention was therapeutic counseling focused primarily on the development of therapeutic relationships to address concerns related to cancer or caregiving. Overall, although these interventions had small to medium effects on reducing caregiver burden and improving caregiver coping, they did increase caregiver self-sufficiency and improve some aspects of quality of life.

Appelbaum and Breitbart (2013) expanded on the meta-analysis conducted by Northouse and colleagues (2010) in a review article that summarized the scope and impact of 49 cancer caregiver intervention studies published between 1980 and 2011. All were classified as psychosocial and were subdivided into eight groups based on primarily therapeutic approaches, such as psychoeducational, problem solving/skill building, supportive therapy, family/couple therapy, cognitive behavioral therapy, interpersonal therapy, complementary and alternative medicine, and existential therapy. They also addressed the unique needs of family caregivers who are faced with a terminal illness of a family member. Although effect sizes were generally not reported, 65 percent of the interventions produced positive improvements in outcomes for caregivers, such as reductions in burden, anxiety, and depression and enhanced problem-solving and caregiving skills. Some interventions, such as interpersonal therapy and family/couples therapy, also resulted in better relationship quality between the caregiver and care recipient and for the care recipient's emotional well-being.

Caregiving for Adults with Other Conditions

The empirical literature on interventions is much less robust for family caregivers of older adults with other conditions such as adults with persistent mental illness (e.g., schizophrenia, major depression) and spinal cord injury. This is an emerging area of need as many adults are living longer with these conditions and many rely on family members for support.

Caregivers of adults with persistent mental illness have some unique challenges such as dealing with the issue of stigma, non-normative illness expectations, cyclic illness trajectory, unpredictable patterns of behavior, and often a lack of available support and resources (Biegel and Schulz, 1999). In general, the available literature suggests that psychoeducational family interventions can be effective in terms of helping families cope with and care for a relative who has a severe mental illness such as schizophrenia. Dixon and colleagues (2000) conducted a review of 15 studies on psychoeducational family interventions and found overall psychoeducational programs for family members are efficacious in terms of family outcomes such as burden and family functioning. However, they concluded that there is incomplete knowledge on how to best design these programs. Overall, the data are quite limited regarding family caregivers of older adults with a mental illness and that which has been conducted is most often on caregivers of individuals with schizophrenia. In addition, programs targeting caregivers of individuals with mental illness are not widely available. This is clearly an area of need as a large number of people with severe and persistent mental illness live with and/or rely on their families for help and support, and literature clearly demonstrates that caring for a family member with mental illness is burdensome for the caregiver (e.g., Biegel and Schulz, 1999).

Caregivers of persons with spinal cord injury also are often confronted with some physical challenges related to lack of mobility of the care recipient and provision of care tasks related to medical complications such as the pressure sores or urinary system disorders. Similar to caregivers of individuals after a stroke, they also have to cope with being suddenly thrust into the caregiving role and the need to provide emotional support to the person with the spinal cord injury who is confronting living with disabilities.

With respect to interventions for these caregivers, the literature generally suggests that psychosocial interventions such as problem-solving therapy, family psychoeducational and dyadic multicomponent psychosocial interventions (e.g., those that combine skills training, stress management techniques) can be beneficial to family caregivers. However, the evidence is limited and some of the studies that have been conducted have involved small samples or lack of a comparison group and most of this work does not focus on older adults. However, the committee chose to include a review of some of this literature to identify strategies that might also be beneficial to older adults. For example, Elliott and Berry (2009) evaluated a brief problem-solving training for family caregivers of recent-onset spinal cord injury. They found that the intervention was beneficial in that the caregivers who received the intervention, as compared to those in the control condition, experienced a decrease in dysfunctional problem-solving styles. In another study, Elliott and colleagues (2008) evaluated a problem-solving intervention delivered via videoconferencing and found that there was a significant decline in depression for caregivers who received the intervention. They also reported an increase in social functioning. However, again the sample was relatively small. Schulz and colleagues (2009) compared a caregiver-focused multicomponent psychosocial intervention to a dual target intervention where the caregiver intervention was complemented by an intervention targeting the care recipient age 35 and older. The intervention conditions were compared to a control condition where caregivers received standard information about caregiving, spinal cord injury, and aging. One hundred and seventy-three dyads were randomized to one of the three conditions. Overall, the results indicated that caregivers who were in the dual-target condition had improved quality of life, significantly fewer health symptoms, and were less depressed. More recently, Molazem and colleagues (2014) investigated the effectiveness of psychoeducational interventions on the life quality of the family caregivers of people with spinal cord injuries. The study, an RCT, involved 72 family caregivers in Iran who were randomized into an intervention or control group. The study results indicated that the intervention resulted in positive outcomes for caregivers who received the intervention; specifically the caregivers experienced improvement in aspects of quality of life.

Generally, the psychosocial interventions for family caregivers of older adults with chronic conditions such as persistent mental illness and spinal cord injury are similar to those targeting caregivers of adults with dementia and cancer and involve strategies such as psychoeducational programs, support groups, problem-solving training, skills training, and stress management techniques. The results are promising with respect to showing positive benefits of these interventions for caregivers and in some cases care recipients. However, the literature is rather sparse and the empirical data are limited especially for caregivers of older adults living with these conditions.

Cost and Cost-Effectiveness of Caregiver Support Programs

Although many caregiver interventions show improvement in caregiver outcomes such as health and well-being, relatively few assess economic impacts of these interventions such as health care savings associated with reduced formal health care utilization by the care recipient. These might include savings associated with delayed nursing home placement and fewer hospitalizations and emergency room visits. Most intervention studies also fail to quantify the cost of delivering the intervention such as the costs of training the interventionists and the time, travel, and monitoring costs of delivering the intervention.

Randomized trials show significant delays in nursing home placement. The New York University Caregiver Intervention, a program of enhanced supportive services for spouse and adult child caregivers of community-dwelling people with dementia (Gaugler et al., 2013; Mittelman et al., 2006) showed significantly delayed nursing home placement for care recipients in the treatment arm. In addition, caregivers who received the intervention experienced fewer depressive symptoms and less distress compared to those in the usual care control group. A simulation analysis of the widespread use of this program suggested that there would be substantial government savings through the delay in nursing home placement (Long et al., 2013).

Several trials have studied the impact of integrating caregivers into discharge planning in a hospital or institutional setting. Compared to usual care, integrating caregivers into the discharge process and providing follow-up support to caregivers and patients resulted in significant reductions in readmissions at 90 and 180 days and overall lower costs of post-discharge care (e.g., Huang and Liang, 2005; Legrain et al., 2011; Naylor et al.. 1999). These findings taken as whole suggest that a relatively modest investment in integrating and supporting family caregivers can potentially generate significant health care cost savings. There is little information however on the long-term impact on the caregiver and the potential savings that might be accrued by preventing adverse downstream effects.

Other studies that have evaluated the cost-effectiveness of individual-level interventions suggest that these interventions can be low cost and result in cost savings to the caregiver in terms of reductions in time spent in caregiving, a highly valuable resource for caregivers (Gitlin et al., 2010a; Jutkowitz et al., 2010; Nichols et al., 2008). However, overall few studies have examined the cost-effectiveness of an intervention.

ORGANIZATIONAL LEVEL

Interventions at the organizational level include those targeting caregivers of older adults but which are embedded in or delivered through a formal organizational structure such as the workplace, primary care or other health care delivery settings, and/or community agencies such as Area Agencies on Aging or adult day services. The implementation of a caregiver program in an organizational structure typically requires adjustments to a workflow of the setting and/or connecting various service delivery and/or community agencies in a coordinated fashion to address family caregiver needs. There is a growing body of research on interventions at this level, although typically programs are in a research or evaluation phase and have not been widely implemented and sustained in organizational settings. Summarized below are some of the most promising by the type of program they represent.

Care Coordination Programs

There is a growing body of research evaluating the effects of care coordination approaches. While care coordination is defined differently across studies/programs, it typically involves an assessment phase to identify unmet needs of family caregivers and then helping families connect to and use local resources and services. The programs are intended to help caregivers and care recipients address the challenges in accessing the range of services that care recipients need and to also help support the caregiver, ameliorate problems with service fragmentation, and enhance communication with care providers. An essential feature tends to be a team approach linking different resources and areas of expertise in a collaborative network to provide caregiver support. Additional elements may include disease education and the provision of coping or stress-reduction strategies. The role of the caregiver in these programs varies. Some programs, such as the Partners in Dementia Care (described below), actively involve the caregiver; in other programs their role is more limited/passive and care coordination primarily occurs through a nurse, case manager, or social worker (Bass et al., 2013). Programs typically last for 1 or more years, follow families over time, and seek to delay nursing home placement, reduce health care utilization, and enhance quality of life at home. However, studies are needed to establish that cost savings can be achieved for LTSS by helping the family caregiver connect to needed resources and services.

Most care coordination programs have been tested for families caring for individuals with dementia because of the lack of a systematic, coordinated care system for persons with dementia and their families and the documented high needs of this group (Black et al., 2013). For example, a survey of 307 caregivers found that only 32 percent of caregivers reported being confident in managing dementia-related problems, only 19 percent knew how to access community services to help provide care, and only 28 percent indicated that the individual's provider helped them work through dementia care problems (Jennings et al., 2015). In response, a wide range of care management programs have been developed and evaluated.

Systematic reviews and meta-analyses of these interventions reveal that the quality of the research is highly variable with only a few being well-controlled studies (Pimouguet et al., 2010; Somme et al., 2012; Tam-Tham et al., 2013). A few studies report positive impacts on institutional delay or admission rate (e.g., nursing home placement). However, there is inconsistent evidence with regard to cost savings in health care or reductions in hospitalization.

One of the earliest care management programs to be tested was the Medicare Alzheimer's Disease Demonstration Project, which was designed to decrease nursing home placement by improving caregiver outcomes through case management and subsidized community services. Unfortunately, although more than 5,300 dyads participated, there were no substantial benefits to families including reductions in caregiver burden and nursing home placement (Miller et al., 1999; Newcomer et al., 1999). While more recent efforts have demonstrated more positive results, the efficacy of these approaches remains inconclusive as it concerns their impact on caregiver well-being, care costs, and health care utilization.

Several more recent and well-designed trials are promising however. The Maximizing Independence at Home (MIND) study is an 18-month care coordination program that addresses dementia-related care needs for the person with dementia and his or her family caregivers through individualized care planning, referral and linkage to services, provision of dementia education and skill-building strategies, and care monitoring. Delivered by non-clinical community workers from participating social agencies trained and overseen by a team of geriatric psychiatrists, the MIND program resulted in a significant delay in time to all-cause transition from home to institutional settings compared to control participants. However, there was no significant group difference in the reduction of total percentage of unmet needs from baseline to 18 months, although families receiving the MIND program did have significant reductions in the proportion of unmet needs in safety and legal/advance care domains relative to controls. Intervention participants (older adults with dementia) had significant improvement in self-reported quality of life relative to control participants but this did not extend to their family caregivers (Samus et al., 2014). Initially tested in a randomized trial with 303 dyads, a variant of this intervention is currently being replicated in a large randomized trial (MIND Plus), which integrates other evidence-based care programs (such as COPE and TAP discussed earlier) and is being tested in a Center for Medicare & Medicaid Innovation grant.

The Partners in Dementia Care (PDC) is another effective care coordination program delivered via a partnership between the U.S. Department of Veterans Affairs (VA) Medical Centers (VAMCs) and Alzheimer's Association chapters. It targets caregivers of veterans with dementia living in the community and who are receiving primary care from the VA. In this approach, care coordinators from VAMCs and Alzheimer's Association chapters work as a team and share computerized records to assess, reassess, develop, and implement action plans and monitor the needs of veteran families via telephone and e-mail for 12 months. A randomized trial involving 486 caregivers demonstrated positive outcomes for caregivers at 6 months and more limited improvements at 12 months in the areas of unmet needs, caregiver strain, depression, and access to support resources (Bass et al., 2013). The care coordination approach also resulted in positive outcomes for the older adult veteran at 6 months that included reduced strain in relationships, depression, and unmet needs as well as less embarrassment about memory problems. At 12 months, more impaired veterans had further reductions in unmet need and embarrassment. The extent and type of improvement appeared to vary by levels of initial need and severity of impairments among veterans, suggesting that segments of the caregiver population need different levels and types of support.

Another care management program is the Alzheimer's and Dementia Care Program (ADC) developed by the University of California, Los Angeles and launched in 2012. The ADC involves a nurse practitioner dementia care manager who partners with primary care physicians and local community-based organizations to provide comprehensive, coordinated, and person-centered care for individuals with dementia and their families (Reuben et al., 2013).

Several care coordination models designed to link primary care to community-based programs are also promising. Using a cluster randomized trial involving 18 primary care clinics and 408 dyads (persons with dementia and their caregivers), Vickrey and colleagues (2006) showed that a 12-month care coordination model that linked families to needed community resources as well as to health care resulted in improved adherence to treatment guidelines, care recipient quality of life and caregiver social support, mastery of caregiving, and confidence. Similarly, Callahan and colleagues (2006) tested a collaborative care intervention led by a nurse practitioner who also used standard protocols, treatment guidelines, and nonpharmacologic management to improve recognition and treatment of Alzheimer's disease in primary care. In a controlled trial involving 153 dyads, the individuals with dementia and their caregivers receiving the collaborative care management approach were more likely to rate the care they received as good or excellent, caregivers reported less distress and depression, and individuals with dementia had significantly fewer behavioral symptoms at 12 months.

In summary, although the evidence is still inconsistent, recent tests of care coordination models targeting family caregivers demonstrate benefits for both persons with dementia and their caregivers. Most of these approaches involve an initial assessment of caregiver and older adult needs, followed by coordination and linkages to address needs. Of importance is that each program differs from the other with regard to assessment used, level of caregiver involvement, case manager level of expertise, outcome measures, and results.

Respite Programs

Respite programs occur in a wide range of settings (e.g., in home and community group settings), are provided by multiple and diverse providers, and are based on the principle that providing caregivers episodic relief from their ongoing care responsibilities benefits caregivers health and well-being and secondarily persons receiving care (Kirk and Kagan, 2015). Respite typically refers to services that provide caregivers some time away from caregiver responsibilities. There is a wide range of respite-type programs. Some provide daily medical and social services to older adults such as adult day services that in turn afford family caregivers opportunities for respite. Respite care services are available in some communities for a few hours, 1 day, or a weekend.

Although the need for respite for many high-intensity or strained caregivers of older adults is widely recognized, families are not always aware of the availability of these services, cannot or do not want to leave their family member, or do not have access to such services (IOM, 2012). Furthermore, it has been challenging to demonstrate that such programs are effective in achieving their goal of reducing the adverse effects of caregiving. This may be due in large part to methodological challenges and the lack of consensus in the design and implementation of these programs. Information is lacking regarding how best to provide respite to maximize its benefits to both caregivers and older adults (Kirk and Kagan, 2015). Initial studies of respite programs found inconclusive results (Reifler et al., 1992). However, a second generation of studies strongly suggests that respite helps to reduce caregiver distress (Zarit et al., 2014).

One especially promising venue for respite for caregivers is adult day services (ADS), which provide out-of-home, supervised, group services with the goals of improving mood, well-being, and quality of life of the caregiver and care recipient and enabling clients to remain at home for as long as possible. ADS also provide caregivers with respite from their day-to-day care responsibilities. Most ADS offer their services during "normal business hours," although some offer flexible hours to meet the needs of working caregivers. Although the number of ADS programs is increasing, not every community/state offers ADS thus limiting access to these programs for families.

A recent integrative review of 19 research studies suggests that ADS benefit both the older adult client and the family caregiver although outcomes depend on the range and quality of services provided. For caregivers the treatment of the person with dementia and the availability of caregiver support services and opportunities for training in dementia care were important indicators of quality and use of the ADS. Collectively, the findings show that caregivers report feeling supported, having improved competency in care provision, and reduced burden associated with care provision (Tretteteig et al., 2016). Another recent study involving 158 family caregivers who were using ADS, demonstrated that use of ADS improved regulation of the stress hormone cortisol. Caregivers' daytime cortisol responses on days they used ADS were compared to the days in which they did not. The study demonstrated that ADS use improved caregiver cortisol regulation, which in turn has potential to enhance long-term health outcomes (Klein et al., 2016). This important study is the first to link a social service program to biomarkers and to show physiological benefits for family caregivers.

Augmenting ADS with a systematic caregiver support program is also promising. The Adult Day Plus Program (ADS Plus) involves ADS staff who provide systematic care management, education, skills training, situational counseling, and ongoing support to family caregivers through face-to-face and telephone contact based on an initial needs assessment. The intervention is intensive over the first 3 months and then ongoing support is provided up to 12 months. Of 106 caregivers participating in a pilot trial that used a cluster RCT design (two sites assigned to an intervention and one to a control condition), at 3 months, caregivers receiving ADS Plus reported less depression, improved confidence managing behaviors, and enhanced well-being compared to caregivers using ADS only. Long-term effects (12 months) showed that compared to the ADS only users, ADS Plus caregivers continued to report less depression and more confidence, used ADS for more days, and had fewer nursing home placements (Gitlin et al., 2006).

Thus, the benefits of respite opportunities, particularly those offered through ADS that provide a safe and secure setting for older adults, appear to be amplified by providing systematic support and education in addition to the time for respite. Research is further needed to determine the added value of respite-type services to existing evidence-based programs for family caregivers. Perhaps a dyadic focus (e.g., services for the older adult coupled with caregiver respite and other forms of support) results in better outcomes for caregivers and older adult recipients of care. Also, the long-term benefits of respite care to caregivers have not yet been demonstrated (Kansagara et al., 2010).

SOCIETAL/POLICY LEVEL

Policies and programs delivered at the societal or policy level such as Medicare payment rules and Medicaid waiver programs can also be viewed as interventions. These are discussed in the previous chapters and include those listed below. The previous chapters describe federal programs that provide direct services to caregivers of older adults (see Chapter 1), state and federal policies regarding unpaid or paid leave for family caregivers (see Chapter 4), and health care and LTSS policies that affect caregivers (see Chapter 6). These policies include

- the NFCSP;
- the VA Caregiver Support Program;
- FMLA;
- state and local paid sick leave statutes;
- various provisions in the Patient Protection and Affordable Care Act related to caregivers' role as decision makers, caregiver assessment, quality metrics, and testing of new care models that promote person- and family-centered care;
- Medicaid's consumer-directed options for home- and community-based services (e.g., Cash and Counseling);
- state-funded caregiver support programs;

- the Caregiver Advise, Record, Enable (CARE) Act;
- the Lifespan Respite Act;
- Medicare hospice benefits that provide interventions for both the person and the family; and
- the National Alzheimer's Project Act (NAPA).

Medicaid policy concerning home- and community-based services for people with disabilities illustrates how state and federal policy can benefit family caregivers. Many state Medicaid programs offer consumer-directed options to Medicaid beneficiaries who are eligible for home- and community-based programs. Cash and Counseling, for example, was evaluated in the original demonstration program in three states (Arkansas, Florida, and New Jersey). While implementation varied in some ways, each demonstration provided consumers a monthly allowance to hire individuals (including family caregivers) or to help them purchase goods and services related to their care (e.g., counseling and related financial recordkeeping). In the demonstration, eligible Medicaid beneficiaries who volunteered to participate were randomly assigned to Cash and Counseling or usual Medicaid services (control group). Overall, the evaluation of the program found beneficial effects for both care recipients and their caregivers. The participants' primary family caregivers reported significantly less physical, emotional, and financial stress than the caregivers assigned to the control group and lower rates of adverse health effects from caregiving (Brown et al., 2007; Carlson et al., 2007). Fifteen states continue to operate Cash and Counseling program and many other states have implemented similar programs.

With respect to cost, although program spending may be higher for those in the Cash and Counseling demonstration group versus usual care (e.g., agency-directed care), a new study by Coe and colleagues (2016) suggests that the program saved costs and led to improved health outcomes for participants when family caregivers were provided pay for their assistance. As anticipated, the treatment group spent significantly more Medicaid dollars on counseling, had more family involvement, and received more paid hours of care and fewer unpaid hours of care compared to the control group. However, paid family care resulted in substantial decreases for inpatient expenditures (emergency room and inpatient use), suggesting that family involvement in home care may be a substitute for hospital care. Family involvement also significantly decreased Medicaid utilization and lowered the likelihood of infections (e.g., urinary tract infections, bedsores, respiratory infections) (Coe, 2016).

THE ROLE OF TECHNOLOGY IN CAREGIVER INTERVENTIONS

In a broad sense, technology refers to the tools, equipment, machines, technical processes, or methods that are used to accomplish a task or activity. Family caregivers interact with technology to access information and support (e.g., via Internet searches, patient portals, electronic medical records, and social media), as a means of accessing or participating in intervention programs (e.g., via videoconferencing, telephone) or to provide care to an older adult. Caregivers may also use technology to monitor the functional status of a care recipient and employ telemedicine technologies to communicate with providers who can monitor the care recipient and/or the caregiver.

The Internet, videophones, videoconferencing, and other communication technologies are increasingly used to support family caregivers. They have several potential advantages including reduced cost (e.g., less travel to providers' offices, fewer home visits by nurses); the ability to offer the intervention to greater numbers of individuals; enhanced flexibility with respect to tailoring and presentation of information; and convenience. Technology applications may be especially beneficial to long-distance caregivers in terms of enhancing access to the care recipient and other care providers. However, Internet-based technologies can also pose challenges to caregivers: not everyone has access; connectivity can be problematic; technology is constantly changing; and technology-based interventions may not be reimbursable. Nor can technology always substitute for face-to-face interactions between interventionist and caregiver (Berkowsky and Czaja, 2015; Czaja et al., 2012). Issues regarding cost and access are important areas for policy makers to consider when crafting state and federal regulations regarding payment for technology.

The range of technologies used for intervention delivery includes simple technology such as the telephone, screen-phones, videophones, touch-screen computers, videoconferencing, GPS systems, and the Internet (Web-based interventions). For example, a recent study used a videophone to deliver a modified version of the REACH II multicomponent intervention to minority family caregivers of individuals with dementia (Czaja et al., 2013). The intervention was compared to an information only/nutrition attention control group. The results indicated that it was feasible to use the videophone to deliver the intervention and that the videophone intervention was efficacious with respect to caregiver outcomes. Caregivers who received the intervention reported a decrease in burden and an increase in perceived social support and positive perceptions of the caregiving experience. Beauchamp and colleagues (2005) evaluated the efficacy of a multimedia caregiver support program delivered over the Internet as compared to a usual care wait list control. They found caregivers who received the intervention had improvements in stress, anxiety, depression, and self-efficacy.

In a systematic review of eight psychosocial interventions (i.e., couples-based cognitive behavior therapy (CBT) via video counseling, CD-based multimedia to enhance treatment decision making, Web-based CBT, Web-based for developing a shared care-plan for managing symptoms, multimedia caregiving training program, Internet combination of CBT and education, Web-based symptom management tool kit, and Web-based supportive education, marital therapy, dyadic coping skills training), Badr and colleagues (2015) found that information technology can be a useful tool for conveying health-related information and support to caregivers. The researchers also suggest that a major research gap is the lack of integration of Web 2.0 technologies such as social media in these intervention programs given that social support and communication serve as frequent targets of interventions for caregivers and individuals with cancer. They also suggest that the use of interactive health communication technologies (IHCT) in dyadic interventions in the cancer space is still in its infancy and that more research is needed to examine impact on outcomes for individuals with cancer and caregivers (e.g., impact on relationship, communication, burden, and distress).

Chodosh and colleagues (2015) compared two modes of delivery for a caregiver management program (ACCESS)—in-person visits plus telephone and mail or telephone and mail only and found that care quality improved substantially in both arms. To date, there are no reports of mobile applications (smartphones and tablet technologies); however, it is likely that these will emerge in the future given the recent focus on mobile health applications.

Caregiver intervention research has focused primarily on caregivers of older adults with ADRD, although a few studies have included caregivers of stroke survivors (Grant et al., 2002), individuals with spinal cord injuries (e.g., Elliot et al., 2008), frail older adults (e.g., Magnusson et al., 2005), persons in hospice (Mooney et al., 2014), individuals with heart failure (Piette et al., 2015), and individuals with depression (Aikens et al., 2015). The types of interventions delivered via technology are varied and include counseling, education, skill building, links to resources and services, support groups, chat rooms, and reminiscence cues. Outcomes are wide ranging and include caregiver knowledge, burden, self-efficacy, psychological morbidity (anxiety/depression), self-efficacy, skills, service utilization, and caregiver satisfaction with the technology. Although limited, these studies suggest that caregiver interventions can be delivered via technology and can improve caregiver outcomes.

Only a few studies have examined costs. Chodosh and colleagues (2015), as noted earlier, found that the telephone only plus mail arm was more cost-effective than the in-person plus mail and telephone arm with respect to costs associated with intervention delivery. This suggests that interventions delivered via telephone or mail may be more economical than in-person clinic-based or home-based visits by health personnel especially with recent developments in technology, which allow for video communication. However, this issue needs to be evaluated more systematically. Dang and colleagues (2008) used videophones to provide support, education, resource access, and enhanced communication to caregivers of veterans with dementia. They found that total facility utilization costs (hospitals and clinic visits) decreased for caregivers who received the intervention. However, there was no comparison group in this study—all caregivers received the intervention. In general, the findings from this study also indicate that technology-based interventions are well received by caregivers and that issues of usability are important as is caregiver training on use of the technology.

Caregivers are also increasingly going online in pursuit of information and support. A recent report by the Pew Research Center (Fox et al., 2013) indicates that 84 percent of caregivers with Internet access go online to access information about a particular treatment or disease, medications, or health insurance. A majority of those caregivers (59 percent) report that the Internet has been helpful to their ability to provide care and support to older adults with disability. There are numerous websites that offer information and support to caregivers such as the websites from the National Alliance for Caregiving, the Family Caregiver Alliance, and the Alzheimer's Association.[1] AARP also includes a section for caregivers on its website. The NIH seniorhealth.gov website provides information on resources for caregivers such as support groups and educational materials as well as tips and videos for Alzheimer's caregivers on topics such as managing medications, safety and driving, and legal issues.

Mobile health apps are also proliferating and can also provide caregivers with support and information. For example, the VA has developed a suite of mobile health apps to support family caregivers (Frisbee, 2014). These apps include the Care4Caregiver App that includes a self-assessment tool for tracking strain, tips for coping with stress, and connections to community resources; the Summary of Care App that allows veterans and their caregivers to receive and view VA medical information; and the Journal App, which is a personal health journal that allows veterans and

[1] See http://www.caregiving.org; https://www.caregiver.org; https://www.alz.org/care; http://www.aarp.org/home-family/caregiving/caregiving-tools; http://nihseniorhealth.gov/alzheimerscare/caregiversupport/01.html; and http://nihseniorhealth.gov/endoflife/supportforcaregivers/01.html (accessed August 23, 2016).

their caregivers to enter, view, and track vital signs and patient-generated data that could be shared with their VA care team as well as several others.

Emerging sensing and monitoring technologies may also prove to be beneficial to caregivers, especially those who work or live apart from their care recipient. These technologies can help caregivers track the health status and activities of the care recipient. Home monitoring systems and tracking systems are currently available and many more are emerging. There are also task management applications that can help with care coordination and medication management. However, to date these programs have not been systematically evaluated.

Very few studies involving the use of technology have examined issues of diversity in terms of differences among subgroups (e.g., race/ethnicity); however several have included diverse populations, primarily African Americans and Latinos (Chodosh et al., 2015; Czaja et al., 2013; Dang et al., 2008; Winter and Gitlin, 2006). Generally, the results of these studies suggest that using technology for intervention delivery is both feasible and acceptable (i.e., are well received by caregivers). It is important to note, however, that currently minorities generally tend to have less Internet access at home; thus, technology access may be an issue for some subgroups of caregivers. Clearly there is a need to include representatives from other ethnic/racial backgrounds, LGBT caregivers, and caregivers in rural locations in technology intervention studies. There is also a need to examine the use of technology to aid caregivers in work settings. For example, monitoring technologies might be useful to working caregivers.

The development, implementation, and evaluation of technology to support caregivers could be enhanced by innovative partnerships between researchers and the technology industry. An example is Oregon Health & Science University and Intel who are partnering in the development and testing of technology products and devices such as unobtrusive intelligent systems, which include unobtrusive sensing and monitoring systems and algorithms and assessment techniques for detecting motor and cognitive changes in older adults in these community settings (Wild et al., 2008). TigerPlace, an innovative independent living environment designed to support aging in place, is another example of an innovative partnership among the University of Missouri, the state of Missouri, and a home care agency (Fergenson, 2013; Rantz et al., 2008). Partnerships between researchers and industry can also support caregiver access to technology. For example, Cisco and AT&T provided support to the VideoCare project through the provision of equipment, technology support, and funding to help defray the Internet costs for the caregivers (Czaja et al., 2013).

THE PIPELINE FOR CAREGIVER INTERVENTIONS

Although a wide range of programs have been tested in randomized clinical trials and have demonstrated small to moderate treatment effects on important outcomes, few caregivers have access to these programs. Unlike the drug discovery pipeline, there is not a similar trajectory for developing, evaluating, and then implementing interventions for families (Gitlin and Czaja, 2016). As most interventions are tested external to service delivery settings and payment mechanisms and/or for specific populations, they need to undergo a translational phase in which the program is adapted, shortened, or modified in some way to fit within the daily routines of an agency or clinic, the current structure of a payment mechanism, and/or the unique situations of diverse caregivers. Interventions that require extensive training of interventionists for their delivery also face challenges of scalability and delivery to reach all family caregivers in need. To move proven interventions for delivery into different health and human service settings, several actions may be required.

First, most individually targeted caregiver interventions have been developed and evaluated in efficacy trials with community-based populations. With few exceptions such as the ADS Plus intervention that was tested for delivery within ADS (Gitlin et al., 2006), the collaborative care model tested for delivery in primary care (Callahan et al., 2006), and the Guided Care program (Wolff et al., 2010), interventions have not been evaluated within a particular delivery context. Thus, most interventions require what has been referred to as a translational phase in which manuals, procedures, and protocols are revised in order to better fit a particular health and human service setting (Burgio et al., 2009; Gitlin et al., 2015; Nichols et al., 2016).

Proven interventions may also need to be adapted to meet the needs of different targeted populations or cultural groups. Adaptations may include changing format, setting, language, and health literacy levels of materials as well as evaluating cultural appropriateness (Nápoles et al., 2010). Even for those interventions tested for efficacy within a delivery setting, pilot testing may be necessary to identify effective implementation processes and strategies (e.g., marketing and referral procedures, workflow, staff training) prior to widespread dissemination and implementation. No studies to date have evaluated the feasibility of sustaining interventions over time and the business plans and associated costs. Remarkably few studies have taken into account the involvement of multiple caregivers and how best to tailor existing interventions and assess outcomes for such circumstances.

More research is needed to understand the best strategies for widespread dissemination and implementation of proven programs. A primary barrier has been the lack of adequate funding for this effort. Notably, only two federal agencies have funded dissemination efforts. The Administration of Community Living (ACL) has funded dissemination efforts, but funding levels for ACL also remain low. The VA's Caregiver Support Program funds dissemination of the REACH individual intervention and telephone support groups through training of VA staff, in addition to funding the online Building Better Caregivers classes. As implementation science provides the theoretical foundation and the evidentiary base for the strategies most effective in moving proven interventions into care settings, there is an opportunity to more rapidly overcome the research-to-practice gap in this area.

Other methodological challenges relate to understanding how interventions that primarily target older adults, such as care coordination or supportive services, impact family caregivers. Such programs are typically developed using embedded designs in which delivery is integrated and examined within mainstream care delivery and often include older adults with variable underlying diseases or conditions. The design and evaluation of such interventions present unique challenges relating to determining eligibility criteria for family caregivers, determining adequate sample to observe desired effects, and outcomes of care in light of the widely varied needs and circumstances of older adults (Wolff et al., 2010; Zarit et al., 2016). For example, caregivers who are not experiencing caregiving-related negative emotions, strain, or stress may nevertheless benefit from education and skills to increase their knowledge, confidence, and skills to provide care, or additional services to better support the older adult they assist that reduce time spent caregiving and caregiver-related work productivity loss. For such caregivers, appropriate outcomes may relate to the ability to participate in valued activities, confidence for the caregiving role, or the perceived quality of care delivered to the person they assist. Few interventions of older adults have developed programs for family caregivers or examined outcomes for family caregivers.

In addition to more federal funding for these efforts, private–public partnerships could be considered to advance the implementation of proven interventions. Exploration of how such interventions may fit within existing and new funding streams, health care organizations such as Accountable Care Organizations, and/or existing programs, such as the NFCSP, would be important to pursue and should be a high priority for helping families and health and human service professionals gain access to evidence-based programs (Lynn and Montgomery, 2015).

CONCLUSIONS

The committee's key findings and conclusions are described in detail in Box 5-5. In summary, the committee concludes that there is a rich body of research assessing a wide range of caregiver interventions designed to help

BOX 5-5
Key Findings and Conclusions:
Programs and Supports for Family Caregivers of Older Adults

A variety of interventions improve caregiver outcomes, especially when provided in combination:

- Most effective interventions begin with an assessment of caregivers' risks, needs, and preferences.
- Education and skills training improve caregiver confidence and ability to manage daily care challenges.
- Counseling, self-care, relaxation training, and respite programs can improve both the caregiver's and care recipient's quality of life.
- Caregiver training strategies that involve the active participation of the caregiver are more effective than didactic approaches.

Randomized controlled trials have demonstrated that interventions that involve caregivers may delay institutionalization, reduce re-hospitalization, and lead to shorter hospital stays:

- Personal counseling and care management programs can delay nursing home admission for older adults with dementia when their family caregivers receive counseling.
- Integrating caregivers into the hospital discharge process can decrease re-hospitalizations and shorten lengths of stay.

Despite the demonstrated effectiveness of some caregiver services and supports, few of these interventions have moved from the research phase to everyday health and social service settings for a variety of reasons:

- The intervention is not reimbursable under Medicare or other coverage sources.
- Organizations do not have the resources to train staff to provide the intervention.
- The intervention is not feasible in rural and low-resource areas if it requires face-to-face sessions or multiple personnel.
- Information about the intervention has not been effectively communicated to relevant provider organizations.

A growing body of evidence indicates that technology can be effectively employed to help caregivers:

- Technology-based caregiver support, education, and skills training may offer effective alternatives for enhancing caregiver and older adult outcomes.
- Limited technology access is an issue for some subgroups, such as minority and rural caregivers.

alleviate the negative consequences of caregiving, especially for caregivers of older adults with dementia. Well-designed trials, conducted in a variety of settings, have demonstrated that caregiver education and skills training, environmental modifications of care recipients' homes, care coordination and management, counseling, self-care and relaxation training, respite programs, and other approaches can improve quality of life for both caregivers and care recipients, increase caregivers' abilities and confidence, and delay care recipients' institutionalization.

Trials have also demonstrated that interventions that involve caregivers may reduce the resource use of care recipients by delaying nursing home placement, reducing rehospitalizations, and shortening hospital stays.

Effective caregiver interventions tend to share several characteristics. They incorporate an assessment of caregivers' needs, tailor the intervention accordingly, and consider the caregivers' preferences. Training programs that actively involve caregivers in learning a particular skill result in better outcomes compared to didactic, prescriptive approaches such as handing out information sheets.

Yet, few of the nation's millions of family caregivers of older adults have access to evidence-based interventions. Numerous barriers have stymied translation of research successes into everyday settings. Many interventions have not been evaluated in or integrated into real-world settings where third-party reimbursement rules and financial and other organizational constraints prevail.

Wider dissemination of effective caregiver interventions will also require attention to the limitations of the available evidence. So far, trials have only rarely included sufficient numbers of diverse caregivers and care recipients to allow an assessment of their effectiveness for Hispanic, African American, and other ethnic and racial groups; long-distance caregivers; LGBT caregivers; and others. Future trials should assess whether existing models are effective across diverse populations to determine if further modifications or cultural adaptations are needed. Additional work is also needed to identify optimal strategies to disseminate and sustain effective models in diverse communities (Nápoles et al., 2013). Most caregiving research has focused primarily on improving outcomes for family caregivers of persons with Alzheimer's disease and often on a single caregiver rather than on situations where multiple family caregivers are involved. Although the lessons learned from these studies likely apply to a variety of caregiving contexts, additional research on caregivers of older adults with other impairments is needed.

REFERENCES

Aikens, J. E., R. Trivedi, A. Heapy, P. N. Pfeiffer, and J. D. Piette. 2015. Potential impact of incorporating a patient-selected support person into mHealth for depression. *Journal of General Internal Medicine* 30(6):797-803.

Alzheimer's Association. 2014. *2014 Alzheimer's disease fact and figures*. https://www.alz.org/downloads/facts_figures_2014.pdf (accessed December 14, 2015).

Appelbaum, A., and W. Breitbart. 2013. Care for the cancer caregiver: A systematic review. *Palliative and Supportive Care* 11(3):231-252.

Badr, H., C. L. Carmack, and M. A. Diefenbach. 2015. Psychosocial interventions for patients and caregivers in the age of new communication technologies: Opportunities and challenges in cancer care. *Journal of Health Communications* 20(3):328-342.

Bakas, T., P. C. Clark, M. Kelly-Hayes, R. B. King, B. J. Lutz, and E. L. Miller. 2014. Evidence for stroke family caregiver and dyad interventions: A statement for healthcare professionals from the American Heart Association and American Stroke Association. *Stroke* 45(9):2836-2852.

Bass, D. M., P. A. Clark, W. J. Looman, C. A. McCarthy, and S. Eckert. 2003. The Cleveland Alzheimer's managed care demonstration: Outcomes after 12 months of implementation. *The Gerontologist* 43(1):73-85.

Bass, D. M., K. S. Judge, A. Lynn Snow, N. L. Wilson, R. Morgan, W. J. Looman, C. A. McCarthy, K. Maslow, J. A. Moye, R. Randazzo, M. Garcia-Maldonado, R. Elbein, G. Odenheimer, and M. E. Kunik. 2013. Caregiver outcomes of Partners in Dementia Care: Effect of a care coordination program for veterans with dementia and their family members and friends. *Journal of the American Geriatrics Society* 61(8):1377-1386.

Beauchamp, N., A. B. Irvine, J. Seeley, and B. Johnson. 2005. Work-site-based Internet multimedia program for family caregivers of persons with dementia. *The Gerontologist* 45(6):793-801.

Belle, S., L. Burgio, R. Burns, D. Coon, S. Czaja, D. Gallagher-Thompson, L. Gitlin, J. Klinger, K. Koepke, C. Lee, J. Martindale-Adams, L. Nichols, R. Schulz, S. Stahl, A. Stevens, L. Winter, and S. Zhang. 2006. Enhancing the quality of life of dementia caregivers from different ethnic or racial groups: A randomized, controlled trial. *Annals of Internal Medicine* 145(10):727-738.

Berkowsky, R. W., and S. J. Czaja. 2015. The use of technology in behavioral intervention research: Advantages and challenges. In *Behavioral intervention research: Designing, evaluating, and implementing*, edited by L. Gitlin and S. J. Czaja. New York: Springer. Pp. 119-136.

Bertrand, R. M., L. Fredman, and J. Saczynski. 2006. Are all caregivers created equal? Stress in caregivers to adults with and without dementia. *Journal of Aging and Health* 18(4):534-551.

Biegel, D. E., and R. Schulz. 1999. Caregiving and caregiver interventions in aging and mental illness. *Family Relations* 48(4):345-354.

Black, B. S., D. Johnston, P. V. Rabins, A. Morrison, C. Lyketsos, and Q. M. Samus. 2013. Unmet needs of community-residing persons with dementia and their informal caregivers: Findings from the Maximizing Independence at Home Study. *Journal of the American Geriatrics Society* 61(12):2087-2095.

Brodaty, H., and C. Arasaratnam. 2012. Meta-analysis of nonpharmacological interventions for neuropsychiatric symptoms of dementia. *American Journal of Psychiatry* 169(9):946-953.

Brodaty, H., A. Green, and A. Koschera. 2003. Meta-analysis of psychosocial interventions for caregivers of people with dementia. *Journal of the American Geriatric Society* 51(5):657-664.

Brown, R., B. L. Carlson, S. Dale, L. Foster, B. Phillips, and J. Schore. 2007. *Cash and Counseling improving the lives of Medicaid beneficiaries who need personal care or home and community-based services.* Princeton, NJ: Mathematica Policy Research.

Burgio, L. D., I. B. Collins, B. Schmid, T. Wharton, D. McCallum, and J. DeCoster. 2009. Translating the REACH caregiver intervention for use by area agency on aging personnel: The REACH OUT program. *The Gerontologist* 49(1):103-116.

Caldwell, J. 2006. Consumer-directed supports: Economic, health, and social outcomes for families. *Mental Retardation* 44(6):405-417.

Callahan, C. M., M. A. Boustani, F. W. Unverzagt, M. G. Austrom, T. M. Damush, A. J. Perkins, B. A. Fultz, S. L. Hui, S. R. Counsell, and H. C. Hendrie. 2006. Effectiveness of collaborative care for older adults with Alzheimer disease in primary care: A randomized controlled trial. *Journal of the American Medical Association* 295(18):2148-2157.

Callahan, C. M., G. Arling, W. Tu, M. B. Rosenman, S. R. Counsell, T. E. Stump, and H. C. Hendrie. 2012. Transitions in care for older adults with and without dementia. *Journal of the American Geriatrics Society* 60(5):813-820.

Carlson, B. L., L. Foster, S. B. Dale, and R. Brown. 2007. Effects of Cash and Counseling on personal care and well-being. *Health Services Research* 42(1p2):467-487.

Chee, Y. K., L. N. Gitlin, M. P. Dennis, and W. W. Hauck. 2007. Predictors of adherence to a skill-building intervention in dementia caregivers. *Journal of Gerontology Medical Sciences* 62(6):673-678.

Cheung, K. S., B. H. Lau, P. W. Wong, A. Y. Leung, V. W. Lou, G. M. Chan, and R. Schulz. 2015. Multicomponent intervention on enhancing dementia caregiver well-being and reducing behavioral problems among Hong Kong Chinese: A translational study based on REACH II. *International Journal of Geriatric Psychiatry* 30(5):460-469.

Chodosh, J., B. A. Colaiaco, K. I. Connor, D. W. Cope, H. Liu, D. A. Ganz, M. J. Richman, D. L. Cherry, J. M. Blank, R. P. Carbone, S. M. Wolf, and B. G. Vickrey. 2015. Dementia care management in an underserved community: The comparative effectiveness of two different approaches. *Journal of Aging and Health* 27(5):864-893.

Clark, P. A., D. M. Bass, W. J. Looman, C. A. McCarthy, and S. Eckert. 2004. Outcomes for patients with dementia from the Cleveland Alzheimer's managed care demonstration. *Aging & Mental Health* 8(1):40-51.

Coe, N. B., J. Guo, R. T. Konetzka, and C. H. Van Houtven. 2016. *What is the marginal benefit of payment-induced family care? National Bureau of Economic Research Working Paper No. 22249.* http://www.nber.org/papers/w22249 (access June 27, 2016).

Czaja, S. J., L. N. Gitlin, R. Schulz, S. Zhang, L. D. Burgio, A. B. Stevens, N. O. Nichols, and D. Gallagher-Thompson. 2009. Development of the Risk Appraisal Measure: A brief screen to identify risk areas and guide interventions for dementia caregivers. *Journal of the American Geriatrics Society* 57(6):1064-1072.

Czaja, S. J., C. C. Lee, and R. Schulz. 2012. Quality of life technologies in supporting family caregivers. In *Quality of life technology handbook*, edited by R. Schulz. Boca Raton, FL: CRC Press. Pp. 245-262.

Czaja, S. J., D. Loewenstein, R. Schulz, S. N. Nair, and D. Perdomo. 2013. A videophone psychosocial intervention for dementia caregivers. *American Journal of Geriatric Psychiatry* 21(11):1071-1081.

Dang, S., N. Remons, J. Harris, J. Malphurs, L. Sandals, A. Lozada Cabrera, and N. Nedd. 2008. Care coordination assisted by technology for multiethnic caregivers of persons with dementia: A pilot clinical demonstration project on caregiver burden and depression. *Journal of Telemedicine and Telecare* 14(8):443-447.

Dassel, K. B., D. C. Carr, and P. Vitaliano. 2015. Does caring for a spouse with dementia accelerate cognitive decline? Findings from the Health and Retirement Study. *The Gerontologist*: Advance Access. http://gerontologist.oxfordjournals.org/content/early/2015/11/18/geront.gnv148.abstract (accessed April 6, 2015).

Dixon, L., C. Adams, and A. Lucksted. 2000. Update on family psychoeducation for schizophrenia. *Schizophrenia Bulletin* 26(1):5-20.

Eisdorfer, C., S. J. Czaja, D. Loewenstein, M. P. Rubert, S. Argüelles, V. B. Mitrani, and J. Szapocznik. 2003. The effect of a family therapy and technology-based intervention on caregiver depression. *The Gerontologist* 43(4):521-531.

Elliott, T. R., and J. W. Berry. 2009. Brief problem-solving training for family caregivers of persons with recent-onset spinal cord injuries: A randomized controlled trial. *Journal of Clinical Psychology* 65(4):406-422.

Elliott, T. R., D. Brossart, J. W. Berry, and P. R. Fine. 2008. Problem-solving training via videoconferencing for family caregivers of persons with spinal cord injuries: A randomized controlled trial. *Behaviour Research and Therapy* 46(11):1220-1229.

Family Caregiver Alliance. 2006. *Caregiver assessment: Principles, guidelines and strategies for change, Vol. I.* San Francisco, CA.

Family Caregiver Alliance. 2012. *Selected caregiver assessment measures: A resource inventory for practitioners, 2nd ed.* https://www.caregiver.org/sites/caregiver.org/files/pdfs/SelCGAssmtMeas_ResInv_FINAL_12.10.12.pdf (accessed April 6, 2016).

Feil, D. G., R. Lukman, B. Simon, A. Walston, and B. Vickrey. 2011. Impact of dementia on caring for patients' diabetes. *Aging & Mental Health* 15(7):894-903.

Feinberg, L. F., and C. Levine. 2015. Family caregiving: Looking to the future. *Generations* 39(4):11-20.

Fergenson, M., 2013. TigerPlace: An innovative "Aging in Place" community. *The American Journal of Nursing* 113(1):68-69.

Fortinsky, R. H., M. Kulldorff, A. Kleppinger, and L. Kenyon-Pesce. 2009. Dementia care consultation for family caregivers: Collaborative model linking an Alzheimer's Association chapter with primary care physicians. *Aging & Mental Health* 13(2):162-170.

Fox, S., M. Duggan, and K. Purcell. 2013. *Family caregivers are wired for health.* Washington, DC: Pew Research Center's Internet & American Life Project. http://www.pewinternet.org/2013/06/20/family-caregivers-are-wired-for-health (accessed March 23, 2016).

Friedman, E. M., R. A. Shih, K. M. Langa, and M. D. Hurd. 2015. U.S. prevalence and predictors of informal caregiving for dementia. *Health Affairs* 34(10):1637-1641.

Frisbee, K. 2014. Assessing the impact of mobile health apps on family caregiver burden levels and the factors predicting mobile health app use. *International Journal of Integrated Care* 14(8):e035.

Gallagher-Thompson, D., W. Haley, D. Guy, M. Rupert, T. Argüelles, L. M. Zeiss, C. Long, S. Tennstedt, and M. Ory. 2003. Tailoring psychological interventions for ethnically diverse dementia caregivers. *Clinical Psychology: Science and Practice* 10(4):423-438.

Gaugler, J. E., M. Reese, and M. S. Mittelman. 2013. Effects of the NYU Caregiver Intervention-Adult Child on residential care placement. *The Gerontologist* 53(6):985-997.

Gearing, R. E., N. El-Bassel, A. Ghesquiere, S. Baldwin, J. Gillies, and E. Ngeow. 2011. Major ingredients of fidelity: A review and scientific guide to improving quality of intervention research implementation. *Clinical Psychology Review* 31(1):79-88.

Gitlin, L. N., and Czaja, S. J. 2016. *Behavioral intervention research: Designing, evaluating and implementing.* New York: Springer.

Gitlin, L., and N. Hodgson. 2015. Caregivers as therapeutic agents in dementia care: The evidence-base for interventions supporting their role. In *Family caregiving in the new normal*, edited by J. E. Gaugler and R. L. Kane. London, UK: Academic Press. Pp. 305-353.

Gitlin, L. N., M. Corcoran, L. Winter, A. Boyce, and W. W. Hauck. 2001. A randomized, controlled trial of a home environmental intervention effect on efficacy and upset in caregivers and on daily function of persons with dementia. *The Gerontologist* 41(1):4-14.

Gitlin, L. N., L. Winter, M. Corcoran, M. P. Dennis, S. Schinfeld, and W. W. Hauck. 2003. Effects of the home environmental skill-building program on the caregiver-care recipient dyad: 6-month outcome from the Philadelphia REACH initiative. *The Gerontologist* 43(4):532-546.

Gitlin, L. N., K. Reever, M. P. Dennis, E. Mathieu, and W. W. Hauck. 2006. Enhancing quality of life of families who use adult day services: Short- and long-term effects of the Adult Day Services Plus program. *The Gerontologist* 46(5):630-639.

Gitlin, L. N., L. Winter, J. Burke, N. Chernett, M. P. Dennis, and W. W. Hauck. 2008. Tailored activities to manage neuropsychiatric behaviors in persons with dementia and reduce caregiver burden: A randomized pilot study. *The American Journal of Geriatric Psychiatry* 16(3):229-239.

Gitlin, L. N., N. Hodgson, E. Jutkowitz, and L. Pizzi. 2010a. The cost-effectiveness of a nonpharmacologic intervention for individuals with dementia and family caregivers: The Tailored Activity Program. *The American Journal of Geriatric Psychiatry* 18(6):510-519.

Gitlin, L. N., L. Winter, M. P. Dennis, N. Hodgson, and W. W. Hauck. 2010b. Targeting and managing behavioral symptoms in individuals with dementia: A randomized trial of a nonpharmacological intervention. *Journal of the American Geriatrics Society* 58(8):1465-1474.

Gitlin, L. N., L. Winter, M. P. Dennis, N. Hodgson, and W. W. Hauck. 2010c. A biobehavioral home-based intervention and the well-being of patients with dementia and their caregivers: The COPE randomized trial. *Journal of the American Medical Association* 304(9):983-991.

Gitlin, L. N., K. Marx, I. H. Stanley, and N. Hodgson. 2015. Translating evidence-based dementia caregiving interventions into practice: State-of-the-science and next steps. *The Gerontologist* 55(2):210-226.

Gitlin, L. N., N. A. Hodgson, and S. S. W. Choi. 2016. Home-based interventions targeting persons with dementia: What is the evidence and where do we go from here? In *Dementia care*, edited by M. Boltz and J. Galvin. New York: Springer. Pp. 167-188.

Grant, J. S., T. R. Elliott, M. Weaver, A. A. Bartolucci, and J. N. Giger. 2002. Telephone intervention with family caregivers of stroke survivors after rehabilitation. *Stroke* 33:2060-2065.

Greenfield, E. A., A. E. Scharlach, A. J. Lehning, J. K. Davitt, and C. L. Graham. 2013. A tale of two community initiatives for promoting aging in place: Similarities and differences in the national implementation of NORC programs and villages. *The Gerontologist* 53(6):928-938.

Heller, T., and J. Caldwell. 2006. Supporting aging caregivers and adults with developmental disabilities in future planning. *Mental Retardation* 44(3):189-202.

Heller, T., A. B. Miller, and K. Hsieh. 1999. Impact of a consumer-directed family support program on adults with developmental disabilities and their family caregivers. *Family Relations* 48(4):419-427.

Hepburn, K. W., J. Tornatore, B. Center, and S. W. Ostwald. 2001. Dementia family caregiver training: Affecting beliefs about caregiving and caregiver outcomes. *Journal of the American Geriatrics Society* 49(4):450-457.

Hepburn, K. W., M. Lewis, C. W. Sherman, and J. Tornatore. 2003. The Savvy Caregiver Program: Developing and testing a transportable dementia family caregiver training program. *The Gerontologist* 43(6):908-915.

Hepburn, K., M. Lewis, J. Tornatore, C. W. Sherman, and K. L. Bremer. 2007. The Savvy Caregiver Program: The demonstrated effectiveness of a transportable dementia caregiver psychoeducation program. *Journal of Gerontological Nursing* 33(3):30-36.

HHS (U.S. Department of Health and Human Services). 2014. *National plan to address Alzheimer's disease: 2014 update.* https://aspe.hhs.gov/national-plan-address-alzheimer%E2%80%99s-disease-2014-update (accessed February 12, 2016).

Hodgson, N., L. N. Gitlin, L. Winter, and W. W. Hauck. 2014. Caregiver's perceptions of the relationship of pain to behavioral and psychiatric symptoms in older community residing adults with dementia. *The Clinical Journal of Pain* 30(5):421-427.

Huang, T., and S. Liang. 2005. A randomized clinical trial of the effectiveness of a discharge planning intervention in hospitalized elders with hip fracture due to falling. *Journal of Clinical Nursing* 14(10):1193-1201.

IOM (Institute of Medicine). 2012. *Living well with chronic illness: A call for public health action.* Washington, DC: The National Academies Press.

Jennings, L. A., D. B. Reuben, L. C. Evertson, K. S. Serrano, L. Ercoli, J. Grill, J. Chodosh, Z. Tan, and N. S. Wenger. 2015. Unmet needs of caregivers of individuals referred to a dementia care program. *Journal of the American Geriatrics Society* 63(2):282-289.

Judge, K. S., D. M. Bass, A. L. Snow, N. L. Wilson, R. Morgan, W. J. Looman, C. McCarthy, and M. E. Kunik. 2011. Partners in dementia care: A care coordination intervention for individuals with dementia and their family caregivers. *The Gerontologist* 51(2):261-272.

Jutkowitz, E., L. N. Gitlin, and L. T. Pizzi. 2010. Evaluating willingness-to-pay thresholds for dementia caregiving interventions: Application to the Tailored Activity Program. *Value in Health* 13(6):720-725.

Kajiyama, B., L. W. Thompson, T. Eto-Iwase, M. Yamashita, J. Di Mario, Y. Marian Tzuang, and D. Gallagher-Thompson. 2013. Exploring the effectiveness of an Internet-based program for reducing caregiver distress using the iCare Stress Management e-Training Program. *Aging & Mental Health* 17(5):544-554.

Kalra, L., A. Evans, I. Perez, A. Melbourn, A. Patel, M. Knapp, and N. Donaldson. 2004. Training carers of stroke patients: Randomised controlled trial. *BMJ* 328(7448):1099-1104.

Kansagara, D., E. Goy, and M. Freeman. 2010. *A systematic evidence review of interventions for non-professional caregivers of individuals with dementia.* Washington, DC: U.S. Department of Veterans Affairs.

Kasper, J. D., V. A. Freedman, B. C. Spillman, and J. L. Wolff. 2015. The disproportionate impact of dementia on family and unpaid caregiving to older adults. *Health Affairs* 34(10):1642-1649.

Kelly, K., N. Wolfe, M. Gibson, and L. F. Feinberg. 2013. *Listening to family caregivers: The need to include caregiver assessment in Medicaid home and community-based service waiver programs.* Washington, DC: AARP Public Policy Institute.

Kirk, R. S., and J. Kagan. 2015. *A research agenda for respite care: Deliberations of an expert panel of researchers, advocates and funders.* http://archrespite.org/images/docs/2015_Reports/ARCH_Respite_Research_Report_web.pdf (accessed March 22, 2016).

Klein, L. C., K. Kim, D. M. Almeida, E. E. Femia, M. J. Rovine, and S. H. Zarit. 2016. Anticipating an easier day: Effects of adult day services on daily cortisol and stress. *The Gerontologist* 56(2):303-312.

Knowles, J. 2006. Donepezil in Alzheimer's disease: An evidence-based review of its impact on clinical and economic outcomes. *Core Evidence* 1(3):195-219.

Kwok, T., I. I. Bel Wong, K. Chui, D. Young, and F. Ho. 2013. Telephone-delivered psychoeducational intervention for Hong Kong Chinese dementia caregivers: A single-blinded randomized controlled trial. *Clinical Interventions in Aging* 8:1191-1197.

Legrain, S., F. Tubach, D. Bonnet-Zamponi, A. Lemaire, J. P. Aquino, E. Paillaud, E. Taillandier-Heriche, C. Thomas, M. Verny, B. Pasquet, A. L. Moutet, D. Lieberherr, and S. Lacaille. 2011. A new multimodal geriatric discharge-planning intervention to prevent emergency visits and rehospitalizations of older adults: The optimization of medication in AGEd multicenter randomized controlled trial. *Journal of the American Geriatrics Society* 59(11):2017-2028.

Levine, C., D. E. Halper, J. L. Rutberg, and D. A. Gould. 2013. *Engaging family caregivers as partners in transitions: TC-QuIC: A quality improvement collaborative.* New York: United Hospital Fund.

Lingler, J. H., L. M. Martire, and R. Schulz. 2005. Caregiver-specific outcomes in antidementia clinical drug trials: A systematic review and meta-analysis. *Journal of the American Geriatrics Society* 53(6):983-990.

Long, K. H., J. P. Moriarty, M.S. Mittelman, and S. S. Foldes. 2013. Estimating the potential cost savings from The New York University Caregiver Intervention in Minnesota. *Health Affairs* 33(4):596-604.

Lynn, J., and A. Montgomery. 2015. Creating a comprehensive care system for frail elders in "age boom" America. *The Gerontologist* 55(2):278-285.

Magnusson, L., E. Hanson, and M. Nolan. 2005. The impact of information and communication technology on family carers of older people and professionals in Sweden. *Ageing and Society* 25(5):693-713.

Martindale-Adams, J., L. O. Nichols, R. Burns, M. J. Graney, and J. Zuber. 2013. A trial of dementia caregiver telephone support. *Canadian Journal of Nursing Research* 45(4):30-48.

Maslow, K. 2011. Dementia, diabetes and family caregiving. *Aging & Mental Health* 15(8): 933-935.

Maslow, K. 2012. *Translating innovation to impact: Evidence-based interventions to support people with Alzheimer's disease and their caregivers at home and in the community.* Washington, DC: Alliance for Aging Research, Administration on Aging, and MetLife Foundation.

Miller, R., R. Newcomer., and P. Fox. 1999. Effects of the Medicare Alzheimer's Disease Demonstration on nursing home entry. *Health Services Research* 34(3):691-714.

Mittelman, M. S. 2008. Psychosocial intervention research: Challenges, strategies and measurement issues. *Aging & Mental Health* 12(1):1-4.

Mittelman, M. S., S. H. Ferris, G. Steinberg, E. Shulman, J. A. Mackell, A. Ambinder, and J. Cohen. 1993. An intervention that delays institutionalization of Alzheimer's disease patients: Treatment of spouse-caregivers. *The Gerontologist* 33(6):730-740.

Mittelman, M. S., S. H. Ferris, E. Shulman, G. Steinberg, A. Ambinder, J. A. Mackell, and J. Cohen. 1995. A comprehensive support program: Effect on depression in spouse-caregivers of AD patients. *The Gerontologist* 35(6):792-802.

Mittelman, M. S., S. H. Ferris, E. Shulman, G. Steinberg, and B. Levin. 1996. A family intervention to delay nursing home placement of patients with Alzheimer disease: A randomized controlled trial. *Journal of the American Medical Association* 276(21):1725-1731.

Mittelman, M. S., W. E. Haley, O. J. Clay, and D. L. Roth. 2006. Improving caregiver well-being delays nursing home placement of patients with Alzheimer disease. *Neurology* 67(9):1592-1599.

Molazem, Z., T. Falahati, I. Jahanbin, P. Jafari, and S. Ghadakpour. 2014. The effect of psycho-educational interventions on the quality of life of the family caregivers of the patients with spinal cord injury: A randomized controlled trial. *International Journal of Community Based Nursing and Midwifery* 2(1):31-39.

Moon, H., C. J. Whitlatch, M. H. Kim, and P. Dilworth-Anderson. 2014. *Predictors of discrepancy between care recipients with early-stage dementia and their caregivers on perceptions of the care recipients' quality of life.* Paper presented at Society for Social Work and Research 18th Annual Conference: Research for Social Change: Addressing Local and Global Challenges, January 17. San Antonio, TX.

Mooney, K., P. Berry, B. Wong, and G. Donaldson. 2014. *Helping cancer-family caregivers with end-of-life home symptom management: Initial evaluation of an automated symptom monitoring and coaching system.* Paper presented at ASCO Annual Meeting, October 24. Chicago, IL.

Nápoles, A. M., L. Chadia, R. Eveersley, and G. Moreno-John. 2010. Developing culturally sensitive caregiver interventions: Are we there yet? *American Journal of Alzheimer's Disorders and Other Dementias* 25(5):389-406.

Nápoles, A. M., J. Santoyo-Olsson, and A. L. Stewart. 2013. Methods for translating evidence-based behavioral interventions for health-disparity communities. *Preventing Chronic Disease* 10:E193.

Navaie, M. 2011. Accessibility of caregiver education and support programs: Reaching hard-to-reach caregivers. *Education and Support Programs for Caregivers: Research, Practice, Policy* 13-28.

Naylor, M. D., D. Brooten, R. Campbell, B. S. Jacobsen, M. D. Mezey, M. V. Pauly, and J. S. Schwartz. 1999. Comprehensive discharge planning and home follow-up of hospitalized elders—A randomized clinical trial. *JAMA* 281(7):613-620.

Newcomer, R., C. Yordi, R. DuNah, P. Fox, and A. Wilkinson. 1999. Effects of the Medicare Alzheimer's Disease Demonstration on caregiver burden and depression. *Health Services Research* 34(3):669-689.

Nichols, L. O., C. Chang, A. Lummus, R. Burns, J. Martindale-Adams, M. J. Graney, D. W. Coon, and S. Czaja. 2008. The cost-effectiveness of a behavior intervention with caregivers of patients with Alzheimer's disease. *Journal of the American Geriatrics Society* 56(3):413-420.

Nichols, L. O., J. Martindale-Adams, R. Burns, M. J. Graney, and J. Zuber. 2011. Translation of a dementia caregiver support program in a health care system—REACH VA. *Archives of Internal Medicine* 171(4):353-359.

Nichols, L. O., J. Martindale-Adams, R. Burns, J. Zuber, and M. J. Graney. 2016. REACH VA: Moving from translation to system implementation. *The Gerontologist* 56(1):135-144.

Northouse, L. L., M. Katapodi, L. Song, L. Zhang, and D. W. Mood. 2010. Interventions with family caregivers of cancer patients: Meta-analysis of randomized trials. *CA: A Cancer Journal for Clinicians* 60(5):317-339.

Ory, M. G., R. R. Hoffman, J. L. Yee, S. Tennstedt, and R. Schulz. 1999. Prevalence and impact of caregiving: A detailed comparison between dementia and nondementia caregivers. *The Gerontologist* 39(2):177-185.

Ostwald, S. K., K. W. Hepburn, W. Caron, T. Burns, and R. Mantell. 1999. Reducing caregiver burden: A randomized psychoeducational intervention for caregivers of persons with dementia. *The Gerontologist* 39(3):299-309.

Piette, J. D., D. Striplin, N. Marinec, J. Chen, and J. E. Aikens. 2015. A randomized trial of mobile health support for heart failure patients and their informal caregivers: Impacts on caregiver-reported outcomes. *Medical Care* 53(8):692-699.

Pimouguet, C., T. Lavaud, J. Dartigues, and C. Helmer. 2010. Dementia case management effectiveness on health care costs and resource utilization: A systematic review of randomized controlled trials. *The Journal of Nutrition, Health and Aging* 14(8):669-676.

Rantz, M., M. Aud, G. L. Alexander, D. P. Oliver, D. Minner, M. Skubic, J. M. Keller, Z. He, M. Popescu, G. Demiris and S. J. Miller. 2008. TigerPlace: An innovative educational and research environment. In *AAAI Fall Symposium: AI in eldercare: New solutions to old problems* Pp. 84-91.

Redfoot, D., L. Feinberg, and A. Houser. 2013. *The aging of the baby boom and the growing care gap: A look at future declines in the availability of family caregivers.* Washington, DC: AARP Public Policy Institute.

Reifler, B. V., R. S. Henry, K. A. Sherrill, and C. H. Asbury. 1992. A national demonstration program on dementia day centers and respite services: An interim report. *Behavior, Health, & Aging* 2(3):199-206.

Reinhard, S. C., R. Montgomery, and M. J. Gibson. 2008. *Informal caregivers: Sustaining the core of long-term services and supports.* Paper presented at Building Bridges: Making a Difference in Long-Term Care Fifth Annual Long-Term Care Colloquium, Washington, DC.

Reuben, D. B., L. C. Evertson, N. S. Wenger, K. Serrano, J. Chodosh, L. Ercoli, and Z. S. Tan. 2013. The University of California at Los Angeles Alzheimer's and Dementia Care program for comprehensive, coordinated, patient-centered care: Preliminary data. *Journal of American Geriatrics Society* 61(12):2214-2218.

Richards, K. C., C. A. Enderlin, C. Beck, J. C. McSweeney, T. C. Jones, and P. K. Roberson. 2007. Tailored biobehavioral interventions: A literature review and synthesis. *Research and Theory for Nursing Practice* 21(4):271-285.

Rosalynn Carter Institute. 2012. *REACH II intervention* (Schulz and colleagues). http://www.rosalynncarter.org/caregiver_intervention_database/dimentia/reach_ii_intervention (accessed February 17, 2016).

Roth, D. L., M. S. Mittelman, O. J. Clay, A. Madan, and W. E. Haley. 2005. Changes in social support as mediators of the impact of a psychosocial intervention for spouse caregivers of persons with Alzheimer's disease. *Psychology and Aging* 20(4):634-644.

Samus, Q. M., D. Johnston, B. S. Black, E. Hess, C. Lyman, A. Vavilikolanu, J. Pollutra, J. M. Leoutsakos, L. N. Gitlin, P. V. Rabins, and C. G. Lyketsos. 2014. A multidimensional home-based care coordination intervention for elders with memory disorders: The Maximizing Independence at Home (MIND) pilot randomized trial. *American Journal of Geriatric Psychiatry* 22(4):398-414.

Schulz, R., S. J. Czaja, A. Lustig, B. Zdaniuk, L. M. Martire, and D. Perdomo. 2009. Improving the quality of life of caregivers of persons with spinal cord injury: A randomized controlled trial. *Rehabilitation Psychology* 54(1):1-15.

Somme, D., H. Trouve, M. Dramé, D. Gagnon, Y. Couturier, and O. Saint-Jean. 2012. Analysis of case management programs for patients with dementia: A systematic review. *Alzheimer's & Dementia* 8(5):426-436.

Stanley, M. A., J. Calleo, A. L. Bush, N. Wilson, A. L. Snow, C. Kraus-Schuman, A. L. Paukert, N. J. Petersen, G. A. Brenes, and P. E. Schulz. 2013. The Peaceful Mind program: A pilot test of a cognitive–behavioral therapy–based intervention for anxious patients with dementia. *The American Journal of Geriatric Psychiatry* 21(7):696-708.

Stevens, A. B., E. R. Smith, L. R. Trickett, and R. McGhee. 2012. Implementing an evidence-based caregiver intervention within an integrated healthcare system. *Translational Behavioral Medicine* 2(2):218-227.

Stevens, A., J. Cho, J. L. Thorud, and M. Ory. 2016 (unpublished). *Live well our health initiative year 6 6 month report.* Fort Worth, TX: United Way of Tarrant County, Scott & White Healthcare, and Texas A&M Health Science Center.

Tam-Tham, H., M. Cepoiu-Martin, P. E. Ronksley, C. J. Maxwell, and B. R. Hemmelgarn. 2013. Dementia case management and risk of long-term care placement: A systematic review and meta-analysis. *International Journal of Geriatric Psychiatry* 28(9):889-902.

Tappen, R. M., and D. Hain. 2014. The effect of in-home cognitive training on functional performance of individuals with mild cognitive impairment and early-stage Alzheimer's disease. *Research in Gerontological Nursing* 7(1):14-24.

Tremont, G., J. D. Davis, G. D. Papandonatos, B. R. Ott, R. H. Fortinsky, P. Gozalo, M. S. Yue, K. Bryant, C. Grover, and D. S. Bishop. 2015. Psychosocial telephone intervention for dementia caregivers: A randomized, controlled trial. *Alzheimer's & Dementia* 11(5):541-548.

Tretteteig, S., S. Vatne, and A. M. M. Rokstad. 2016. The influence of day care centres for people with dementia on family caregivers: An integrative review of the literature. *Aging & Mental Health* 20(5):450-462.

Vickrey, B. G., B. S. Mittman, K. I. Connor, M. L. Pearson, R. D. Della Penna, T. G. Ganiats, J. R. W. DeMonte, J. Chodosh, X. Cui, S. Vassar, N. Duan, and M. Lee. 2006. The effect of a disease management intervention on quality and outcomes of dementia care: A randomized, controlled trial. *Annals of Internal Medicine* 145(10):713-726.

Whitlatch, C. J., K. Judge, S. H. Zarit, and E. Femia. 2006. Dyadic intervention for family caregivers and care receivers in early-stage dementia. *The Gerontologist* 46(5):688-694.

Wild, K., L. Boise, J. Lundell, and A. Foucek. 2008. Unobtrusive in-home monitoring of cognitive and physical health: Reactions and perceptions of older adults. *Journal of Applied Gerontology* 27(2):181-200.

Winter, L., and L. N. Gitlin. 2006. Evaluation of a telephone-based support group intervention for female caregivers of community-dwelling individuals with dementia. *American Journal of Alzheimer's Disease and Other Dementias* 21(6):391-397.

Wolff, J. L., E. R. Giovannetti, C. M. Boyd, L. Reider, S. Palmer, D. Scharfstein, J. Marsteller, S. T. Wegener, K. Frey, B. Leff, K. D. Frick, and C. Boult. 2010. Effects of guided care on family caregivers. *The Gerontologist* 50(4):459-470.

Zarit, S., and E. Femia. 2008. Behavioral and psychosocial interventions for family caregivers. *American Journal of Nursing* 108(9 Suppl):47-53.

Zarit, S. H., K. Kim, E. E. Femia, D. M. Almeida, and L. C. Klein. 2014. The effects of adult day services on family caregivers' daily stress, affect, and health: Outcomes from the Daily Stress and Health (DaSH) study. *The Gerontologist* 54(4):570-579.

Zarit, S. H., L. R. Bangerter, Y. Liu, and M. J. Rovine. 2016. Exploring the benefits of respite services to family caregivers: Mmethodological issues and current findings. *Aging & Mental Health* (E-publication ahead of print). http://www.tandfonline.com/doi/abs/10.1080/13607863.2015.1128881 (accessed April 8, 2016).

6

Family Caregivers' Interactions with Health Care and Long-Term Services and Supports

ABSTRACT: Building on the findings of the previous chapters' descriptions of family caregivers' roles and responsibilities, this chapter examines caregivers' experiences in health care and long-term services and supports as they try to fulfill these roles. The committee concludes that despite their critical role, family caregivers of older adults are often marginalized or ignored by providers and systems of care. Yet, providers assume that caregivers are not only available but also skilled and knowledgeable enough to provide the tasks prescribed in older adults' care plans. Numerous barriers impede systematic recognition and partnership with family caregivers, including payment rules that discourage providers from spending time to communicate with caregivers, misinterpretations of privacy regulations, and a health insurance model oriented to individual coverage. The chapter describes the opportunities for advancing high-quality care, focusing in four priority areas: (1) identification, assessment, and support of family caregivers in the delivery of care; (2) inclusion of family caregiver experiences in quality measurement; (3) supporting family caregivers through health information technology; and (4) preparing care professionals to provide person- and family-centered care.

Although not formally recognized as such, family caregivers[1] of older adults are often key players in health care settings and long-term services and supports (LTSS)—along with physicians, nurses, nurse practitioners, physician assistants, social workers, psychologists, pharmacists, home care aides and other direct care workers, hospice workers, physical and occupational therapists, and others. Chapter 3 described the varied roles that caregivers play in coordinating, managing, and indeed providing older adults' health care and LTSS. Chapter 5 described the types of caregiver services and supports that have been tested and shown to be effective at improving caregiver outcomes. The focus in this chapter is on caregivers' experiences as they try to fulfill their roles in today's health care and social services settings. The objective is twofold: first, to describe how the "current paradigm" for providing health care and LTSS serves more as a barrier than facilitator for effective caregiver involvement in older adults' care and, second, to review ways to move to a "new paradigm" of person- and family-centered care and services with the potential to optimize caregivers' support of older adults. The latter includes four priority areas: systematic identification, assessment, and support of family caregivers; including both family and caregiver experiences in quality measurement; supporting family caregivers through health information technology; and preparing the health care and social services workforce to provide person- and family-centered care.

THE CURRENT PARADIGM AND ITS CONSEQUENCES

It is well established that health care in the United States is often of low value, poor quality, or results in harm (IOM, 2000, 2001, 2012b). The experiences of caregivers in advocating for older adults mirror the difficulties that many Americans face in obtaining high-quality, high-value health care services. Care delivery is fragmented; there is little, if any coordination between the health care and LTSS sectors; provider reimbursement policies discourage providers from taking the time to speak with individuals about their preferences, needs, and values; services are costly; and individual's access to understandable and timely health information is often elusive.

In some ways, the challenges that individuals encounter in navigating the health care system are amplified for caregivers who are acting on behalf of an older adult. Under the status quo, care delivery simultaneously ignores and relies heavily on family caregivers to provide ongoing support to older adults with cognitive and/or physical impairments. There is a lack of shared understanding and expectations among older adults, family care-

[1] This report uses the terms "family caregiver" and "caregiver" interchangeably to refer specifically to family caregivers of older adults. See Chapter 1 for a definition of these terms.

givers, and providers regarding the roles and responsibilities of family caregivers. The current paradigm has significant negative consequences for all stakeholders—older adults, families, providers, and systems of care—and presents critical ethical challenges for providers (Barnard and Yaffe, 2014; Hinton et al., 2007; Mitnick et al., 2010). These consequences include impeding information sharing between family caregivers and providers of care (Crotty et al., 2015; Petronio et al., 2004), tense and adversarial health system interactions, and expensive and unwanted care that is inconsistent with older adults' preferences (Abadir et al., 2011; Levine and Zuckerman, 1999; Srivastava, 2010). One national survey found that only one in three family caregivers (32 percent) reported that a doctor, nurse, or social worker had ever asked them about what was needed to care for their relative. Only half as many (16 percent) said a health provider had asked them what they needed to care for themselves (NAC and AARP Public Policy Institute, 2015a). Taken together these factors contribute to the emotional, physical, and financial distress of caregivers described in in the previous chapters (Adelman et al., 2014; Wolff et al., 2016b).

Family Caregivers and Systems of Care

In order to fulfill the numerous roles that they play (as Chapter 3 describes), family caregivers must interact with a wide range of providers and navigate within a variety of systems. For example, family caregivers often attend older adults' medical visits with physicians (Wolff and Roter, 2008, 2011; Wolff and Spillman, 2014), facilitate the hospital discharge process (Almborg et al., 2009; Hickey, 1990; Levine et al., 2013), interact with home health care agency professionals and paraprofessionals after hospital discharge (Levine et al., 2006), and coordinate and deliver LTSS (Kaye et al., 2010; Newcomer et al., 2012). Although many older adults seek help from their family in making health care decisions (Price et al., 2012; Wolff and Boyd, 2015), there are few evidence-based strategies for effectively involving families in health care encounters.

Although some clinicians have attributed strained, concerned, or overprotective family caregivers as contributing to older adults' risk for potentially preventable hospitalization (Davies et al., 2011; Freund et al., 2013), evidence to substantiate this relationship does not exist. In fact, the impact of specific caregiver characteristics on older adults' health outcomes is limited and not well understood. As a result, little is known about what might be achieved by better integration and support of family caregivers.

The Impact of Family Caregivers on Older Adults' Care

Table 6-1 provides examples of optimal family caregiver involvement in older adults' care as well as barriers to their optimal involvement. For example, physicians, nurses, social workers, therapists, and other providers routinely initiate an encounter with a new patient by asking about their health history, the medications they are on, past diagnoses, previous treatments and surgeries, adverse reactions to any drugs, and so on. When family caregivers accompany an older adult, as they often do, they help provide or supplement this information particularly if the patient is forgetful or has dementia (Bookman and Harrington, 2007). The family caregiver may encourage the older person to ask questions and actively engage the provider, thus increasing his or her involvement in his or her own health

TABLE 6-1 Barriers to Optimal Caregiver Involvement in Older Adults' Care

Aspect of Care	Optimal Caregiver Involvement	Barriers to Optimal Caregiver Involvement
Shared decision making	When caregivers (CGs) prompt older adults to ask questions and tell a physician, nurse, social worker, or other provider their concerns, the provider may take more time to help resolve any confusion and, thus, foster decisions that best reflect the care recipient's values and priorities.	CGs can undermine older adults' decision making if the CG inappropriately speaks for, interrupts, or criticizes the older adult during health care or social service encounters. Providers can likewise undermine decision making if they inappropriately direct their advice to the CG instead of the older adult—or when providers exclude CGs whose involvement is desired by the older adult.
Appropriate use of medications	CGs can inform providers' therapeutic advice if they help fill in missing details from older adults' health history (e.g., current and past medications, allergies, past treatments). If providers ensure that CGs understand the appropriate use and potential side effects of medications, CGs can facilitate appropriate use and recognize adverse effects if they occur.	CGs may not be able to access timely and accurate information about older adults' prescribed medications—or may not receive adequate training to manage or administer them. As a result, they may unintentionally make medication mistakes, or they may not be able to detect medication errors or side effects.

TABLE 6-1 Continued

Aspect of Care	Optimal Caregiver Involvement	Barriers to Optimal Caregiver Involvement
Coordinated care	CGs often play an integral role in arranging medical visits, coordinating home- and community-based services, facilitating older adults' transitions between settings of care, and transmitting critical health and other information across settings of care.	When CGs do not have access to up-to-date, understandable, and comprehensive information about care recipients' health and treatments, they cannot coordinate older adults' care and services effectively.
Assuring adequate personal care and safety	CGs are the main providers of older adults' personal care services and may also supervise LTSS provided by others. As such, they are critical to older adults' safety and receipt of appropriate services.	When CGs lack necessary skills, resources, or knowledge of care recipients' treatments, they may unintentionally place older adults at heightened risk of adverse health events such as medication mistakes or failure to report emerging side effects.
Transitional care	CGs can help ensure that critical information is transmitted correctly to new providers and care settings during transitions, monitor the appropriate delivery of services in the new care setting, and inform providers of symptoms or problems that arise.	When CGs do not have access to up-to-date, understandable, and comprehensive information from providers, they cannot help ensure older adults' safety and well-being during critical care transitions.
Emergency care	CGs can help older adults avoid unnecessary emergency room visits—or help obtain emergency care when needed.	Without adequate preparation, CGs may fail to recognize or act in emergency situations or overuse emergent care services when they are anxious.
Home safety	CGs often arrange for modifications to older adults' homes (e.g., ramps, grab bars) that prevent accidents and injury.	When CGs are overwhelmed or lack resources, they may be unable to ensure that older adults are living in a safe environment.

NOTE: Shared decision making refers to older adults' understanding of their choices and ability to make decisions with their care team to the extent that they want or are able.
SOURCES: Clayman et al., 2005; Greene et al., 1994; IOM and NRC, 2014; Ishikawa et al., 2005, 2006; Laidsaar-Powell et al., 2013; Silver et al., 2004; Thorpe et al., 2006; Wolff and Roter, 2011, 2012; Wolff et al., 2015, 2016a; Zulman et al., 2011.

care decisions (Clayman et al., 2005; Wolff et al., 2015). However, the caregiver may help or hinder the quality of communication with providers (Laidsaar-Powell et al., 2013; Wolff and Roter, 2011, 2012). For example, family caregivers who bring their own agenda to the visit, criticize the older adult, or dominate the conversation with the provider may diminish an individual's participation in his or her own care (Clayman et al., 2005; Greene et al., 1994; Ishikawa et al., 2005, 2006; Wolff et al., 2015).

Reducing Health Care Utilization

The availability of a family caregiver is associated with fewer and shorter hospital stays for older adults (McClaran et al., 1996; Picone et al., 2003). The converse is true as well—complex family dynamics, providers' unfounded assumptions regarding families' ability to provide assistance, and caregiver burden and depression are also associated with delayed or otherwise problematic hospital discharges (Procter et al., 2001; Shugarman et al., 2002; vom Eigen et al., 1999; Wolff and Kasper, 2004), readmissions (Lotus Shyu et al., 2004; Schwarz and Elman, 2003), and more hospitalization (Dong and Simon, 2013).

Longitudinal descriptive studies have found that the availability of caregivers reduces home health care use and delays nursing home entry (Van Houtven and Norton, 2004). Using data from a nationally representative sample of older adults, Charles and Sevak (2005) also found that receiving a family caregiver's help substantially reduces the risk of nursing home entry. These effects are strongest for adult children providing care to a single older adult (Van Houtven and Norton, 2008).

Moreover, as noted in Chapter 5, several randomized controlled trials have demonstrated that when older adults' caregivers receive a standard assessment, training, respite, and other supports, caregiver outcomes improve. In addition, older adults' nursing home placement is delayed, they have fewer hospital readmissions, decreased expenditures for emergency room visits, and decreased Medicaid utilization (Gaugler et al., 2013; Lavelle et al., 2014; Long et al., 2013; Mittleman et al., 2006). More recent findings from the Washington State Family Caregiver Support Program further suggest that providing screening and support for caregivers lowers overall use of Medicaid long-term care services (Lavelle et al., 2014; Miller, 2012). Additional research is needed to determine the associated cost savings (Gaugler et al., 2005; Lavelle et al., 2014; Miller and Weissert, 2000; Mittleman et al., 2006; Spillman and Long, 2009).

The Importance of Caregiver Assessment

Chapter 3 described how caregivers and the caregiving experience are uniquely individual. Caregivers may share many common experiences, but individual caregiver's roles are highly variable and dependent on numerous factors that affect his or her availability, capacity, and willingness to assume critical responsibilities. Thus, providers cannot develop an individualized care plan for older adults—if a caregiver's help is needed—without assessing or knowing who the primary caregiver is and what his/her capabilities are. As Chapter 5 finds, the most effective caregiver interventions begin with an assessment of caregivers' risks, needs, strengths, and preferences. Research also suggests that primary care settings can be appropriate venues for assessing caregivers and providing them needed supports (Callahan et al., 2006; Burns et al., 2003).

A note of caution: caregiver assessments can have unintended consequences if they are used primarily to determine an older adult's eligibility for services. Anecdotal reports suggest that agencies with limited resources have used the availability of caregivers to deny older adults services that they need and are eligible for.

Overall, these findings suggest that investments in family caregiver services and supports may generate savings in both health care and social services. However, there is much to learn. Despite research showing the benefits, providers, payers, and health care organizations have yet to establish mechanisms to capitalize on or optimize the role of caregivers in the health care of older adults. A workable mechanism for documenting the identity of the family caregiver in older adults' medical records needs to be developed. For example, providers may need to create a new field in the demographic section of the electronic health record to capture caregiver information and also develop an alert to ask for updates at each new encounter.

The lack of research and investment in developing systems for routinely identifying, assessing, and engaging older adults' caregivers is striking. Moreover, although important research by the Agency for Healthcare Research and Quality, Centers for Disease Control and Prevention, Centers for Medicare & Medicaid Services (CMS), Patient-Centered Outcomes Research Institute, National Institutes of Health, and other federal agencies is assessing the effectiveness of innovations in health care delivery and payment, most of these efforts do not explicitly involve family caregivers.

Decision Making

Older adults and their families confront a wide range of decisions in care delivery and planning for future care needs. Such decisions range from whether to adjust, stop, or start a prescribed medication, the selection of alternative treatment options or procedures when confronting a major life event or diagnosis, whether to continue life-sustaining support, and making choices about residential care such as whether to move to a nursing home. A considerable research literature has focused on shared decision making in health care. Research on individual or family decisions regarding nursing home placement or other LTSS issues is scare. The term "shared decision making" is generally used to describe the process of communication, deliberation, and decision making in which one or more professionals

- share information about testing or treatment options including severity and probability of potential harms and benefits and alternatives of options given individual circumstances;
- elicit individual preferences regarding harms, benefits, and potential outcomes; and
- engage in an interactive process of reflection and discussion until a mutual decision is reached about the subsequent treatment or plan of action (Braddock et al., 1999; Charles et al., 1999; Clayman et al., 2012; Dy and Purnell, 2012).

Given that the vast majority of individuals prefer to participate in decisions about their health (Chewning et al., 2012) and that optimal decisions rely on an understanding of care recipients' values and priorities, strategies to engage people in their care have received great attention (Alston et al., 2014; Edwards and Elwyn, 2009; Fried, 2016; Stacey et al., 2012). Although the importance of family in older adults' decision making is well appreciated (Price et al., 2012; Vladeck and Westphal, 2012), relatively little attention has been directed at developing interventions to support older adults and their family members when confronting difficult decisions (Garvelink et al., 2016). The gap in knowledge is significant given variability in individual preferences for participating in medical decision making (Brom et al., 2014; Kiesler and Auerbach, 2006; Levinson et al., 2005). Moreover, older individuals who lack the capacity to make informed decisions are likely to prefer or rely on the help of family members (Stacey et al., 2012; Wolff and Boyd, 2015).

Family involvement in decision making is distinct from patient–provider decision making in numerous ways. Such decisions may occur during the course of care when older adults and their family members communicate face to face with providers or they may occur during routine conversations, such as at the dinner table or in discussions among family members that do not involve the older adult. The decisions may be made in a crisis situation or over time.

Not all family members may share the same views or possess the same information to guide decision making, leading to disagreement or conflict regarding the optimal course of care. Such differences in perspectives is an important feature of family involvement in care (Lobchuk, 2006; Urbanik and Lobchuk, 2009) as both older adults and families commonly value and expect family involvement in decision making, but that congruence regarding attitudes, decisions, and behaviors may be low (Kitko et al., 2015; Moon et al., 2016; Shin et al., 2013). As differences between older adults' and family members' perspectives are inversely associated with effective illness management and care planning (Brom et al., 2014; Kiesler and Auerbach, 2006; Kitko et al., 2015; Moon et al., 2016), strategies to more effectively involve and better support the role of family caregivers in decision making could be beneficial for both older adults and their family caregivers. The nuances and range of considerations in decision making vary widely by specific circumstances but the process and effects may be highly consequential. For example, the challenges of surrogate decision making have been widely documented and may include stress, anxiety, or emotional burdens that persist for years (Vig et al., 2007; Wendler and Rid, 2011; Whitlach and Feinberg, 2007).

Access to Older Adults' Health Information

The Health Insurance Portability and Accountability Act (HIPAA) has provisions that govern access to an older adult's health information by his or her family caregiver, other family members, or friends. The HIPAA Privacy Rule provides family caregivers three avenues of access to an older adult's protected health information (HHS, 2016):

- First, every state allows people to designate a "personal representative" via a health care advance directive (health care power of attorney). If the person has not designated a representative, most states have a statute that determines the process for identifying an authorized surrogate decision maker. If the person lacks the capacity to manage his or her affairs, a guardian may be appointed through judicial proceedings.
- Second, people can name the individual with access to their protected health information through a formal HIPAA authorization document or a signed "directed right to access."
- Third, if there is no formally appointed representative or authorized surrogate, health care providers can share a person's information with a family caregiver if (a) the person gives permission; (b) the person is present and does not object; or (c) the person is not present and the provider determines that it is in his or her best interest to share the information. In these discretionary disclosure situations, the Privacy Rule directs providers to limit the disclosed

information to that which the involved third party reasonably needs to know about the person's care or payment.

It appears that the HIPAA Privacy Rule is commonly misinterpreted as a barrier to caregivers' access to older adults' health information (Levine, 2006). Although there is no published research on the impact of HIPAA on older adults and their caregivers, anecdotal reports suggest that many providers misunderstand the law and its regulations. Providers may tell caregivers that they cannot share any health information even when the individual older adult has authorized it. Or, providers may be overly restrictive in discretionary disclosures. Institutional culture may also affect the sharing of information with caregivers.

See Appendix H for further details regarding HIPAA and caregivers' access to older adults' protected health information.

COMMITTING TO A NEW PARADIGM: PERSON- AND FAMILY-CENTERED CARE

The National Strategy for Quality Improvement ("The National Quality Strategy"), developed by the U.S. Department of Health and Human Services (HHS), calls for more transparent, accountable, and higher quality care through broad partnerships that extend beyond individual providers and settings and that actively involve individuals *and their families* (HHS, 2013). The strategy also calls for using quality measures to help achieve person- and family-centered care. However, this vision is not reflected in current approaches to quality measurement or care delivery and financing reform efforts.

The quest for higher quality and more affordable care has led to a growing appreciation of the impact of the broader social and physical environments in which individuals are born and their lives unfold. The World Health Organization has characterized family as "the primary social agent in the promotion of health and well-being" (WHO, 1991). As providers, payers, and society work toward higher value systems of care to support population health, the need has never been greater for delivery systems to more effectively partner with and support family caregivers of older adults with complex needs.

The committee agreed that a new vision for health care and LTSS—in which family caregivers are better supported in the care of older adults—is needed now. This vision, described in Chapter 1, requires fundamental change in the delivery of health care and LTSS, including a reorientation of care systems to a focus on family-centeredness. Family-centered care has been variably defined, but is best characterized by the National Quality Forum (NQF) as

> an approach to the planning and delivery of care across settings and time that is centered in collaborative partnerships among individuals, their defined family, and providers of care. It supports health and well-being by being consistent with, respectful of, and responsive to an individual's priorities, goals, needs, and values. (NQF, 2014a p. 2)

The core concepts of person- and family-centered care, illustrated in Figure 6-1, include the support and involvement of family, as defined by each individual (NQF, 2014a). The "care team" is defined as including individuals, families, and the health care and supportive services workers who interact with individuals. Person- and family-centered care recognizes that many people—including older adults—desire or require the involvement of family members or trusted friends to obtain health and supportive

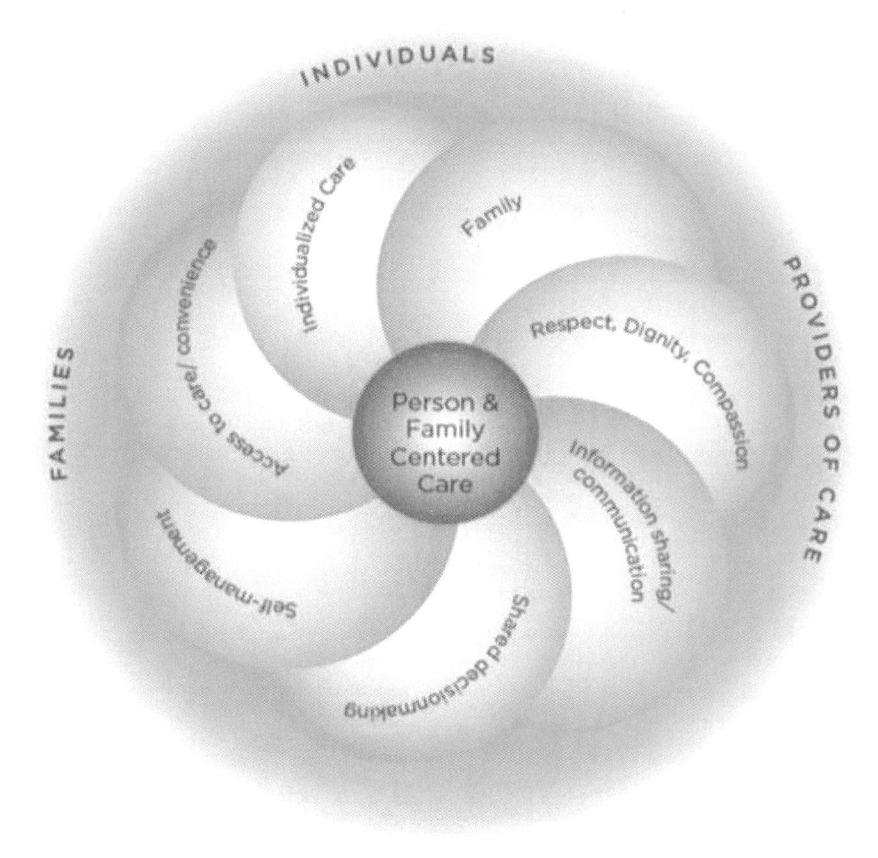

FIGURE 6-1 Core concepts of person- and family-centered care.
SOURCE: NQF, 2014a.

services, to meet health system demands, to communicate with providers, to make health care decisions, and to help with daily health-related and other activities of daily living (Feinberg, 2012; Price et al., 2012; Torke et al., 2012; Wolff and Boyd, 2015). NQF notes that the concept of "family" specifically addresses involvement in care and need for support, but that all the core concepts extend to the family, especially when individuals are those for whom decisions must be made in full or in part by surrogates (NQF, 2014a).

Table 6-2 describes five domains of person- and family-centered care. It notes the distinction between person-centered and person- and family-centered care and emphasizes that the family should not simply be viewed as a "resource" for a particular individual, but rather as individuals who themselves may need information, training, or support (Feinberg, 2012).

TABLE 6-2 Elements of Person- and Family-Centered Care

Element	Implications for Care Delivery
Respect and dignity for the older person and family	Health and social service professionals listen to and honor the person's and family's needs, values, preferences, and goals for care.
Recognition of the whole person	Emphasizes the person's and the family's well-being, taking into account physical and mental health, spiritual and cultural traditions, social supports, and engagement with community.
Assessing and addressing both the individual's and family caregiver's information, care, and support needs and their experience of care	A plan of care reflects the goals, values, and preferences of the person and his or her family. The plan of care is based on wants and needs that are meaningful to the person and the support needs of family members or friends to enable them to continue to provide support without being overstressed.
Promotion of communication, shared decision making, and empowerment	The individual, family, and providers have access to timely, complete, and accurate information and tools to make shared and informed decisions and plan for future needs that respect individuals and families.
Emphasis on coordination and collaboration across settings of care	Collaborative care integrates families in the care team, engaging them as partners in care, and providing tools for family caregivers themselves. Care and supportive services are accessible, comprehensive, continuous over time, and coordinated across providers and settings.

SOURCE: Feinberg, 2012.

Elevating the family alongside person-centered care in health delivery reform will require identifying involved family caregivers; assessing their capabilities; addressing their needs for education, training, and supportive services (e.g., counseling, respite care); and facilitating their involvement in delivery processes. Opportunities exist within the uptake of electronic health records to better capture people's health care encounters, and to incorporate person-reported and family-reported measures in clinical care. Likewise, accreditation activities related to the Patient-Centered Medical Home and Accountable Care Organizations involve documenting core elements of quality care processes, with commensurate measurement opportunities. Person- and family-centered care is a natural link between delivery innovations and the major priorities of the National Quality Strategy (National Priorities Partnership, 2011). Opportunities for the inclusion of family caregivers exist in numerous federally sponsored demonstrations, contracts, and payment reforms, yet practical approaches for inclusion and engagement of family caregivers remain poorly defined.

The need to explicitly clarify and support family caregivers in care delivery has never been greater. Transforming delivery processes so as to purposefully recognize, involve, and address the needs of family caregivers will not be a simple process, but the potential benefits to older adults and their family caregivers could be significant. Achieving this report's vision will, at a minimum, require acknowledging that older adults and family caregivers are often interdependent and that current delivery systems rely too much on family caregivers in some areas, while too little in others. Addressing these issues will require stakeholders to be catalysts for broad-based change. To this end, the committee identified four priority areas for action:

1. Identification, assessment, and support of family caregivers in the delivery of care
2. Inclusion of both family and caregiver experiences in quality measurement
3. Supporting family caregivers through health information technology
4. Preparing care professionals to provide person- and family-centered care.

Identify, Assess, and Support Family Caregivers in the Delivery of Care to Older Adults

A pivotal first step toward supporting family caregivers will be a sustained effort to assess and address caregiver needs. Systematic identification of caregivers is an essential part of delivering care to older adults in virtually every setting. To make this happen, documenting when older adults need a family caregiver to enact their care plan should become routine. Caregivers' contact information should be collected as a regular part of the medical record and in the care planning process for LTSS. The purpose should be to not only support appropriate care by professionals, but to serve as a mechanism for identifying caregivers who serve in critical and demanding roles. Caregivers may also be identified directly (and their data similarly recorded) through their own interaction with the system, including annual wellness exams, visits to physicians and other health care providers, and both admissions and discharges from hospitals and emergency rooms. Fundamental to the improvement of caregiving will be the development and adoption of caregiver assessment tools that can be used in practice. Without such tools it is very difficult to determine what roles caregivers can and cannot accomplish, how to appropriately engage them as team members in care and treatment, and how to best meet their own health and support needs.

The organization, delivery, and financing of health care and LTSS are designed to provide needed services to individuals not families. Yet older adults who rely on a family caregiver by definition need help to successfully navigate the complex service delivery environment or manage daily care needs. When older adults rely on a family caregiver to engage in health care decision making or enact their treatment or personal care plan, identifying the presence and ensuring the capacity of the family caregiver is foundational to quality care (FCA, 2006; McDaniel et al., 2005; NQF, 2014b). Stated differently, when family caregivers and older adults are engaged in a reciprocal and interdependent relationship, delivery of care benefits from a broader orientation that recognizes that the older adult and family caregiver together constitute a "unit of care," as articulated in the concept of person- and family-centered care (NQF, 2014a,b). Reorienting service delivery to reflect this reality will require the adoption of processes throughout the health care and LTSS systems to systematically identify, assess, engage, and support family caregivers, including talking with caregivers directly to better understand and address their needs, problems, resources, and strengths.

Paying for Recognition, Involvement, and Support of Family Caregivers

As the predominant payers of care for older adults, Medicare and Medicaid payment and regulatory policies are critical to motivating and changing provider practice. Private payers that provide supplemental coverage to Medicare beneficiaries also have a role in creating incentives for providers to engage caregivers. Some recent innovations in Medicare and Medicaid provide the potential, although quite limited, for family- and person-centeredness in coverage, payment, and delivery of services (see Table 6-3). Recent updates to hospital conditions of participation, for example, encourage engagement and support of family caregivers in the discharge planning process. New integrated care models, such as the Financial Alignment Initiative, promote better coordinated care and support family caregivers of older adults who are dually eligible for Medicare

TABLE 6-3 Selected Examples of How Medicare and Medicaid Provide Incentives for Person- and Family-Centered Care for Older Adults

Incentive	Description
Annual wellness visit	A Medicare benefit; offers coverage for providers to evaluate and document beneficiaries' demographic characteristics, family history, self-assessed health status, psychosocial and behavioral risks, and functional status.
Balancing incentive program	A financial incentive for state Medicaid programs; provides an enhanced federal match to states spending less than 50 percent of long-term services and supports care expenditures on home- and community-based settings and that implement structural changes, including use of a core standardized assessment instrument. Family caregiver assessment is recommended, but not required in core standardized assessment.
Medicare billing codes	Several new billing codes can be used by specified fee-for-service providers to bill Medicare for services that may involve contact with family caregivers. CPT code 99490 (Chronic Care Management Services) covers *non*-face-to-face care coordination services (e.g., by telephone, secure messaging, or Internet) for beneficiaries with two or more chronic conditions (including time spent communicating with family caregivers). CPT codes 99495 and 99496 (Transitional Care Management Services) cover providers' time spent communicating with family caregivers by phone, e-mail, or in person (within 2 days of discharge from an inpatient facility) during the beneficiary's transition from an inpatient stay to a community setting. CPT codes 99497 and 9948 (Advance Care Planning Services) cover face-to-face conversations with family members regarding advance directives.
Financial alignment initiative	States may elect to establish integrated care models that promote care coordination for dually eligible Medicare and Medicaid enrollees. Some models allow for the involvement of caregivers, use caregiver surveys to assess satisfaction (e.g., Consumer Assessment of Health Care Providers and Systems or CAHPS), and encourage family members/caregivers to participate in the care and evaluation process.

continued

TABLE 6-3 Continued

Incentive	Description
Home- and community-based services (HCBS)	A financial incentive for state Medicaid programs; HCBS programs may cover respite care, caregiver education and training, environmental modifications, bereavement services, family counseling, and other services that facilitate community living. States must provide for independent assessments of care recipients that include the need for physical, cognitive, or behavioral services and supports; strengths and preferences; available services and housing options; and whether an unpaid caregiver will provide any elements of the person-centered service plan (if yes, a caregiver assessment is required).
Home health	Skilled nursing care and medical social services provided by home health agencies to Medicare beneficiaries can include caregiver supportive services (e.g., teaching/training activities that require skilled nursing personnel to teach a beneficiary's caregivers how to provide the treatment regimen).
Hospice benefit	A Medicare benefit that includes counseling to patient and family caregiver for loss or grief counseling, respite, and a medical social worker to facilitate effective palliation and management of a patient's illness or related condition. Continuous home care is available under certain conditions when the caregiver is unable or unwilling to continue to provide a skilled level of care for the patient.
Hospital discharge planning	The Centers for Medicare & Medicaid Services (CMS) set Conditions of Participation (COPs) that health providers must meet to be eligible for payment under the Medicare and Medicaid programs. CMS provides interpretative guidelines for meeting COPS to promote better individual outcomes (they are not required for compliance, however). The guidelines for hospitals emphasize the importance of engaging both the individual and family during hospital discharge planning.
Innovative payment and delivery models	Financial incentives for providers; eligible providers and other entities can receive awards if they meet specified standards for high-quality and coordinated care for a particular population. Some standards may implicitly encourage providers to actively engage caregivers as a resource in the care delivery process. CMS is testing these models to inform potential changes in health care payment rules.
Meaningful use criteria	CMS criteria for how providers use electronic health records, including the information and functionality that is available to individuals.

SOURCES: Alley et al., 2016; CMS, 2013, 2014, 2015, 2016; Justice et al., 2014; Komisar and Feder, 2011; Mission Analytics Group, 2013; Rajkumar et al., 2014.

and Medicaid. Other CMS initiatives, such as the Transitional Care Management Services Program and innovative payment and delivery models, implicitly encourage providers to actively engage or support caregivers (Alley et al., 2016; Komisar and Feder, 2011; Rajkumar et al., 2014).

Medicare

In 2015, Medicare introduced a billing code that physicians, clinical nurse specialists, nurse practitioners, and physician assistants may use to be paid for *non*-face-to-face care coordination services for beneficiaries with multiple chronic conditions (CMS, 2015). Providers can use the code to provide 20 minutes (per month) of care management services including time spent communicating with the beneficiary's caregiver. It is a small step toward formal recognition of the value of involving family caregivers in older adults' care. However, CMS requires that the 20 minutes of service include numerous mandatory components and providers appear to be unaware that the code is available. Moreover, because Medicare payment is intended to reimburse for the beneficiaries' care only, it does not cover the supports that caregivers often need. Providers cannot bill, for example, for a comprehensive assessment of caregivers' needs (Gitlin et al., 2010). In addition, if the care recipient's treatment is completed, the provider cannot bill for any additional supports that the caregiver needs.

As this report went to press, CMS was finalizing a set of proposed revisions to Medicare regulations governing the home health benefit (CMS, 2014). The proposed revisions would require home health agencies to identify the care recipient's primary family caregiver, develop the Medicare beneficiary's plan of care in partnership with not only the older adult but also the caregiver, include education and training for the caregiver specific to the older adult's needs in the plan of care, and other measures involving caregivers.

Medicaid

The Medicaid program has a significant role in the financing of LTSS (Favreault and Dey, 2015). In contrast to Medicare, Medicaid recognizes the role of family caregivers in care planning and delivery in some circumstances (Newcomer et al., 2012; O'Keefe et al., 2010; Sands et al., 2012), particularly with respect to the delivery of home- and community-based services (HCBS) (Kelly et al., 2013; Miller, 2012). For example, federal law requires that state Medicaid HCBS waiver programs include a plan of care that could include the role of caregivers, although states have considerable latitude regarding the specific components of the care plan. Only about 30 percent of states require an assessment of family caregivers' needs (Kelly et al., 2013). In these states, the information that is collected from the family caregiver affects the individualized care plan for the Medicaid beneficiary and is also used to connect family caregivers to services and supports to meet their own needs. Questions posed in the family caregiver assessment may address domains such as family caregivers' skills, abilities, knowledge, or training needs to assist the Medicaid beneficiary; questions directly asked of the family caregiver to assess his/her well-being (e.g., self-rated health and a depression screen); and resources that the family caregiver can choose to use to address support needs of the caregiver.

In 2014, CMS released a new rule on community living for Medicaid HCBS programs. For the first time, CMS required that family caregivers' needs be addressed if their involvement is part of the care plan for persons with disabilities. However, only the 1915(i) HCBS state plan option has the new requirement for caregiver assessment (Feinberg and Levine, 2015). Moreover, anecdotal reports suggest that some state Medicaid-managed care organizations often compel unpaid assistance from a family caregiver even though federal rules require that unpaid supports be provided voluntarily (Carlson, 2016).

One example of state policy change through Medicaid is Rhode Island's Family Caregivers Support Act of 2013. The Act requires a family caregiver assessment if the Medicaid beneficiary's plan of care includes a role for the family caregiver. If a family caregiver is involved, the plan of care must address the needs of both the care recipient and the family caregiver.

As discussed in Chapter 5, individuals who need LTSS who are enrolled in Medicaid may self-direct personal care through HCBS waiver programs or personal care optional benefits, including the hiring of relatives, friends, or independent providers whose compensation is covered by the Medicaid program. Needs assessment and service planning are critical processes used to safeguard participant health and welfare and to ensure that services and supports enable participants to meet individual community living goals. States have considerable latitude in establishing the process and qualifications to ensure that providers possess necessary competencies and skills. States also increasingly require individuals who would provide personal care services to undergo background checks against abuse/neglect registries (Galantowicz et al., 2010). Little information is now available about how states evaluate qualifications of family caregivers who are paid personal care attendants, although the 2013 National Inventory Survey on Participant Direction reported that about one-third of programs require certification and that about half of programs require training of workers in skills or knowledge such as cardiopulmonary resuscitation or HIPAA (NRCPDS, 2014).

Some policies of state Medicaid programs may undermine effective caregiving (Carter, 2015). Federal Medicaid person-centered care planning rules require written service plans identifying not only the services a beneficiary will receive, but who will provide them—whether they are family caregivers or Medicaid-financed paid care. Some regulations also specify that family-provided services should be voluntary. In practice, however, some states or managed care plans reduce Medicaid-provided services based on the presence of a family caregiver, also referred to as "natural supports" (Sands et al., 2012).

Despite attention to policies and services that recognize, support, and compensate family caregivers, Medicaid policy still falls short of commitment to a systematic approach to person- and family-centered care that takes into account the needs of both the care recipient and the family caregiver—at either the state or federal level. A meaningful approach would—at a minimum—entail requirements for caregiver assessment in all HCBS options (as well as for the managed care plans that increasingly provide them) for care plans that depend on family caregivers for their enactment. A meaningful commitment to the identification and support of family caregivers would also involve oversight and review of assessment tools to assure their appropriateness and effectiveness in serving both beneficiaries and caregivers.

Administration for Community Living

Chapter 1 described the federal programs that are relevant to the adequacy of caregiver support albeit on a much smaller scale. The Administration for Community Living, for example, oversees several programs that support family caregivers. The largest is the National Family Caregiver Support Program, which distributes about $150 million to states and territories to provide caregivers with information, help in accessing services, individual counseling, education, respite care, and other services. Some states have also moved forward in supporting the assessment of family caregivers through state-funded support programs. For example, in 2012, Washington state increased its funding for the Family Caregiver Support Program by $3.45 million to expand eligibility and to increase the level of services for caregivers including more comprehensive assessment of their needs. A legislatively mandated evaluation of the expanded program found that it delayed the use of Medicaid long-term care services (Lavelle et al., 2014).

Many states have enacted legislation to raise awareness and better support family caregivers. For example, the Caregiver Advise, Record, Enable (CARE) Act, now law in 29 states, mandates that the name of the family caregiver is recorded when an individual is admitted to a hospital or rehabilitation facility, that the family caregiver is notified at the time of discharge, and that the family caregiver is afforded an explanation and is given instruction prior to discharge of medical tasks he or she is expected to perform at home. CARE Act legislation is being considered by many other states as well.

Identify, Assess, and Support Caregivers: Conclusions

Although recent policy initiatives have created incentives for stronger partnership with family caregivers, initiatives stop short of making an explicit commitment to systematic identification and meaningful support. The implications of available knowledge and the principles of good practice support the importance of identifying, assessing, and addressing the main concerns that family caregivers are a necessary and essential part of working with older people in all care settings. In light of available knowledge and existing infrastructure, making a commitment to systematically identify and explicitly support family caregivers will require purposeful attention in the reform of federal entitlement programs and state benefit programs, as well as significant investment to develop and broadly implement metrics, tools, and policies that facilitate systematic identification, assessment, and support of caregivers in payment and delivery of care. Investments in research will be needed to determine how to identify at-risk older adults and family caregivers who are likely to benefit from assessments, as well as how to appropriately distinguish and address older adults' needs from those of their caregivers. Investments in performance measures will be needed to make possible the inclusion of family caregivers' perspectives on and experiences with care. Investments will need to be made to enhance health information technology and to expand provider competencies to recognize and support family caregivers by facilitating appropriate information disclosure of an older adult's health information when the involvement of a family member is desired by the older adult or required to enact the individual's care plan. Although changes to organizational culture and provider workflows are not inconsequential, the financial outlays required to bring about these changes are likely to be relatively modest. Although subsequent sections of this chapter address these topics in greater detail, these activities collectively rest on the ability to identify family caregivers who are now largely invisible in systems of care.

Establishing approaches to systematically identify and meaningfully support family caregivers will require resources and motivation to undertake changes in provider practice. Financing arrangements could reward providers for the explicit identification and support of family caregivers. Likewise, performance standards should hold providers accountable for supporting family caregivers when the plan of care rests on their involvement. Achieving the vision laid out of involving family caregivers in care will require that changes be made to clarify HIPAA regulations and guidance so as to support, rather than inhibit, appropriate information exchange and communication among providers, caregivers, and care recipients. Care coordination, especially in new Medicare and Medicaid payment mechanisms designed to pay for it, should encourage referrals that enable caregivers to access LTSS and other social supports through Area Agencies on Aging and other agencies.

Inclusion of Family Caregiver-Reported Experiences in Quality Measurement

Recent initiatives to reward the provision of high-value care have elevated the prominence of performance measurement in care delivery and payment reform. The Institute of Medicine report *Vital Signs: Core Metrics for Health and Health Care Progress* found that thousands of performance measures are now in use to assess the quality of care delivery (IOM, 2015). Although the report concluded that many measures provide useful information, the large number and lack of focus, consistency, and organization were recognized as limiting effectiveness in measuring and improving health system performance. Against this backdrop, there is a growing appreciation that the utility of performance measures rests on measuring elements of care that matter, that are outcomes oriented, and that reflect system performance (Blumenthal and McGinnis, 2015). For those with complex care needs or multiple chronic conditions, technical quality may not align with the care or outcomes that matter most based on individual values, priorities, and goals of care (Boyd et al., 2005; Lynn et al., 2015). For older adults with significant and complex needs, performance measures should encompass person- and family-centered care in recognizing goals of comfort, the care setting of choice, and preferences for actively engaging or delegating care to others (NQF, 2014a; Wolff and Boyd, 2015). For many older adults, high-quality care involves supporting their family caregivers—by respecting their values and preferences without imposing financial burden, physical strain, or undue anxiety regarding lack of experience or knowledge to perform tasks expected of them.

Although the number of health care performance measures has dramatically increased in recent years, so too has recognition of the gaps of existing measures in important domains of quality. Although the field is rapidly evolving, the perspectives of family caregivers have not been extensively included in performance measurement to date (Gage and Albaroudi, 2015). In light of existing measurement gaps, HHS contracted with NQF to conduct environmental scans, identify priority areas for potential measures and measurement concepts, and develop multistakeholder recommendations for future measure development and endorsement. A theme throughout this work is that it is both individuals and families who engage in the planning, delivery, and evaluation of care across all levels of performance measurement. For example, work by NQF conceptualizes support and involvement of family as a core concept of person- and family-centered care (NQF, 2014a), and support of caregivers as an overarching theme for performance measurement in the care of persons with Alzheimer's disease and related disorders, as well as crosscutting measures that span any given disease category (NQF, 2014b).

As core measures are identified to assess the performance of the health care system, a similar effort is underway with respect to LTSS. A 2-year process to prioritize opportunities to address gaps in HCBS quality measurement is now underway (NQF, 2015). A conceptual framework has been agreed on by a multistakeholder committee that includes Caregiver Support as 1 of 11 measurement domains. In its description of this domain, financial, emotional, and technical support are listed as examples of measures that apply to both paid and unpaid caregivers. Other characteristics that fall under the Caregiver Support domain include caregiver assessment, training and skill building, respite care, and supports for well-being.

Although the inclusion of caregiver measures is increasingly supported in principle, the development, validation, and endorsement of such measures will require resources and prioritization. For these reasons, the committee urges HHS to establish a process for identifying, prioritizing, and harmonizing caregiver-related measures across sites and models of care. This effort will be important to achieving better outcomes for the care receiver and caregiver, as well as for improving system properties that influence quality and efficiency of care delivery. Moreover, consensus processes for measure identification, selection, and prioritization takes time—years in many instances. The inclusion of caregiver perspectives in performance measures would send a strong signal to providers that for some older adults—especially those with complex care needs—caregivers are a key element in care planning and delivery, and that their experiences provide important insight in the quality of service delivery.

Supporting Family Caregivers Through Health Information Technology

Health information technology (IT) is now being widely diffused throughout health care delivery systems due in part to its promise of promoting more timely, accurate, and transparent exchange of information, improved quality and efficiency of care, and more active involvement of individual and family "consumers" (Hsiao et al., 2013; Kellermann and Jones, 2013). One broad class of these technologies includes systems that enhance the efficiency and coordination of care, including the integration of health care with LTSS services. For example, the IEP (Information Exchange Portal) is a recently developed electronic platform designed to facilitate seamless integration across social and health systems. Specifically, the system integrates critical clinical and social data (individual support needs) to predict adverse events in vulnerable people and help facilitate the delivery of targeted interventions.

A second broad class of health IT is directed at the consumer to facilitate access to health information and services, involvement in health management activities, and health decision making (Bobinet and Petito, 2015). These technologies include secure Internet portals that are tethered to the individual's health information in electronic health records (EHRs), personal monitoring devices, secure e-mail messaging between consumer and health care providers, and Internet-based resources for health education, information, and advice. The Office of the National Coordinator for Health Information Technology defines consumers to include individuals, their families, and other caregivers (Ricciardi et al., 2013).

EHR vendors and care providers have focused primarily on increasing the older adult's registration for and use of patient portals. The role of family members and friends in the use of these systems has not been well defined. Many EHR vendors support functionality to allow individuals to explicitly share access to their patient portal account with family members or friends through a consumer-facing "proxy" portal. The U.S. Department of Veterans Affairs, for example, is currently modifying "My Health*e*Vet" to allow veterans to delegate electronic access to a caregiver.[2] National information about provider adoption and consumer uptake of shared access to the proxy portal is limited, but suggests it is far from widespread (Osborn et al., 2011; Sarkar and Bates, 2014; Wolff et al., 2016a). Implementation barriers to proxy portal registration are numerous and include lack of availability (e.g., limitations on who may register for the proxy portal [e.g., Kaiser restricts registration for the proxy portal to Kaiser members]) (Sarkar and Bates, 2014); lack of transparency in registration processes; poor awareness that the proxy portal exists (Zulman et al., 2013); lack of technology skills and usability difficulties (Czaja et al., 2014); and lack of understanding of benefits to justify the effort of initiating and navigating proxy portal registration protocols. Variability in state privacy laws (Pope, 2012) and provider implementation decisions may also influence consumer uptake of a proxy portal (PSTT, 2014; Strong et al., 2014). In one survey, nearly half (48.6 percent) of family caregivers reported that health system privacy rules and restrictions were the most common barrier to their using technology to access care recipients' health information (Zulman et al., 2013).

Although most people want control over their electronic health information, preferences for sharing personal information vary widely (Caine et al., 2015; Zulman et al., 2011). Current technology allows people to select

[2] Information about the My Health*e*Vet program is available at: https://www.myhealth.va.gov/index.html (accessed August 23, 2016).

who has permission to access their electronic health information as well as the limits of that access (Leventhal et al., 2015; Osborn et al., 2011; Tierney et al., 2015; Zulman et al., 2011). For example, someone might authorize a paid caregiver to schedule appointments or refill prescribed medications but bar his or her access to personal health information. In one survey, veterans were twice as likely to support allowing someone to request prescription refills (87 percent) than to communicate with health care providers (40 percent) on their behalf (Zulman et al., 2011). Giving older adults the option to authorize a family caregiver's access to their electronic health information would facilitate the caregiver's engagement and management of their care (Wolff et al., 2016a).

Several issues will require careful attention if family caregivers are to be more widely and purposefully engaged in the use of patient portals of EHRs. First, system designers and vendors should better accommodate the reality that individuals' information-sharing preferences are nuanced and evolve over time (Caine and Hanania, 2013; Crotty et al., 2015). Second, designers should incorporate user-centered design principles in system design to develop shared access functionality that better reflects caregiver and individual preferences (Nath and Sharp, 2015). Third, best practice implementation strategies are needed to guide provider policies and processes for credentialing and registering family members to access their older relatives' health information. To this end, the Office of the National Coordinator for Health Information Technology is well positioned to disseminate best practices through education and outreach via Regional Extension Centers, through HIT.gov, and by partnering with professional societies and credentialing organizations. Finally, organizations and federal and state governmental agencies tasked with monitoring the implementation and use of consumer-facing health information technologies should provide equal weight and attention to individual and family adoption in tracking diffusion and use. Accreditation organizations such as the National Committee for Quality Assurance should incorporate proxy portal availability and rates of registration for particular subgroups (e.g., persons with dementia) or programs (e.g., individual-centered medical homes) to serve as quality measures that pertain to person and family engagement. Adoption of a secure online identity ecosystem to guarantee private credentials, now in development (White House, 2011), could also facilitate broader electronic credentialing and registration of family caregivers.

A third category of technology-based systems that is potentially useful for family caregivers as well as health care providers is embedded in-home activity-monitoring systems with unobtrusive sensors that can track behaviors, such as movement patterns (e.g., trips to the bathroom) or sleep behaviors, and allow for real-time transfer of information to family caregivers or health care providers. These types of systems can alert caregivers to emergency situations such as a fall or changes in activity patterns that may signal a potential health issue or functional decline. This can enable caregivers to stage an early intervention and potentially avoid catastrophic health events or hospitalization. Numerous technical and ethical issues need to be resolved regarding implementation of these systems, however. One set of issues relates to monitoring protocols—when monitoring should occur (e.g., 24 hours, intermittently) and what types of behaviors should be monitored. Other issues relate to privacy concerns and data-sharing privileges; data coding and integration (how to make the information meaningful and user-friendly to end users); and potential problems with false alarms. Attention to usability issues and caregiver training in the use of these systems is also paramount. Finally, there are questions regarding cost, reimbursement, and system maintenance/sustainability. One recent study found that caregivers are receptive to using technologies to help them monitor care recipients (Schulz et al., 2015). They are also willing to pay for these technologies, but at a limited amount. The authors of that study suggested that a combination of private pay and government subsidy may enhance the development and dissemination of these technologies to family caregivers. Overall, broader inclusion of family caregivers in the use of health IT would further National Quality Strategy priorities, including ensuring that each person and family is engaged as partners in their care, promoting effective communication and coordination of care, and reducing avoidable harm (HHS, 2013).

Preparing Care Professionals to Provide Person- and Family-Centered Care

For more than a decade, the National Academies of Sciences, Engineering, and Medicine has called for urgent attention to the inadequate preparation of the health care and/or social services workforce to meet the needs of older adults (IOM, 2003, 2008, 2012a, 2014). It is beyond the scope of this report to assess the curricula and licensing requirements of the relevant professions. Nevertheless, it is clear that preparing providers to deliver person- and family-centered care to older adults will require a broad-based effort—across the educational continuum and in an interdisciplinary manner—to address and ensure the competence of their respective professions to work with family caregivers of older adults. Many disciplines are likely to encounter family caregivers of older adults, including physicians; physician assistants; nurses (including advanced practice nurses); social workers; psychologists; physical, occupational, and speech therapists; pharmacists; and direct care workers (e.g., certified nursing assistants, home health aides, and personal care aides). Primary care physicians, nurse practitioners, and social workers serve an especially important role as communicator with

BOX 6-1
Perspectives of Primary Care Physicians Who Care for Older Adults with Dementia

In 2006, a team of University of California researchers conducted qualitative interviews with 40 primary care physicians in northern California to learn about practice constraints that interfere with their clinical management of older adult patients with dementia. The study also examined how such barriers affected the quality of care—for the persons with dementia and also their caregivers. Below are selected excerpts from the interviews.

Insufficient Time

"Most of the time when they come in to see me there may be some specific concerns like, you know, they're [patient] wetting the bed all the time, or they're [patient] wandering, or you know, whatever, but the majority of the visit is hand-holding and listening, that sort of thing. It takes a long time."

Low Reimbursement

"When you deal with a patient who has dementia, maybe depression, as well as hypertension and diabetes, it's a lot more complicated than the intact 50-year-old hypertensive diabetic but the reimbursement is the same."

Difficulties with Specialists

"We have good neurologists, but they are generally scheduled far in advance so it takes a least a month, two months to get an appointment unless the patient's hospitalized. Psychiatrists are more of a problem. There aren't enough of them."

families and caregivers. Examples of the challenges they face are presented in Box 6-1.

Although few standards for health and social services professionals' engagement with family caregivers have been developed, the priority areas for training the workforce to provide person- and family-centered care include

- recognizing family caregivers' involvement in older adults' care;
- assessing caregivers' willingness and ability to take on the tasks in older adults' care plans;
- engaging family caregivers as respected members of the care team;

"It's hard, bottom line is it's hard. The feedback is slow [from specialists] . . . So you don't get anything and then the patient comes back and they are usually, they don't have any idea, and then they're kind of frustrated too."

Poor Connections with Social Services

"Since I'm not a licensed clinical social worker and I don't know what's available in the community, and I don't know how to, nor do I have time to call up and make arrangements for Meals on Wheels, or call up and find out what they need for a choreworker, or call up and find out how to access daycare. All I can do is say, you know, these things exist and here's some ways to contact them, there's a green booklet that the county put out a couple of years ago."

Lack of Interdisciplinary Teams

"I just feel, I don't have the network we need, so, because for the dementia care it's a team care, dietician, social work, psychiatry, psychologist, and pharmacist. . . . I feel I don't have this. I don't think anybody has this luxury, but the gist of care should be that."

SOURCE: Hinton et al., 2007, pp. 1489-1490.

- providing and communicating information to the family caregiver; and
- recognizing family caregivers' health care and support needs and helping them obtain caregiver supportive services (e.g., training, counseling, respite care) where appropriate, and referral to the caregiver's primary care physician.

Some promising efforts to identify needed standards and facilitate their implementation are under way, especially in nursing and social work (Kelly et al., 2008; Mast et al., 2012; Messecar, 2012; Mitnick et al., 2010; National Association of Social Workers, 2010; Parker et al., 2016; Rabow et al., 2010). For example, a State of the Science Symposium on Professional Partners Supporting Family Caregivers identified a set of recommended standards for social workers and nurses related to communication, assessment and practice, collaboration, and leadership. However, the standards are generally stated and lack necessary specifics regarding essential knowledge and skills. Whether any of the recommendations have been implemented in practice is uncertain.

Little attention has been paid to understanding family systems, changing family structures, and identifying, assessing, and addressing family caregiver needs as a growing area of practice in physician training. *Family-Oriented Primary Care*, a textbook for primary care physicians originally published in 1990, has long advocated for full inclusion of family in primary care through all stages of a person's life (McDaniel et al., 2005). It does not, however, address the skills and competencies for providers that would be required. Similarly, although the American Geriatrics Society (AGS) has defined person-centered care to include family, the AGS recommendations do not address the challenges that family caregivers face or treat caregivers as central to the care team (AGS Expert Panel, 2012). The American College of Physicians' Ethics, Professionalism and Human Rights Committee has done promising work on bioethics related to family caregivers, recognizing the evolving need for consideration of the role of family caregivers while protecting individual rights (Mitnick et al., 2010). It goes further than the AGS Panel in recognizing physicians' responsibility to plan for necessary caregiver training and to attend to caregiver stress.

Cultural competence in working with family caregivers is also essential, given the growing diversity of the older adult population and family caregivers.[3] The concept of cultural competence has gained wide acceptance in health care and social services. While the importance of preparing providers for working with diverse caregivers is recognized for LTSS and the health care system, few guidelines exist on the core competencies for working with diverse caregivers and the best strategies for implementing these in systems of care. Cultural competence standards, such as the National Standards on Culturally and Linguistically Appropriate Services developed by the Office of Minority Health, are widely regarded as important for reducing health disparities in diverse populations, including access to and quality of care, and have been incorporated into professional training and continuing education. However, these cultural competence guidelines focus primarily on the individual, although competence in working with family caregivers is often noted. Many approaches to cultural competence have been developed, but evidence for the effectiveness of these approaches is modest and mixed. For example, while there is modest evidence for the effectiveness of cultural competence training interventions on provider attitudes, knowledge, and

[3] See Chapter 2 for demographic data on the makeup of the caregiver and care recipient populations.

skills and individual adherence to a treatment regimen, the impact on other individual outcomes is weaker (Beach, 2007; Bhui et al., 2007; Clifford et al., 2015; Horvat et al., 2014). Few training programs have included specific content on how to work with diverse caregivers or have measured the impact of cultural competence on relevant caregiver outcomes (e.g., satisfaction or adherence).

Organizational Change and New Models of Care

Given the current state of interactions between family caregivers and the health care and LTSS systems, new models of person- and family-centered care are clearly needed (Lewis, 2008). Individual organizations and systems of care will need to change their cultures in order to successfully ensure that the health care and LTSS systems adequately recognize and support family caregivers.

There are resources to guide organizations committed to developing person- and family-centered practices. For example, the Roadmap for Patient + Family Engagement in Healthcare Practice and Research, developed by the American Institutes for Research, offers practical strategies that organizations can use to help clinicians and health care leaders partner with older adults and their families at both the direct care and organizational levels (Carman et al., 2014). The roadmap emphasizes that to achieve this aim, organizations and systems of care have to be held accountable to the core principle of family-centeredness. The Institute for Healthcare Improvement's "Always Events" initiative provides another framework to help health care leaders achieve person- and family-centered care service delivery (Bowie et al., 2015; IHI, 2014). The framework defines "always events" as evidence-based practices or sets of behaviors that provide the following: "a foundation for partnering with individuals and their families; actions that will ensure optimal individual experiences and improved outcomes; and a unifying force for all that demonstrates an ongoing commitment to person- and family-centered care" (IHI, 2014, p. 4).

The extent to which providers encounter family caregivers of older adults and the nature of their interaction varies substantially depending on the care setting and other factors. Regardless, family-centered care is achievable to some degree across different care settings and providers. For example, physicians working in emergency departments may often encounter family caregivers of older adults, but are likely to have limited opportunity to engage and support them. By contrast, family practice physicians who care for older adults are likely to have more frequent opportunities to engage with and provide ongoing support to the caregivers they encounter. Nurses and social workers in hospitals, nursing homes, or home care programs have frequent contact with family caregivers. Home health aides, personal care aides, and certified nursing assistants working in homes or residential settings also commonly serve older adults who have family caregivers. In fact, they are often in the best position to understand the challenges of caregiving, but may lack sufficient training or authority to support the family caregiver. Providers who are engaged in palliative or end-of-life care often view family caregivers as an essential part of the care team and can play an important role in supporting them. Whatever the setting or professional discipline, organizations and systems of care should be held accountable for providing family-centered services and care.

Evaluation of the effectiveness of efforts to prepare health care and social service professionals with the skills and competencies to actively engage and support both older individuals and their family caregivers is needed. Rigorous evaluation of metric-based family caregiver outcomes will be critical to making competence in family-centered care a standard practice. No metrics have been developed, however, and significant work is required to develop them. The committee urges CMS to take on this challenge.

CONCLUSIONS

The committee's key findings and conclusions are described in detail in Box 6-2. In summary, the committee concludes that despite the integral role that family caregivers play in the lives of older adults with complex care needs, they are often marginalized or ignored in the delivery of health

BOX 6-2
Key Findings and Conclusions: Regarding Family Caregivers of Older Adults' Interactions with Health Care and Long-Term Services and Supports Systems

To fulfill the numerous roles that they play, family caregivers must interact with a wide range of providers and navigate within a variety of systems. For example:

- They communicate with physicians, physician assistants, nurses, nurse practitioners, social workers, psychologists, pharmacists, physical and occupational therapists, direct care workers (e.g., certified nursing assistants, home health aides, and personal care aides), and others.
- They help provide or supplement providers' information about older adults' health histories, the medications they take, past diagnoses, previous treatments and surgeries, and adverse reactions to any drugs (especially if the older adult is forgetful or has dementia).

BOX 6-2 Continued

- They communicate with home health care agency professionals and paraprofessionals and other community-based service providers who offer services to older adults.

Health care and long-term services and supports (LTSS) organizations and providers expect and depend on family caregivers to coordinate and help carry out older adults' care plans, but at the same time:

- The organization, delivery, and financing of health care and LTSS are designed to serve the beneficiary or care recipient.
    - o As a result, providers have little or no financial incentive to spend time with caregivers, seek their input, or provide the support they need to carry out older adults' care plans.
- Health care and social service providers do not routinely identify older adults' family caregivers and do not assess caregivers' availability, capacity, and willingness to assume critical responsibilities.
    - o Providers need training and appropriate tools to assess caregiver's capacity to provide care assigned to them.
- Caregivers have difficulty getting access to timely and reliable health information about the older adult for whom they are caring—at times because providers misinterpret the privacy requirements of the Health Insurance Portability and Accountability Act.

Several studies have found that when older adults have a family caregiver, they use fewer health care resources. For example:

- Randomized controlled trials have demonstrated that when older adults' caregivers receive a standard assessment, training, respite, and other supports, hospital readmissions and expenditures for emergency room visits decline and nursing home placement is delayed.

Centers for Medicare & Medicaid Services (CMS) payment policies are critical to motivating changes in provider practice with respect to family caregivers:

- Some recent Medicare and Medicaid reforms are encouraging, but are not enough to ensure that caregivers are routinely identified by providers and given needed supports. For example:
    - o Although CMS is using quality measures to encourage quality improvement, family caregivers are not included in these efforts.

care and LTSS, and are often ignored in public policy as well. Paradoxically, family caregivers may be excluded from treatment decisions and care planning while the providers who exclude them assume their availability to perform the wide range of tasks prescribed in the older adults' care plan. Numerous barriers impede systematic recognition and partnership with family caregivers, including the bioethical emphasis on individual autonomy, payment rules that discourage care providers from spending time to communicate with caregivers, legal issues related to individual privacy, and a health insurance model oriented to individual coverage.

REFERENCES

Abadir, P. M., T. E. Finucane, and M. K. McNabney. 2011. When doctors and daughters disagree: Twenty-two days and two blinks of an eye. *Journal of the American Geriatrics Society* 59(12):2337-2340.

Adelman, R. D., L. L. Tmanova, D. Delgado, S. Dion, and M. S. Lachs. 2014. Caregiver burden: A clinical review. *JAMA* 311(10):1052-1060.

AGS Expert Panel (American Geriatrics Society Expert Panel on the Care of Older Adults with Multiple Morbidity). 2012. Patient-centered care for older adults with multiple chronic conditions: A stepwise approach from the American Geriatrics Society. *Journal of the American Geriatrics Society* 60(10):1957-1968.

Alley, D. E., C. N. Asomugha, P. H. Conway, and D. M. Sanghavi. 2016. Accountable Health Communities—Addressing social needs through Medicare and Medicaid. *New England Journal of Medicine* 374(1):8-11.

Almborg, A. H., K. Ulander, A. Thulin, and S. Berg. 2009. Discharge planning of stroke patients: The relatives' perceptions of participation. *Journal of Clinical Nursing* 18(6): 857-865.

Alston, C., Z. D. Berger, S. Brownlee, G. Elwyn, F. J. Fowler, L. K. Hall, V. M. Montori, B. Moulton, L. Paget, B. H. Shebel, R. Singerman, J. Walker, M. K. Wynia, and D. Henderson. 2014. *Shared decision-making strategies for best care: Patient decision aids.* Discussion paper. Washington, DC: Institute of Medicine.

Barnard, D., and M. J. Yaffe. 2014. What is the physician's responsibility to a patient's family caregiver? *The Virtual Mentor* 16(5):330-338.

Beach, M. C., M. M. Rosner, L. A. Cooper, M. P. S. Duggan, and J. Shatzer. 2007. Can patient-centered attitudes reduce racial and ethnic disparities in care? *Academic Medicine* 82(2):193-198.

Bhui, K., N. Warfa, P. Edonya, K. McKenzie, and D. Bhugra. 2007. Cultural competence in mental health care: A review of model evaluations. *BMC Health Services Research* 7(15):1.

Blumenthal, D., and J. M. McGinnis. 2015. Measuring vital signs: An IOM report on core metrics for health and health care progress. *JAMA* 313(19):1901-1902.

Bobinet, K. and J. Petito. 2015. *White paper. Designing the consumer-centered telehealth & eVisit experience. Considerations for the future of consumer healthcare.* https://www.healthit.gov/sites/default/files/DesigningConsumerCenteredTelehealtheVisit-ONC-WHITEPAPER-2015V2edits.pdf (accessed July 12, 2016).

Bookman, A., and M. Harrington. 2007. Family caregivers: A shadow workforce in the geriatric health care system. *Journal of Health Politics, Policy and Law* 32(6):1005-1041.

Bowie, P., D. McNab, J. Ferguson, C. de Wet, G. Smith, M. MacLeod, J. McKay, and C. White. 2015. Quality improvement and person-centeredness: A participatory mixed methods study to develop the "always event" concept for primary care. *BMJ Open* 5(4):e006667.

Boyd, C. M., J. Darer, C. Boult, L. P. Fried, L. Boult, and A. W. Wu. 2005. Clinical practice guidelines and quality of care for older patients with multiple comorbid diseases: Implications for pay for performance. *JAMA* 294(6):716-724.

Braddock, C., K. Edwards, N. M. Hasenberg, T. L. Laidley, and W. Levinson. 1999. Informed decision making in outpatient practice: Time to get back to basics. *JAMA* 282(24):2313-2320.

Brom, L., W. Hopmans, H. R. Pasman, D. R. Timmermans, G. A. Widdershoven, and B. D. Onwuteaka-Philipsen. 2014. Congruence between patients' preferred and perceived participation in medical decision-making: A review of the literature. *BMC Medical Informatics and Decision Making* 14(1):25.

Burns, R., L. O. Nichols, J. Martindale-Adams, M. J. Graney, and A. Lummus. 2003. Primary care interventions for dementia caregivers: 2-year outcomes from the REACH study. *The Gerontologist* 43(4):547-555.

Caine, K., and R. Hanania. 2013. Patients want granular privacy control over health information in electronic medical records. *Journal of the American Medical Informatics Association* 20(1):7-15.

Caine, K., S. Kohn, C. Lawrence, R. Hanania, E. M. Meslin, and W. M. Tierney. 2015. Designing a patient-centered user interface for access decisions about EHR data: Implications from patient interviews. *Journal of General Internal Medicine* 30(Suppl 1):7-16.

Callahan, C., M. Boustani, F. Unverzagt, M. Austrom, T. Damush, A. Perkins, B. Fultz, S. Hui, S. Counsell, and H. Hendrie. 2006. Effectiveness of collaborative care for older adults with Alzheimer disease in primary care: A randomized controlled trial. *JAMA* 295(18):2148-2157.

Carman, K. L., P. Dardess, M. E. Maurer, T. Workman, D. Ganachari, and E. Pathak-Sen. 2014. *A roadmap for patient and family engagement in healthcare practice and research.* http://patientfamilyengagement.org/#sthash.ZTrTAqkA.dpuf (accessed March 13, 2016).

Carlson, E. 2016. *Voluntary means voluntary: Coordinating Medicaid HCBS with family assistance.* http://www.justiceinaging.org/wp-content/uploads/2016/05/Voluntary-Means-Voluntary-Coordinating-Medicaid-HCBS-with-Family-Assistance.pdf (accessed June 26, 2016).

Carter, J. 2015. *Person-centered planning? Not without family caregivers!* http://www.americanbar.org/publications/bifocal/vol_37/issue_1_october2015/person_centered_planning.html (accessed December 2, 2015).

Charles, C., A. Gafni, and T. Whelan. 1999. Decision-making in the physician-patient encounter: Revisiting the shared treatment decision-making model. *Social Science & Medicine* 49(5):651-661.

Charles, K. K., and P. Sevak. 2005. Can family caregiving substitute for nursing home care? *Journal of Health Economics* 24(6):1174-1190.

Chewning, B., C. L. Bylund, B. Shah, N. K. Arora, J. A. Gueguen, and G. Makoul. 2012. Patient preferences for shared decisions: A systematic review. *Patient Education and Counseling* 86(1):9-18.

Clayman, M., D. Roter, L. Wissow, and K. Bandeen-Roche. 2005. Autonomy-related behaviors of patient companions and their effect on decision-making activity in geriatric primary care visits. *Social Science & Medicine* 60(7):1583-1591.

Clayman, M. L., G. Makoul, M. M. Harper, D. G. Koby, and A. R. Williams. 2012. Development of a shared decision making coding system for analysis of patient-healthcare provider encounters. *Patient Education and Counseling* 88(3):367-372.

Clifford, A., J. McCalman, R. Bainbridge, and K. Tsey. 2015. Interventions to improve cultural competency in health care for Indigenous peoples of Australia, New Zealand, Canada and the USA: A systematic review. *International Journal for Quality in Health Care* 27(2):89-98.

CMS (Centers for Medicare & Medicaid Services). 2013. *Revision to State Operations Manual (SOM), Hospital Appendix A—Interpretive guidelines for 42 CFR 482.43, discharge planning.* https://www.cms.gov/Medicare/Provider-Enrollment-and-Certification/Survey CertificationGenInfo/Downloads/Survey-and-Cert-Letter-13-32.pdf (accessed December 4, 2015).

CMS. 2014. Medicare and Medicaid program: Conditions of participation for home health agencies; proposed rule. *Federal Register* 79(196):61164-61213.

CMS. 2015. *Chronic care management services.* https://www.cms.gov/Outreach-and-Education/Medicare-Learning-Network-MLN/MLNProducts/Downloads/ChronicCare Management.pdf (accessed December 4, 2015).

CMS. 2016. *Frequently asked questions about billing the physician fee schedule for advance care planning services.* https://www.cms.gov/Medicare/Medicare-Fee-for-Service-Payment/PhysicianFeeSched/Downloads/FAQ-Advance-Care-Planning.pdf (accessed August 11, 2016).

Crotty, B. H., J. Walker, M. Dierks, L. Lipsitz, J. O'Brien, S. Fischer, W. V. Slack, and C. Safran. 2015. Information sharing preferences of older patients and their families. *JAMA Internal Medicine* 175(9):1492-1497.

Czaja, S. J., C. Zarcadoolas, W. L. Vaughon, C. C. Lee, M. L. Rockoff, and J. Levy. 2014. The usability of electronic personal health record systems for an underserved adult population. *Human Factors: The Journal of the Human Factors and Ergonomics Society* 57(3):491-506.

Davies, S., K. M. McDonald, E. Schmidt, E. Schultz, J. Geppert, and P. S. Romano. 2011. Expanding the uses of AHRQ's prevention quality indicators: Validity from the clinician perspective. *Medical Care* 49(8):679-685.

Dong, X., and M. A. Simon. 2013. Elder abuse as a risk factor for hospitalization in older persons. *JAMA Internal Medicine* 173(1):911-917.

Dy, S. M., and T. S. Purnell. 2012. Key concepts relevant to quality of complex and shared decision-making in health care: A literature review. *Social Science & Medicine* 74(4):582-587.

Edwards, A., and G. Elwyn, eds. 2009. *Shared decision-making in health care: Achieving evidence-based patient choice.* 2nd ed. New York: Oxford University Press.

Favreault, M., and J. Dey. 2015. *Long-term services and supports for older Americans.* http://aspe.hhs.gov/daltcp/reports/2015/ElderLTCrb.pdf (accessed December 4, 2015).

FCA (Family Caregiver Alliance). 2006. *Caregiver assessment: Report from a national consensus development conference (Volume 1-2).* San Francisco, CA: Family Caregiver Alliance.

Feinberg, L. F. 2012. *Moving toward person- and family-centered care.* Washington, DC: AARP Public Policy Institute.

Feinberg, L. F., and C. Levine. 2015. Family caregiving: Looking to the future. *Generations* 39(4):11-20.

Freund, T., S. M. Campbell, S. Geissler, C. U. Kunz, C. Mahler, F. Peters-Klimm, and J. Szecsenyi. 2013. Strategies for reducing potentially avoidable hospitalizations for ambulatory care-sensitive conditions. *Annals of Family Medicine* 11(4):363-370.

Fried, T. R. 2016. Shared decision making—Finding the sweet spot. *New England Journal of Medicine* 374(2):104-106.

Gage, B., and A. Albaroudi. 2015. The Triple Aim and the movement toward quality measurement of family caregiving. *Generations* 39(4):28-33.

Galantowicz, S., S. Crisp, N. Karp, and J. Accius. 2010. *Safe at home? Developing effective criminal background checks and other screening policies for home care workers.* http://assets.aarp.org/rgcenter/ppi/ltc/2009-12.pdf (accessed June 24, 2016).

Garvelink, M. M., P. A. Ngangue, R. Adekpedjou, N. T. Diouf, L. Goh, L. Blair, and F. Legare. 2016. A synthesis of knowledge about caregiver decision making finds gaps in support for those who care for aging loved ones. *Health Affairs* 35(4):619-626.

Gaugler, J. E., R. A. Kane, R. L. Kane, and R. Newcomer. 2005. Early community-based utilization and its effects on institutionalization in dementia caregiving. *The Gerontologist* 42(2):175-185.

Gaugler, J. E., M. Reese, and M. S. Mittelman. 2013. Effects of the NYU Caregiver Intervention-Adult Child on residential care placement. *The Gerontologist* 53(6):985-997.

Gitlin, L. N., M. Jacobs, and T. V. Earland. 2010. Translation of a dementia caregiver intervention for delivery in homecare as a reimbursable Medicare service: Outcomes and lessons learned. *The Gerontologist* 50(6):847-854.

Greene, M., R. Adelman, E. Friedmann, and R. Charon. 1994. Older patient satisfaction with communication during an initial medical encounter. *Social Science & Medicine* 38(9):1279-1288.

HHS (U.S. Department of Health and Human Services). 2013. *Working for Quality: 2013 annual progress report to Congress: National Strategy for Quality Improvement in Health Care.* http://www.ahrq.gov/workingforquality/nqs/nqs2013annlrpt.htm#improvequal (accessed June 20, 2014).

HHS. 2016. *HIPAA guidance materials.* http://www.hhs.gov/hipaa/for-professionals/privacy/guidance/index.html (accessed August 1, 2016).

Hickey, M. 1990. What are the needs of families of critically ill patients? A review of the literature since 1976. *Heart & Lung: The Journal of Acute and Critical Care* 19(4):401-415.

Hinton, L., C. E. Franz, G. Reddy, Y. Flores, R. L. Kravitz, J.C. Barker. 2007. Practice constraints, behavioral problems, and dementia care: Primary care physicians' perspectives. *Journal of General Internal Medicine* 22(11):1487-1492.

Horvat, L., D. Horey, P. Romios, and J. Kis-Rigo. 2014. Cultural competence education for health professionals. *Cochrane Database of Systematic Reviews* 5.

Hsiao, C. J., A. K. Jha, J. King, V. Patel, M. F. Furukawa, and F. Mostashari. 2013. Office-based physicians are responding to incentives and assistance by adopting and using electronic health records. *Health Affairs* 32(8):1470-1477.

IHI (Institute for Healthcare Improvement). 2014. *Always events getting started kit.* http://www.ihi.org/resources/Pages/Tools/AlwaysEventsGettingStartedKit.aspx (accessed April 5, 2016).

IOM (Institute of Medicine). 2000. *To err is human: Building a safer health system.* Washington, DC: National Academy Press.

IOM. 2001. *Crossing the quality chasm: A new health system for the 21st century.* Washington, DC: National Academy Press.

IOM. 2003. *Health professions education: A bridge to quality.* Washington, DC: The National Academies Press.

IOM. 2008. *Retooling for an aging America: Building the health care workforce.* Washington, DC: The National Academies Press.

IOM. 2012a. *The mental health and substance use workforce for older adults: In whose hands?* Washington, DC: The National Academies Press.

IOM. 2012b. *Best care at lower cost: The path to continuously learning health care in America.* Washington, DC: The National Academies Press.

IOM. 2014. *Graduate medical education that meets the nation's health needs.* Washington, DC: The National Academies Press.

IOM. 2015. *Vital signs: Core metrics for health and health care progress.* Washington, DC: The National Academies Press.

IOM and NRC (National Research Council). 2014. *Elder abuse and its prevention: Workshop summary.* Washington, DC: The National Academies Press.

Ishikawa, H., D. Roter, Y. Yamazaki, and T. Takayama. 2005. Physician-elderly patient-companion communication and roles of companions in Japanese geriatric encounters. *Social Science & Medicine* 60(10):2307-2320.

Ishikawa, H., D. Roter, Y. Yamazaki, H. Hashimoto, and E. Yano. 2006. Patients' perceptions of visit companions' helpfulness during Japanese geriatric medical visits. *Patient Education and Counseling* 61(1):80-86.

Justice, D., S. Holladay, T. Waidmann, E. G. Walsh, A. M. Greene, M. Morley, and W. Anderson. 2014. *Measurement, monitoring, and evaluation of state demonstrations to integrate care for dual eligible individuals' Washington managed fee-for-service evaluation design plan.* Waltham, MA: RTI International.

Kaye, H., C. Harrington, and M. LaPlante. 2010. Long-term care: Who gets it, who provides it, who pays, and how much? *Health Affairs* 29(1):11-21.

Kellermann, A. L., and S. S. Jones. 2013. What it will take to achieve the as-yet-unfulfilled promises of health information technology. *Health Affairs* 32(1):63-68.

Kelly, K., S. C. Reinhard, and A. Brooks-Danso. 2008. Professional partners supporting family caregivers. *American Journal of Nursing* 108(9):6-12.

Kelly, K., N. Wolfe, M. Gibson, and L. Feinberg. 2013. *Listening to family caregivers: The need to include caregiver assessment in Medicaid home and community-based service waiver programs.* Washington, DC: AARP.

Kiesler, D., and S. Auerbach. 2006. Optimal matches of patient preferences for information, decision-making and interpersonal behavior: Evidence, models and interventions. *Patient Education and Counseling* 61(3):319-341.

Kitko, L. A., J. E. Hupcey, C. Pinto, and M. Palese. 2015. Patient and caregiver incongruence in advanced heart failure. *Clinical Nursing Research* 24(4):388-400.

Komisar, H. L., and J. Feder. 2011. *Transforming care for Medicare beneficiaries with chronic conditions and long-term care needs: Coordinating care across all services.* http://www.thescanfoundation.org/sites/default/files/Georgetown_Trnsfrming_Care.pdf (accessed October 2, 2015).

Laidsaar-Powell, R. C., P. N. Butow, S. Bu, C. Charles, A. Gafni, W. W. T. Lam, J. Jansen, K. J. McCaffery, H. L. Shepherd, M. H. N. Tattersall, and I. Juraskova. 2013. Physician–patient–companion communication and decision-making: A systematic review of triadic medical consultations. *Patient Education and Counseling* 91(1):3-13.

Lavelle, B., D. Mancuso, A. Huber, and B. E. M. Felver. 2014. *Expanding eligibility for the Family Caregiver Support Program in SFY 2012: Updated findings (RDA Report 8.31).* https://www.dshs.wa.gov/sites/default/files/SESA/rda/documents/research-8-31.pdf (accessed March 13, 2016).

Leventhal, J. C., J. A. Cummins, P. H. Schwartz, D. K. Martin, and W. M. Tierney. 2015. Designing a system for patients controlling providers' access to their electronic health records: Organizational and technical challenges. *Journal of General Internal Medicine* 30(Suppl 1):17-24.

Levine, C. 2006. HIPAA and talking with family caregivers. *The American Journal of Nursing* 106(8):51-53.

Levine, C., and C. Zuckerman. 1999. The trouble with families: Toward an ethic of accommodation. *Annals of Internal Medicine* 130(2):148-152.

Levine, C., S. Albert, A. Hokenstad, D. Halper, A. Hart, and D. Gould. 2006. "This case is closed": Family caregivers and the termination of home health care services for stroke patients. *Milbank Quarterly* 84(2):305-331.

Levine, C., D. Halper, J. Rutberg, and D. A. Gould. 2013. *Engaging family caregivers as partners in transitions. TC–QuIC: A quality improvement collaborative.* https://www.uhfnyc.org/assets/1111 (accessed March 13, 2016).
Levinson, W., A. Kao, A. Kuby, and R. Thisted. 2005. Not all patients want to participate in decision making. A national study of public preferences. *Journal of General Internal Medicine* 20(6):531-535.
Lewis, L. 2008. Supporting family caregivers. Discussion and recommendations. *American Journal of Nursing* 108(9 Suppl):83-87.
Lobchuk, M. 2006. Concept analysis of perspective-taking: Meeting informal caregiver needs for communication competence and accurate perception. *Journal of Advanced Nursing* 54(3):330-341.
Long, K. H., J. P. Moriarty, M.S. Mittelman, and S. S. Foldes. 2013. Estimating the potential cost savings from the New York University Caregiver Intervention in Minnesota. *Health Affairs* 33(4):596-604.
Lotus Shyu, Y., M. Chen, and H. Lee. 2004. Caregivers' needs as predictors of hospital readmission for the elderly in Taiwan. *Social Science & Medicine* 58(7):1395-1403.
Lynn, J., A. McKethan, and A. K. Jha. 2015. Value-based payments require valuing what matters to patients. *JAMA* 314(14):1003-1004.
Mast, M. E., E. M. Sawin, and K. A. Pantaleo. 2012. Life of a caregiver simulation: Teaching students about frail older adults and their family caregivers. *Journal of Nursing Education* 51(7):396-402.
McClaran, J., R. Berglas, and E. Franco. 1996. Long hospital stays and need for alternate level of care at discharge. *Canadian Family Physician* 42:449-461.
McDaniel, S., T. Campell, J. Hepworth, and A. Lorenz. 2005. *Family-oriented primary care*, 2nd ed. New York: Springer.
Messecar, D. C. 2012. *Nursing Standard of Practice Protocol: Family caregiving.* https://consultgeri.org/geriatric-topics/family-caregiving (accessed March 13, 2016).
Miller, E., and W. Weissert. 2000. Predicting elderly people's risk for nursing home placement, hospitalization, functional impairment, and mortality: A synthesis. *Medical Care Research Review* 57(3):259-297.
Miller, M. 2012. Did expanding eligibility for family caregiver support program pay for itself by reducing the use of Medicaid-paid long-term care? Olympia: Washington State Institute for Public Policy.
Mission Analytics Group. 2013. *The Balancing Incentive Program: Implementation manual.* https://www.medicaid.gov/medicaid-chip-program-information/by-topics/long-term-services-and-supports/balancing/downloads/bip-manual.pdf (accessed December 4, 2015).
Mitnick, S., C. Leffler, and V. Hood. 2010. Family caregivers, patients and physicians: Ethical guidance to optimize relationships. *Journal of General Internal Medicine* 25(3):255-260.
Mittleman, M. S., W. E. Haley, O. J. Clay, and D. L. Roth. 2006. Improving caregiver well-being delays nursing home placement of patients with Alzheimer's disease. *Neurology* 67(9):1592-1599.
Moon, H., A. L. Townsend, C. J. Whitlatch, and P. Dilworth-Anderson. 2016. Quality of life for dementia caregiving dyads: Effects of incongruent perceptions of everyday care and values. *The Gerontologist* Epub April 5.
NAC (National Alliance for Caregiving) and AARP Public Policy Institute. 2015a. *Caregivers of older adults: A focused look at those caring for someone age 50+.* http://www.aarp.org/content/dam/aarp/ppi/2015/caregivers-of-older-adults-focused-look.pdf (accessed August 5, 2015).
Nath, P. A., and C. D. Sharp. 2015. A user-centered design approach to information sharing for older patients and their families. *JAMA Internal Medicine* 175(9):1498-1499.

National Association of Social Workers. 2010. *NASW standards for social work practice with family caregivers of older adults.* http://www.socialworkers.org/practice/standards/Family_Caregivers_Older_Adults.aspNational (accessed October 6, 2016).

National Priorities Partnership. 2011. *Priorities for the National Quality Strategy.* http://www.qualityforum.org/Setting_Priorities/NPP/National_Priorities_Partnership.aspx (accessed December 4, 2015).

Newcomer, R. J., T. Kang, and P. Doty. 2012. Allowing spouses to be paid personal care providers: Spouse availability and effects on Medicaid-funded service use and expenditures. *The Gerontologist* 52(4):517-530.

NQF (National Quality Forum). 2014a. *Priority setting for healthcare performance measurement: Addressing performance measure gaps in person-centered care and outcomes.* http://www.qualityforum.org/Publications/2014/08/Priority_Setting_for_Healthcare_Performance_Measurement__Addressing_Performance_Measure_Gaps_in_Person-Centered_Care_and_Outcomes.aspx (accessed December 4, 2015).

NQF. 2014b. *Priority setting for health care performance measurement: Addressing performance measure gaps for dementia, including Alzheimer's disease.* http://www.qualityforum.org/priority_setting_for_healthcare_performance_measurement_alzheimers_disease.aspx (accessed April 19, 2016).

NQF. 2015. *Addressing performance measure gaps in home and community-based services to support community living: Initial components of the conceptual framework: Interim report.* http://www.qualityforum.org/Projects/h/Home_and_Community-Based_Services_Quality/Interim_Report.aspx (accessed March 13, 2016).

NRCPDS (National Resource Center for Participant-Directed Services). 2014. *Facts and figures. 2013 National Inventory Survey of Participant Direction.* https://nrcpds.bc.edu/details.php?entryid=445 (accessed December 4, 2015).

O'Keefe, J., P. Saucier, B. Jackson, R. Cooper, E. McKenney, S. Crisp, and C. Moseley. 2010. *Understanding Medicaid home and community services: A primer.* http://aspe.hhs.gov/daltcp/reports/2010/primer10.pdf (accessed December 14, 2015).

Osborn, C. Y., S. T. Rosenbloom, S. P. Stenner, S. Anders, S. Muse, K. B. Johnson, J. Jirjis, and G. P. Jackson. 2011. MyHealthAtVanderbilt: Policies and procedures governing patient portal functionality. *Journal of the American Medical Informatics Association* 18(Suppl 1):i18-i23.

Parker, M. W., J. S. Greenberg, M. R. Malick, G. M. Simpson, E. H. Namkung, and R. Toseland. 2016. Caregivers to older and disabled adults. In *The Oxford Handbook of Social Work in Health and Aging*, 2nd ed., edited by D. Kaplan and B. Berkman. Oxford, UK: Oxford University Press. Pp. 443-452.

Petronio, S., J. Sargent, L. Andea, P. Reganis, and D. Cichocki. 2004. Family and friends as healthcare advocates: Dilemmas of confidentiality and privacy. *Journal of Social and Personal Relationships* 21(1):33-52.

Picone, G., R. M. Wilson, and S. Chou. 2003. Analysis of hospital length of stay and discharge destination using hazard functions with unmeasured heterogeneity. *Health Economics* 12(12):1021-1034.

Pope, T. M. 2012. Legal fundamentals of surrogate decision making. *CHEST Journal* 141(4):1074-1081.

Price, E. L., S. Bereknyei, A. Kuby, W. Levinson, and C. H. Braddock, 3rd. 2012. New elements for informed decision making: A qualitative study of older adults' views. *Patient Education Counseling* 86(3):335-341.

Procter, S., J. Wilcockson, P. Pearson, and V. Allgar. 2001. Going home from the hospital: The carer/patient dyad. *Journal of Advanced Nursing* 35(2):206-217.

PSTT (HealthIT Privacy & Security Tiger Team). 2014. *Epic patient portal use by proxies.* Washington, DC: Health Information Technology Policy Committee, Privacy and Security Tiger Team. http://www.healthit.gov/FACAS/calendar/2014/02/10/policy-privacysecurity-tiger-team (accessed June 4, 2014).

Rabow, M. W., S. Goodman, S. Chang, M. Berger, and S. Folkman. 2010. Filming the family: A documentary film to educate clinicians about family caregivers of patients with brain tumors. *Journal of Cancer Education* 25(2):242-246.

Rajkumar, R., A. Patel, K. Murphy, J. M. Colmers, J. D. Blum, P. H. Conway, and J. M. Sharfstein. 2014. Maryland's all-payer approach to delivery-system reform. *New England Journal of Medicine* 370(6):493-495.

Ricciardi, L., F. Mostashari, J. Murphy, J. G. Daniel, and E. P. Siminerio. 2013. A national action plan to support consumer engagement via e-health. *Health Affairs* 32(2):376-384.

Sands, L. P., H. Xu, J. Thomas, S. Paul, B. A. Craig, M. Rosenman, C. C. Doebbeling, and M. Weiner. 2012. Volume of home- and community-based services and time to nursing-home placement. *Medicare & Medicaid Research and Review* 2(3):E1-E20.

Sarkar, U., and D. W. Bates. 2014. Care partners and online patient portals. *JAMA* 311(4): 357-358.

Schulz R., S. R. Beach, J. T. Matthews, K. Courtney, A. DeVito Dabbs, L. Person Mecca. 2015. Caregivers' willingness to pay for technologies to support caregiving. *The Gerontologist* Epub April 9.

Schwarz, K., and C. Elman. 2003. Identification of factors predictive of hospital readmissions for patients with heart failure. *Heart & Lung: The Journal of Acute and Critical Care* 32(2):88-99.

Shin, D. W., J. Cho, D. L. Roter, S. Y. Kim, S. K. Sohn, M. S. Yoon, Y. W. Kim, B. Cho, and J. H. Park. 2013. Preferences for and experiences of family involvement in cancer treatment decision-making: Patient-caregiver dyads study. *Psychooncology* 22(11):2624-2631.

Shugarman, L., A. Buttar, B. Fries, T. Moore, and C. Blaum. 2002. Caregiver attitudes and hospitalization risk in Michigan residents receiving home- and community-based care. *Journal of the American Geriatrics Society* 50(6):1079-1085.

Silver, H., N. Wellman, D. Galindo-Ciocon, and P. Johnson. 2004. Family caregivers of older adults on home enteral nutrition have multiple unmet task-related training needs and low overall preparedness for caregiving. *Journal of the American Dietetic Association* 104(1):43-50.

Spillman, B. C., and S. K. Long. 2009. Does high caregiver stress predict nursing home entry? *INQUIRY: The Journal of Health Care Organization, Provision, and Financing* 46(2):140-161.

Srivastava, R. 2010. The power proxy. *New England Journal of Medicine* 363(19):1786-1789.

Stacey, D., J. Kryworuchko, C. Bennett, M. A. Murray, S. Mullan, and F. Legare. 2012. Decision coaching to prepare patients for making health decisions: A systematic review of decision coaching in trials of patient decision aids. *Medical Decision Making* 32(3):E22-E33.

Strong, D. M., S. A. Johnson, B. Tulu, J. Trudel, O. Volkoff, L. R. Pelletier, I. Bar-On, and L. Garber. 2014. A theory of organization-EHR affordance actualization. *Journal of the Association for Information Systems* 15(2):53.

Thorpe, J. M., B. L. Sleath, C. T. Thorpe, C. H. Van Houtven, S. J. Blalock, L. R. Landerman, W. H. Campbell, and E. C. Clipp. 2006. Caregiver psychological distress as a barrier to influenza vaccination among community-dwelling elderly with dementia. *Medical Care* 44(8):713-721.

Tierney, W. M., S. A. Alpert, A. Byrket, K. Caine, J. C. Leventhal, E. M. Meslin, and P. H. Schwartz. 2015. Provider responses to patients controlling access to their electronic health records: A prospective cohort study in primary care. *Journal of General Internal Medicine* 30(Suppl 1):31-37.

Torke, A. M., S. Petronio, C. E. Purnell, G. A. Sachs, P. R. Helft, and C. M. Callahan. 2012. Communicating with clinicians: The experiences of surrogate decision-makers for hospitalized older adults. *Journal of the American Geriatrics Society* 60(8):1401-1407.

Urbanik, C., and M. Lobchuk. 2009. Encouraging family caregivers to "step inside the patient's shoes." *Home Healthcare Now* 27(4):213-218.

Van Houtven, C. H., and E. C. Norton. 2004. Informal care and health care use of older adults. *Journal of Health Economics* 23(6):1159-1180.

Van Houtven, C. H., and E. C. Norton. 2008. Informal care and Medicare expenditures: Testing for heterogeneous treatment effects. *Journal of Health Economics* 27(1):134-156.

Vig, E., H. Starks, J. Taylor, E. Hopley, and K. Fryer-Edwards. 2007. Surviving surrogate decision-making: What helps and hampers the experience of making medical decisions for others. *Journal of General Internal Medicine* 22(9):1274-1279.

Vladeck, B. C., and E. Westphal. 2012. Dignity-driven decision making: A compelling strategy for improving care for people with advanced illness. *Health Affairs* 31(6):1269-1276.

vom Eigen, K., J. Walker, S. Edgman-Levitan, P. Cleary, and T. Delbanco. 1999. Care partner experiences with hospital care. *Medical Care* 37(1):33-38.

Wendler, D., and A. Rid. 2011. Systematic review: The effect on surrogates of making treatment decisions for others. *Annals of Internal Medicine* 154(5):336-346.

White House. 2011. *National strategy for trusted identities in cyberspace: Enhancing online choice, efficiency, security, and privacy.* http://www.whitehouse.gov/sites/default/files/rss_viewer/NSTICstrategy_041511.pdf (accessed July 12, 2014).

Whitlatch, C. J. and L. F. Feinberg. 2007. Family care and decision making. In *Dementia and social work practice: Research and interventions*, edited by C. Cox. New York: Springer. Pp. 129-148.

WHO (World Health Organization). 1991. *Statistical indices of family health.*

Wolff, J. L., and C. M. Boyd. 2015. A look at person- and family-centered care among older adults: Results from a national survey. *Journal of General Internal Medicine* 30(10):1497-1504.

Wolff, J. L., and J. D. Kasper. 2004. Informal caregiver characteristics and subsequent hospitalization outcomes among recipients of care. *Aging Clinical and Experimental Research* 16(4):307-313.

Wolff, J. L., and D. L. Roter. 2008. Hidden in plain sight: Medical visit companions as a quality of care resource for vulnerable older adults. *Archives of Internal Medicine* 168(13):1409-1415.

Wolff, J. L., and D. L. Roter. 2011. Family presence in routine medical visits: A meta-analytical review. *Social Science & Medicine* 72(6):823-831.

Wolff, J. L., and D. L. Roter. 2012. Older adults' mental health function and patient-centered care: Does the presence of a family companion help or hinder communication? *Journal of General Internal Medicine* 27(6):661-668.

Wolff, J. L., and B. C. Spillman. 2014. Older adults receiving assistance with physician visits and prescribed medications and their family caregivers: Prevalence, characteristics, and hours of care. *The Journals of Gerontology Series B, Psychological Sciences and Social Sciences* 69(Suppl 1):S65-S72.

Wolff, J. L., M. Clayman, P. Rabins, M. Cooke, and D. Roter. 2015. An exploration of patient and family engagement in routine primary care visits. *Health Expectations* 18(2):188-198.

Wolff, J. L., J. D. Darer, and K. L. Larsen. 2016a. Family caregivers and consumer health information technology. *Journal of General Internal Medicine* 31(1):117-121.

Wolff, J. L., B. C. Spillman, V. A. Freedman, and J. D. Kasper. 2016b. A national profile of family and unpaid caregivers who assist older adults with health care activities. *JAMA Internal Medicine* 176(3):372-379.

Zulman, D. M., K. M. Nazi, C. L. Turvey, T. H. Wagner, S. S. Woods, and L. C. An. 2011. Patient interest in sharing personal health record information: A Web-based survey. *Annals of Internal Medicine* 155(12):805-810.

Zulman, D. M., J. D. Piette, E. C. Jenchura, S. M. Asch, and A. M. Rosland. 2013. Facilitating out-of-home caregiving through health information technology: Survey of informal caregivers' current practices, interests, and perceived barriers. *Journal of Medical Internet Research* 15(7):e123.

7

Recommendations to Support Family Caregivers of Older Adults

AN URGENT NEED FOR ACTION

This report raises serious concerns about the current state of family caregiving of older adults in the United States. A confluence of social and demographics trends along with the increasing complexity of our health care and long-term services and supports (LTSS) systems have substantial implications for the nation's family caregivers. These trends, described in the previous chapters, indicate not only a growing demand for families to provide eldercare but also growing evidence that caregiving itself poses risks—mental, physical, and economic—for some people.

A number of factors underscore the urgency of addressing the needs of family caregivers of older adults. The committee's review of the older population and their caregivers, presented in Chapter 2, indicates a growing gap between the demand for and supply of family caregivers for older adults. The demand for caregivers is increasing significantly not only because of sheer numbers but also because the fastest growing cohort of older adults in the United States are those age 80 and older—the age when people are most likely to have a significant physical or cognitive impairment or both. At the same time, the size of American families is shrinking and the makeup of families is changing as more people do not have children, never marry, divorce, or blend families through remarriage. Moreover, half of family caregivers are employed.

Chapter 3 described the increasingly complex and demanding roles that caregivers are expected to take on. Family caregivers—especially women—have always provided the lion's share of LTSS to older adults with impairments. Today, they are also tasked with managing difficult technical and medical procedures and equipment in older adults' homes, overseeing medications, and monitoring symptoms and side effects. Caregiving's impact is highly individual and dependent on personal and family circumstances. For some people, caregiving can instill confidence, provide meaning and purpose, enhance skills, and bring the caregiver closer to the older adult. For others, caregiving takes a toll. An extensive literature finds that, compared to non-caregivers, family caregivers of older adults are more likely to experience emotional distress, depression, anxiety, or social isolation. Some caregivers, compared to others, are more likely to report being in poor physical health and have elevated levels of stress hormones or higher rates of chronic disease. The intensity and duration of caregiving and the older adult's level of impairment are consistent predictors of negative health effects. Family members who spend long hours caring for older relatives with advanced dementia, for example, are especially at risk. Other risk factors include low socioeconomic status, high levels of perceived suffering of the care recipient, living with the care recipient, lack of choice in taking on the caregiving role, poor physical health of the caregiver, lack of social support, and a physical home environment that makes care tasks difficult.

Chapter 4 reviewed the economic risks associated with family caregiving of older adults—finding that research consistently shows that family caregivers of significantly impaired older adults are particularly vulnerable to financial harm. Caregivers may lose income, Social Security and other retirement benefits, and career opportunities if they have to cut back on work hours or leave the workforce. They may also incur substantial out-of-pocket expenses that may undermine their own future financial security.

Chapter 5 described the growing body of research providing important insights into how to effectively support family caregivers. The most effective interventions begin with an assessment of caregivers' risks, needs, strengths, and preferences. Education and skills training can improve caregiver confidence and ability to manage daily care challenges. Counseling, self-care, relaxation training, and respite programs can improve both the caregiver's and care recipient's quality of life. Some research also suggests that providing services, such as personal counseling and care management, may delay the care recipient's institutionalization and reduce re-hospitalization.

In order to fulfill the numerous roles that they play, family caregivers must interact with a wide range of providers and navigate within a variety of systems. They interact with physicians, physician assistants, nurses, nurse practitioners, social workers, psychologists, pharmacists, physical and occupational therapists, direct care workers (e.g., certified nursing assistants, home health aides, and personal care aides), and others. They serve as key sources of information about older adults' health histories, the medications they are taking, past diagnoses, previous treatments and surgeries, and adverse reactions to any drugs (especially if the older adult is forgetful or has dementia). They represent older adults in dealings with home health care agencies, physicians' and other providers' offices, hospitals, pharmacies, assisted living facilities, and nursing homes. Yet, the organizations and systems that serve older adults—and the third-party payers that finance most care—too often act as barriers to caregivers' effective engagement even when the caregiver is expected to coordinate and provide care.

RECOMMENDATIONS

The committee's review of family caregiving for older Americans confirms how essential family caregivers are to both health care and LTSS for older Americans. The committee recognizes that family caregiving for older adults is, and will always be, an intensely personal issue. But the committee also recognizes that family caregiving has become a critical issue of public policy. The committee's work calls into question practices that too often assume the availability of family caregiving without adequate support services that take into account both the individual and the family. In fact, family caregivers often feel invisible, isolated, and unprepared for the tasks they are expected to perform, and caregiving—especially when it involves an intensive commitment over the long term—carries significant costs. Furthermore, the nation faces a growing gap between the numbers of older people in need of support and the numbers of family members able and willing to support them.

The time has come for public acknowledgment of caregiving families—to make caregiving an integral part of the nation's collective responsibility for caring for its older adult population. Family caregivers are the mainstay of support for older persons with a chronic, disabling, or serious health condition. In today's world, family caregivers cannot be expected to provide complex care and support on their own. Family caregivers need greater recognition, information, and meaningful support to help them care for older relatives or friends, and to maintain their own health, financial security, and well-being.

To that end, the committee calls for a transformation in the policies and practices affecting the role of families in the support and care of older adults. Today's emphasis on person-centered care needs to evolve into a focus on person- and family-centered care. The committee's recommendations are presented in Box 7-1 and described below.

The committee recognizes that a strategy to effectively engage and support family caregivers of older Americans cannot be adopted and implemented overnight. In many cases, policy initiatives will have to be developed and evaluated. Implementation will require substantial administrative

BOX 7-1
Recommendations

RECOMMENDATION 1: The committee calls upon the Administration that takes office in January 2017 to take steps to address the health, economic, and social issues facing family caregivers of older Americans. Specifically, the committee recommends that:

The Secretary of the U.S. Department of Health and Human Services, in collaboration with the Secretaries of the U.S. Departments of Labor and Veterans Affairs, other federal agencies, and private-sector organizations with expertise in family caregiving, develop and execute a National Family Caregiver Strategy that, administratively or through new federal legislation, explicitly and systematically addresses and supports the essential role of family caregivers to older adults. This strategy should include specific measures to adapt the nation's health care and long-term services and supports (LTSS) systems and workplaces to effectively and respectfully engage family caregivers and to support their health, values, and social and economic well-being, and to address the needs of our increasingly culturally and ethnically diverse caregiver population.

The Secretaries should publicly announce and begin to implement the strategy by

1. executing steps allowable under current statutory authority;
2. proposing specific legislative action, where appropriate, to address additional steps;
3. convening and establishing partnerships with appropriate government (federal, state, and local) and private-sector leaders to implement the strategy throughout education, service delivery, research, and practice; and
4. addressing fully and explicitly the needs of our increasingly culturally and ethnically diverse caregiver population.

The Secretaries should issue biannual reports on progress and actions of the National Family Caregiver Strategy.

This strategy should include the following steps:

RECOMMENDATION 1-a: Develop, test, and implement effective mechanisms within Medicare, Medicaid, and the U.S. Department of Veterans Affairs to ensure that family caregivers are routinely identified and that their needs are assessed and supported in the delivery of health care and long-term services and supports.

RECOMMENDATION 1-b: Direct the Centers for Medicare & Medicaid Services to develop, test, and implement provider payment reforms that motivate providers to engage family caregivers in delivery processes, across all modes of payment and models of care.

RECOMMENDATION 1-c: Strengthen the training and capacity of health care and social service providers to recognize and to engage family caregivers and to provide them evidence-based supports and referrals to services in the community.

RECOMMENDATION 1-d: Increase funding for programs that provide explicit supportive services for family caregivers such as the National Family Caregiver Support Program and other relevant U.S. Department of Health and Human Services programs to facilitate the development, dissemination, and implementation of evidence-based caregiver intervention programs.

RECOMMENDATION 1-e: Explore, evaluate, and, as warranted, adopt federal policies that provide economic support for working caregivers.

RECOMMENDATION 1-f: Expand the data collection infrastructures within the U.S. Departments of Health and Human Services, Labor, and Veterans Affairs to facilitate monitoring, tracking, and reporting on the experience of family caregivers.

RECOMMENDATION 1-g: Launch a multi-agency research program sufficiently robust to evaluate caregiver interventions in real-world health care and community settings, across diverse conditions and populations, and with respect to a broad array of outcomes.

RECOMMENDATION 2: State governments that have yet to address the health, economic, and social challenges of caregiving for older adults should learn from the experience of states with caregiver supports, and implement similar programs.

RECOMMENDATION 3: The Secretaries of the U.S. Departments of Health and Human Services, Labor, and Veterans Affairs should work with leaders in health care and long-term services and supports delivery, technology, and philanthropy to establish a public–private, multi-stakeholder innovation fund for research and innovation to accelerate the pace of change in addressing the needs of caregiving families.

RECOMMENDATION 4: In all the above actions, explicitly and consistently address families' diversity in assessing caregiver needs and in developing, testing, and implementing caregiver supports.

time and managerial investment. Effectiveness over time will depend on continued improvement through research, evaluation, and experience. And new policies will carry new costs that should be recognized and accounted for. Caregiver supports, like paid family leave, will entail new expenditures that should be financed. Evidence indicates that some portion of new investments will be offset by savings—from reductions in use of nursing home, home health, emergency room, and inpatient hospital care. The committee does not assume, however, that these savings will be sufficient to fully support this report's recommendations. Fundamental to the strategy we call for should be both rigorous evaluation and transparency as to costs as well as benefits and, as appropriate, sufficient financing should be secured to support investments that improve family caregivers' health, economic, and social well-being.

The committee also recognizes that the context for this report is a time of economic constraints, concerns about future financing of Medicare and Social Security, a wide range of competing demands for public dollars, and deep divisions among Americans about the role and size of government. Nevertheless, the rapid aging of the U.S. population and its impact on families and health care expenditures should not be ignored. If the needs of our older adults' caregivers are not addressed, we, as a society, risk compromising the well-being of our elders and their families. Failure to take on these challenges also means a lost opportunity to discover the potential societal benefits of effectively engaging and supporting family caregivers in the care of older adults—both economic and otherwise. The public's investment in family caregiving for older adults should be carefully considered and public dollars shepherded responsibly. As federal and state agencies move to develop new programs and supports to address the needs of family caregivers, it will be important to prioritize the needs of the most vulnerable caregivers and tailor eligibility appropriately.

RECOMMENDATION 1: The committee calls upon the Administration that takes office in January 2017 to take steps to address the health, economic, and social issues facing family caregivers of older Americans. Specifically, the committee recommends that:

The Secretary of the U.S. Department of Health and Human Services, in collaboration with the Secretaries of the U.S. Departments of Labor and Veterans Affairs, other federal agencies, and private-sector organizations with expertise in family caregiving, develop and execute a National Family Caregiver Strategy that, administratively or through new federal legislation, explicitly and systematically addresses and supports the essential role of family caregivers to older adults. This strategy should include specific measures to

adapt the nation's health care and long-term services and supports (LTSS) systems and workplaces to effectively and respectfully engage family caregivers and to support their health, values, and social and economic well-being, and to address the needs of our increasingly culturally and ethnically diverse caregiver population.

The Secretaries should publicly announce and begin to implement the strategy by

1. executing steps allowable under current statutory authority;
2. proposing specific legislative action, where appropriate, to address additional steps;
3. convening and establishing partnerships with appropriate government (federal, state, and local) and private-sector leaders to implement the strategy throughout education, service delivery, research, and practice; and
4. addressing fully and explicitly the needs of our increasingly culturally and ethnically diverse caregiver population.

The Secretaries should issue biannual reports on progress and actions of the National Family Caregiver Strategy.

This strategy should include the following steps:

RECOMMENDATION 1-a: Develop, test, and implement effective mechanisms within Medicare, Medicaid, and the U.S. Department of Veterans Affairs to ensure that family caregivers are routinely identified and that their needs are assessed and supported in the delivery of health care and long-term services and supports.

Despite the integral role that family caregivers play in the care of older adults with disabilities and complex health needs, they are often marginalized or ignored in the delivery of health care, in LTSS, and in public policy. Paradoxically, family caregivers may be excluded from treatment decisions and care planning but at the same time implicitly assumed to be available and expected to perform necessary health management and personal tasks, and care coordination activities to implement older adults' care plans. Providers' assumptions that family caregivers have the requisite knowledge, skills, and resources to administer care may put family caregivers and the adults they care for in harm's way.

The research reviewed in this report provides compelling evidence of the need for caregiver assessment. Caregiver's circumstances vary widely and in ways that affect their availability, capacity, and willingness to assume critical responsibilities. Evidence from randomized clinical trials indicates that most effective interventions begin with an assessment of the caregiver's risks, needs, strengths, and preferences. Yet, most health and LTSS providers do not assess the health, skills, employment, and willingness of family caregivers and provide them little, if any, training to carry out the complicated medical procedures, personal care, and care coordination tasks they are expected to provide. Indeed, the lack of systematic assessment of family participation in health and LTSS not only affects the experience of family caregivers and care recipients, it also precludes knowledge of how their involvement influences the quality of clinical care and social services, limits the spread of evidence-based interventions that strengthen the well-being of family caregivers and their ability to promote and provide quality care, and undermines credible accounting of the value family caregivers bring to the health care delivery system and to society.

Given the growing national commitment to accountability and efficiency in care delivery, the committee concludes that the time is ripe to elevate family-centered care alongside person-centered care to the forefront of delivery system reform—rationalizing the roles of family caregivers and better supporting their involvement in the delivery process. Achieving that goal will require systematic attention to the identification, assessment, and support of family caregivers throughout the care delivery process by

- identifying family caregivers in both the care recipient's and the caregiver's medical record;
- screening family caregivers to identify those who are at risk themselves, or whose circumstances place the older adults they assist in harm's way;
- assessing family caregivers' strengths, limits, needs, and risks across the full range of expected tasks—medical care, personal care, and coordination—and that, at a minimum, asks family caregivers about their own health and well-being, level of stress, and types of training and supports they might need to continue their role; and
- assuring that identification, screening, and appropriate caregiver assessment occurs at each point in care delivery for the care recipient—including delivery of publicly funded LTSS, annual wellness exams, physician visits, admission and discharge for hospitals and emergency rooms, and chronic care coordination and care transition programs.

Key initial steps to implementing this recommendation will require identification and refinement of caregiver assessment tools appropriate to the care delivery context of the care recipient, identification and training of assessors, and evaluation of provider workflow to determine where and when assessments take place.

RECOMMENDATION 1-b: Direct the Centers for Medicare & Medicaid Services to develop, test, and implement provider payment reforms that motivate providers to engage family caregivers in delivery processes, across all modes of payment and models of care.

As the predominant payers of care for older adults, Medicare and Medicaid are essential to motivating appropriate provider practice. Under the status quo, there are few financial incentives for providers to identify, engage, or support an older adult's caregiver. The organization, delivery, and financing of health care and LTSS are designed to provide needed services to individuals not families. Caregiver interventions shown to be effective, and potentially cost saving (in the aggregate), will not proliferate if payment policy discourages identification of caregivers who might benefit from their use.

Chapter 6 described the encouraging steps that the Centers for Medicare & Medicaid Services (CMS) has made to advance recognition of family caregivers in Medicare and Medicaid coverage, payment, and delivery policies. For example, as a condition of participation in Medicare, hospitals are now expected to engage and support family caregivers in the discharge planning process. However, Medicare is rapidly moving away from fee-for-service (FFS) payment to managed care and other models of payment and care delivery.

Innovative delivery mechanisms, such as accountable care organizations and other models of integrated health care services, and value-based payment methods implicitly encourage providers (through shared savings for quality care at lower costs) to actively engage family caregivers as a resource in the care delivery process. In some state Medicaid programs, assessment of family caregivers' needs is part of care planning for beneficiaries eligible for home- and community-based services. Yet, neither CMS nor the states have paid explicit attention to evaluating the effect of these innovations on caregiving. The Center for Medicare & Medicaid Innovation (CMMI), for example, is specifically charged with testing new payment and service delivery models, but its evaluations neither measure nor assess important caregiver and care recipient outcomes. In the U.S. Department of Veterans Affairs (VA), the Caregivers and Veterans Omnibus Health Services Act of 2010[1] established a mechanism for reimbursement/workload credit for services provided to family caregivers but the focus is primarily on caregivers of younger veterans.

---

[1] Public Law 111-163.

Thus, for the most part, these advances create the potential for, rather than a commitment to, developing effective payment practices that support provider engagement with family caregivers. That commitment requires

- the development and application of payment mechanisms to promote providers' interaction with family caregivers when care recipients are not present;
- the development and application of performance standards that hold providers accountable for caregiver engagement, training, and support in accessing the full range of health care and LTSS they require, by explicitly including caregiver outcomes in quality measures;
- the inclusion of family caregivers in CMS payment and service delivery demonstrations; and
- adherence to the National Standards for Culturally and Linguistically Appropriate Services in Health and Health Care to provide quality care that is effective, equitable, understandable, respectful, and responsive to older adults' and caregivers' cultural health beliefs and practices, preferred languages, health literacy, and other communication needs.

RECOMMENDATION 1-c: **Strengthen the training and capacity of health care and social service providers to recognize and to engage family caregivers and to provide them evidence-based supports and referrals to services in the community.**

To ensure high-quality person- and family-centered care by the health and LTSS workforce, providers should see family caregivers not just as a resource in the treatment or support of an older person, but also as both a partner in that enterprise and as someone who may need information, training, care, and support. Achieving and acting on that perspective requires that providers have the skills to recognize a caregiver's presence, assess whether and how the caregiver can best participate in overall care, engage and share information with the caregiver, recognize the caregiver's own health care and support needs, and refer caregivers to needed services and supports.

It is also important that providers understand that the Health Insurance Portability and Accountability Act (HIPAA) does not preclude sharing older adults' health records with caregivers. Misinterpretation of the statute appears to be common and may prevent caregivers from obtaining timely information about care recipients' health status and treatment.

A wide range of professionals and direct care workers are likely to serve older adults with family caregivers—physicians, nurses, social workers, psychologists, pharmacists, occupational therapists, physical and other rehabilitation therapists, certified nursing assistants, physician assistants, and others. Professional organizations in social work and nursing have led the way in taking steps to establish standards for person- and family-centered care. Similar efforts are needed across the health care and social service professions. The Health Resources and Services Administration's Geriatric Workforce Enhancement Program (GWEP) provides some needed training in geriatrics among health professionals as well as family caregivers and direct care workers. However, with current funding, the GWEP caregiver curriculum focuses primarily on dementia and reaches only a small fraction of the relevant providers. Work to date falls far short of a systematic and comprehensive effort that should include

- identification of specific competencies, by provider type, to demonstrate effective practice, including competencies related to working with diverse family caregivers;
- development of educational curricula and training to instill those competencies;
- incorporation of those competencies into requirements for licensure, certification, and accreditation;
- articulation of standards of practice; and
- evaluation of practice using standardized quality-of-care metrics.

The federal government, in collaboration with professional societies, education programs, licensure and certification bodies, accrediting bodies, and other organizations, should move this effort forward. Specifically, action requires

- federal support for the development and enforcement of competencies for identifying, assessing, and supporting family caregivers by health care and human service professionals and regulatory and accrediting organizations;
- the U.S. Department of Health and Human Services (HHS) Office for Civil Rights to clarify caregivers' access to information by providing administrative guidance to health care and social service providers regarding the permitted uses and disclosures of protected health information to family caregivers and encourage providers to train their workforce regarding that clarification;
- convening professional societies, training programs, accrediting bodies, and other organizations to develop educational curricula and to support their systematic evaluation and implementation; and

- convening and collaborating with state agencies and professional organizations to incorporate competencies into standards for licensure and certification.

RECOMMENDATION 1-d: Increase funding for programs that provide explicit supportive services for family caregivers such as the National Family Caregiver Support Program and other relevant U.S. Department of Health and Human Services programs to facilitate the development, dissemination, and implementation of evidence-based caregiver intervention programs.

National policy regarding family caregivers exists mainly in narrowly focused programs. Most of the related federal programs have more indirect than direct implications for family caregivers of older adults because the caregivers are not the primary intended beneficiaries. In 2000, Congress explicitly recognized the importance of caregivers by creating the National Family Caregiver Support Program (NFCSP) under the Older Americans Act, the first and only federal program to specifically address the needs of family caregivers of older individuals and help them access services. The NFCSP is a program of the Administration for Community Living (ACL). In 2015, the program served more than 900,000 individual family caregivers of older adults, providing counseling, training, respite care, and information about available services and supports or assistance with getting access to services. The annual appropriation for the program is around $150 million and has not increased since 2000 despite the marked growth in the older adult population and the increasingly complex services that caregivers are expected to provide. The funding is inadequate and Congress should consider increasing its appropriation. The evaluation of the NFCSP that is currently underway may provide guidance in defining priorities for targeting increased funding.

The Secretary should direct not only ACL but other HHS agencies to develop, disseminate, and implement evidence-based caregiver intervention programs—many of which have been developed with funding from the National Institutes of Health (NIH) and other federal research agencies. A robust body of research demonstrates that interventions aimed at supporting caregivers can significantly improve well-being, quality of life, and quality of care for both family caregivers and care recipients. Interventions that have been tested through well-designed trials have involved (separately or in combination) a broad range of therapeutic techniques, been applied in a variety of settings, and been evaluated for a broad set of impacts for the caregiver and the care recipient. As noted earlier, key findings from this research are that

- education and skills training can improve caregiver confidence in managing daily care challenges;
- caregiver skill building and environmental modifications can improve quality of life for family caregivers and care recipients; and
- interventions to support caregivers have been shown to decrease resource use including reduced care recipient readmissions, shorter lengths of hospital stay, and delayed institutionalization.

Research also provides important lessons regarding what distinguishes effective from ineffective interventions. Specifically, caregiver interventions are more likely to be effective when they

- address multiple areas of caregiver risk or need, including their own self-care and preventive care needs;
- actively involve, rather than simply instruct, caregivers in learning and applying a particular skill; and
- continue over an extended period of time or provide episodic "booster" support over the duration of caregiving.

Although some progress has been made in integrating research-based caregiver intervention strategies into existing health and LTSS systems, policy makers, managers, and practitioners should implement more intensive strategies to promote the dissemination and adoption of evidence-based caregiver supports throughout the health and LTSS delivery system. The NFCSP is one example of a federal program that incorporates elements of evidence-based caregiver interventions into broad-based service programs for caregivers. With increased funding, the NFCSP could serve as an important vehicle for disseminating effective caregiver interventions.

Efficacy trials aimed at developing and refining intervention strategies to support caregivers should continue to be supported, particularly for diverse populations, but an even greater emphasis should be placed on efforts to scale up effective intervention strategies so that they become widely available. ACL and other HHS agencies such as NIH, the Agency for Healthcare Research and Quality, and the Centers for Disease Control and Prevention are uniquely positioned to promote this agenda.

RECOMMENDATION 1-e: Explore, evaluate, and, as warranted, adopt federal policies that provide economic support for working caregivers.

Caregiving and employment are increasingly intertwined. Already about half of the nation's family caregivers for older adults are employed. But the proportion is projected to increase substantially, as older women increasingly participate in the work force and retire at older ages. These working caregivers—especially those who care for people with dementia or with substantial personal care needs—are at risk of significant economic costs: immediately reduced income as they work fewer hours, take time off, or leave jobs altogether; increased expenses to support their relatives; and lower lifetime earnings, savings, and retirement benefits as a result of less time spent in the workforce. Low-wage and part-time workers are most vulnerable to economic harm of family caregiving.

At the same time, job discrimination may affect family caregivers' job security when caregivers are rejected for hire, denied a promotion, or otherwise penalized based on assumptions about the impact of caregiving, without regard to their actual work performance.

Passage of the Family and Medical Leave Act (FMLA) in 1993 was an important step toward providing working caregivers with help in balancing job and family responsibilities. However, FMLA limits participation to only certain family relationships, excluding daughters- and sons-in-law, step-children, grandchildren, siblings, nieces and nephews, and other relatives who care for older adults; and it does not apply to employers with fewer than 50 employees. Perhaps even more important, eligible family caregivers may be unable to afford the unpaid leave that FMLA protects, and many American workers—especially low-wage workers—lack access to paid time off of any kind.

In 2015, President Obama took two new steps to expand access to paid leave, including care of an ill family member. In January, the White House issued a Presidential Memorandum directing federal agencies to advance up to 6 weeks of paid sick leave for federal employees in connection with the birth or adoption of a child, or to care for ill family members, including spouses and parents. Later, in September, the President signed an Executive Order requiring federal contractors to offer their employees up to 7 days of paid sick leave annually, including paid leave allowing for family care.

Four states—California, New Jersey, New York, and Rhode Island—have established access to paid family leave, and five states—California, Connecticut, Massachusetts, Oregon, and Vermont—have enacted paid sick leave statutes that require employers to allow workers a specific number of earned sick days to deal with personal illness or to take certain family members (including older adults) to medical appointments. States finance paid family leave through an insurance model that relies on minimal payroll taxes paid by employees. Public financing mechanisms have the potential to extend protections to contract workers who do not qualify as employees. Although some employers report additional costs, initial evidence suggests that many report that they have adapted to family leave requirements. In recent years, a growing number of city and county governments have similarly required that employers provide access to paid sick leave to their employees. The U.S. Department of Labor has also recently initiated a program that promotes paid leave policies.

Although current awareness and use of family leave programs seem far more focused on new parents than on family caregivers with eldercare responsibilities, these programs have the potential both to facilitate family caregiving and to alleviate its economic hardships.

Furthermore, actions to assure family caregivers' immediate and long-term economic security are not limited to leave policies. A range of worthy proposals merit serious consideration including, for example, Social Security caregiving credits to reduce the impact of foregone wages on retirement benefits; including family caregiver status as a protected class under federal employment discrimination laws; and providing employers with guidance and training on best practices to support workers with caregiving responsibilities. Exploring the feasibility of these proposals will require economic impact assessments that include not only the caregiver but also employers and federal and state agencies such as the Social Security Administration. Evaluating feasibility will also require that policy analysis takes into account unintended consequences, including the impact on a caregiver's labor force participation after they receive economic support from a given program.

RECOMMENDATION 1-f: Expand the data collection infrastructures within the U.S. Departments of Health and Human Services, Labor, and Veterans Affairs to facilitate monitoring, tracking, and reporting on the experience of family caregivers.

The challenges facing family caregivers result more from policy default than from policy design. Indeed, the nation lacks the data infrastructure and knowledge base that policy makers need to design and implement responsible policies and to monitor progress in their implementation and impact over time. Effective protection of the nation's family caregivers and their families requires a data collection system that consistently identifies care recipients and their caregivers and regularly monitors how many there are, who they are, what they do, how much they do, and the impact of their experience on health, economic, and social outcomes for both family caregivers and care recipients.

A number of existing annual population surveys have the potential to contribute to this system. If consistently funded and properly used, potential resources go beyond the combination of the National Survey of Caregivers and the National Health and Aging Trends Study the committee relied on in this report. These efforts should be continued and expanded as they provide a fine-grained assessment of the nature and impact of caregiving.

Other surveys such as the Behavioral Risk Factor Surveillance System and the American Community Survey could be useful in monitoring the prevalence of caregivers at the local, state, and national levels. Having reliable estimates of the number and types of family caregivers in communities and their racial/ethnic makeup would be valuable in planning for needed supportive programs and approaches. To make appropriate use of survey findings, survey instruments should, when appropriate, use common language and definitions, and analysis plans should carefully monitor changes in caregiver prevalence over time.

Chapter 2 noted the difficulties in interpreting the wide range of estimates of the caregiver population coming from various national surveys. Future population surveys should use standardized definitions to allow researchers to develop comparable estimates. There is no "one-size-fits-all" definition of a family caregiver, however. Definitions should vary depending on the context. For example, it may be appropriate to define family caregivers differently for the purposes of program eligibility, in developing payment incentives (including quality measures), or for assessing the effectiveness of an intervention in a specific population.

To provide effective policy support, surveys should address family caregivers and older adults not just at a point in time, but over time, and should have sufficient reach to assess diverse groups of family caregivers—who vary in numerous ways likely to affect caregiving challenges. Key variations likely include age, race and ethnicity, sexual orientation, rural or urban location, employment status, geographic proximity to care recipients, and care recipient condition.

Alongside population data, generating knowledge to guide and evaluate policy requires data collected in the routine delivery of care—data that can only come from adoption of the caregiver identification and assessment practices recommended above. Data from both sources can be used to identify policy targets for intervention that can reduce preventable illness and unnecessary service use and promote better health outcomes for family caregivers and care recipients alike.

The systematic development of a multisource data collection system would require a wide range of expertise and input from survey methodologists, statisticians, health care and LTSS providers, researchers, family caregivers themselves, and policy makers from federal, state, and local agencies such as the Agency for Healthcare Research and Quality, Area Agencies on Aging, Bureau of Labor Statistics, Centers for Medicare & Medicaid Services (CMS), Centers for Disease Control and Prevention, National Center for Health Statistics, and National Institute on Aging. Planning for this effort could be informed by a series of consensus conferences, which could be spearheaded by the Secretary of the U.S. Department of Health and Human Services.

RECOMMENDATION 1-g: Launch a multi-agency research program sufficiently robust to evaluate caregiver interventions in real-world health care and community settings, across diverse conditions and populations, and with respect to a broad array of outcomes.

Despite the valuable lessons learned from research on caregiver interventions, there are significant barriers to moving existing evidence-based interventions from the test phase into implementation in actual practice. Challenges begin with limitations to existing evidence—due in particular to the predominance of interventions focused on specific diagnoses (especially Alzheimer's disease), a particular disease stage, a homogeneous population, and a limited set of outcomes. Knowledge advancement is further hampered by insufficient funding for translation as well as for dissemination and implementation activities; lack of knowledge among providers, health and human service organizations, and administrators of available evidence-based programs; and programmatic barriers to accommodation of new practices.

Progress in caregiver support requires a new approach to research across federal agencies including the Agency for Healthcare Research and Quality, Centers for Disease Control and Prevention, CMS, and NIH; the Patient-Centered Outcomes Research Institute; and private foundations to support large-scale, multisite research studies to evaluate efficacy and cost-effectiveness of a range of caregiver intervention strategies. Research should be guided by consensus among key stakeholders regarding the priority interventions to test. This research ideally would

- include a diverse population of caregivers, varied in socioeconomic status, culture, race, health literacy, gender, and sexual orientation, as well as caregivers with multiple caregiving responsibilities (e.g., two parents or parent and child);
- encompass the needs of caregivers across the trajectory of care;
- be conducted in diverse geographic contexts;
- include metrics related to psychological, physical, and social well-being as well as health care use and cost implications for caregivers and care recipients, as appropriate; and
- explore the efficacy, feasibility, acceptability, usability, and cost-effectiveness of technology-based intervention strategies—including assessment of mechanisms to facilitate caregiver access to broadband or other technical requirements and to teach skills for using technology-based interventions.

ADDITIONAL ACTIONS

Concerted federal leadership will be essential to effectively promote the health, economic, and social well-being of the nation's caregivers and their families. However, the committee's call for the development of a National Family Caregiving Strategy should not in any way impede currently planned or ongoing federal initiatives, or—equally important—inhibit the progress that state and local policy makers and others are making consistent with the reforms proposed in this report. On the contrary, alongside the recommendation for a national strategy, the committee recommends that:

> **RECOMMENDATION 2: State governments that have yet to address the health, economic, and social challenges of caregiving for older adults should learn from the experience of states with caregiver supports, and implement similar programs.**

Some states are well ahead of the federal government in recognizing, valuing, and supporting family caregivers. Twenty-nine states have enacted the Caregiver Advise, Record, Enable (CARE) Act, which requires hospitals to ask individuals—when they are admitted—whether they wish to designate a family caregiver, and, if so, to record the name of the caregiver in the medical record; to notify the family caregiver if the person is to be discharged to another facility or back home; and to provide effective explanation of and instruction on the medical/nursing tasks (e.g., medication management, injections, wound care) that the family caregiver will need to perform at home.

With regard to unpaid leave, 14 states[2] have extended eligibility for the protections of FMLA to family members not covered by the federal status, including domestic partners, grandchildren, daughters- and sons-in-law, or siblings. Six states (including Washington, DC) extended eligibility to workers in businesses with fewer than 50 employees and two states allow broader use of FMLA leave by allowing workers to take family members to medical appointments. Several states, as noted earlier, have enacted paid family or sick leave laws that enable workers to take time off to care for an older family member.

Some states have acted on other fronts, including caregiver assessment in Medicaid LTSS and Medicaid payments to family caregivers providing home- and community-based care.

All the above state experiences are likely to provide important insights to other states seeking to adopt caregiver supports. Not only can the federal government build on these lessons in developing and implementing the committee's recommended National Family Caregiver Strategy, but states

[2] Includes the District of Columbia.

can independently advance caregiver and care recipient well-being by learning these lessons and adopting best practices.

RECOMMENDATION 3: The Secretaries of the U.S. Departments of Health and Human Services, Labor, and Veterans Affairs should work with leaders in health care and long-term services and supports delivery, technology, and philanthropy to establish a public–private, multi-stakeholder innovation fund for research and innovation to accelerate the pace of change in addressing the needs of caregiving families.

Addressing caregiver issues will require not only changes in the public sector, but also the support and guidance of the private sector to achieve maximum impact. Employers of all types have a vested interest in supporting family caregivers. Insurance, health care, and technology companies, among others, can bring to bear both financial resources and expertise to address current and emerging challenges for caregivers. Multiple national and local private foundations, as well as nonprofit organizations, have already invested in moving forward the caregiver agenda. The public sector cannot achieve all necessary progress on its own; a public–private innovation fund could leverage private funding to complement public resources and fill gaps in public funding.

The fund could sponsor the development of market-driven approaches for lessening the strain of caregiving on families—targeting innovative services and products that are scalable and sustainable. Potential products include assistive technologies, remote monitoring and sensing systems, telehealth applications, and other tools to assist family caregivers and to enable older adults to continue living in their home and communities. These systems could also be linked to health care and social service providers to aid in care coordination efforts. The fund could also invest in marketing evidence-based services and products, research to improve the evidence base, and widespread adoption.

The fund might also foster dialogue and collaboration between health care and LTSS organizations to improve coordination among hospitals, local Area Agencies on Aging, and other community-based organizations to improve the older adults' discharge from hospital to home and better support caregivers as they manage the transition and provide or arrange for home care.

The Obama Administration has established two innovation funds that could serve as possible models for a caregiver innovation fund: the Investing in Innovation Fund and the Social Innovation Fund (Office of Social Innovation and Civic Participation, 2016a,b). The Investing in Innovation Fund is administered by the U.S. Department of Education (DOE) and collaborates with school districts and nonprofits to distribute $650 million in grants to develop, validate, and scale-up innovations in education (DOE, 2016). The Social Innovation Fund is administered by the Corporation for National and Community Service and has distributed $50 million in grants to nonprofits looking to evaluate evidence-based programs that address economic opportunity, youth development and school support, and promoting healthy lifestyles. The Social Innovation Fund has also examined issues relevant to older adults as one of the grants looked at the Improving Mood–Promoting Access to Collaborative Treatment (IMPACT) model for treating depression in older adults.

Nonprofit innovation funds have found success investing in projects that cover similar topics to the recommended caregiver innovation fund. The Innovation Fund of the California Health Care Foundation, for example, is investing in existing health care technologies with the potential to significantly improve the quality of care, lower costs of care, or improve Californians access to care (CHCF, 2016). The Brigham Care Redesign Incubator and Startup Program, an innovation initiative sponsored by Brigham and Women's Health Care is exploring ways to improve care during transition from intensive hospital care to long-term rehabilitation (Laskowski and Dudley, 2015). The program has funded projects aimed at improving the transition to long-term acute care rehabilitation, increasing vaginal births after Cesarean section, and addressing emergency department "super users."

The future of caregiving for older Americans will be shaped not only by the growing number of older people needing care but also by the increasing ethnic and racial diversity of older people and their families. In less than 15 years, nearly 3 in 10 older Americans will identify as a member of a minority group. Sometime after 2040, no racial or ethnic group will constitute a majority of people aged 65 and older.

Differences in culture, along with differences in income, education, neighborhood environments, lifetime access to health care, and occupational hazards will have a significant impact on the need for care, the availability and willingness of family caregivers to provide it, and the most effective and appropriate ways to provide caregiver support. Developing programs and services that are accessible, affordable, and tailored to the needs of diverse communities of caregivers presents significant challenges.

In its final recommendation, the committee therefore calls on all parties to:

RECOMMENDATION 4: In all the above actions, explicitly and consistently address families' diversity in assessing caregiver needs and in developing, testing, and implementing caregiver supports.

Our older adult and caregiver population is becoming increasingly diverse, a trend that will continue for decades to come. Specific steps are needed to ensure that our national strategy is developed and implemented so that it addresses the needs and values of diverse family caregivers. This will require specific actions, including oversight to ensure progress, in providing support that is both accessible and effective for all family caregivers. Federal and state governments and philanthropic organizations all have a critical role in achieving this goal. Specific steps that can be taken include the following:

- Related to each of the recommendations above, the strategy will include specific goals for advancing support for diverse family caregivers and the biannual report will specifically address progress of the strategy in meeting these goals.
- Cultural competence is included as a core aspect of provider competencies in working with family caregivers.
- Critical gaps in our knowledge about the effectiveness of interventions for diverse populations are addressed through both research and implementation efforts.
- Monitoring is conducted in a way that allows for meaningful data on the health, well-being, quality, and outcomes of care for diverse family caregivers.

REFERENCES[3]

CHCF (California Health Care Foundation). 2016. *Health innovation fund.* http://www.chcf.org/innovation-fund/investment-criteria (accessed June 16, 2016).

DOE (U.S. Department of Education). 2016. *Investing in innovation fund (i3).* http://www2.ed.gov/programs/innovation/index.html (accessed June 16, 2016).

Haskins, R., and J. Baron. 2011. *The Obama Administration's evidence-based social policy initiatives: An overview.* http://www.brookings.edu/~/media/research/files/articles/2011/4/obama-social-policy-haskins/04_obama_social_policy_haskins.pdf (accessed June 16, 2016).

Laskowski, K., and J. Dudley. 2015. *How Brigham & Women's funds health care innovation.* Harvard Business Review. https://hbr.org/2015/10/how-brigham-s-funds-health-care-innovation (accessed June 16, 2016).

Office of Social Innovation and Civic Participation. 2016a. *Innovation funds.* https://www.whitehouse.gov/administration/eop/sicp/initiatives/innovation-funds (accessed June 16, 2016).

Office of Social Innovation and Civic Participation. 2016b. *Social innovation fund.* https://www.whitehouse.gov/administration/eop/sicp/initiatives/social-innovation-fund (accessed June 16, 2016).

Shah, S. M., and M. Jolin. 2012. *Social sector innovation funds: Lessons learned and recommendations.* https://www.americanprogress.org/issues/education/report/2012/11/20/45110/social-sector-innovation-funds (accessed June 16, 2016).

[3] The citations presented here refer only to new material presented in this chapter. Please refer to the previous chapters for citations related to the findings in Chapters 1 through 6.

Appendix A

Acronyms and Glossary

ACRONYMS

AAA	Area Agencies on Aging
ACA	Affordable Care Act
ACL	Administration for Community Living
AD	Alzheimer's disease
ADL	activity of daily living
ADRD	Alzheimer's disease and related disorders
AoA	Administration on Aging
CG	caregiver
CHD	coronary heart disease
ChEI	cholinesterase inhibitor
CMS	Centers for Medicare & Medicaid Services
COPE	care of older persons in the home environment
CR	care recipient
DOL	U.S. Department of Labor
EHR	electronic health record
FMLA	Family and Medical Leave Act
FRD	family responsibilities discrimination
HCBS	home- and community-based services

HHS	U.S. Department of Health and Human Services
HRS	Health and Retirement Survey
HRSA	Health Resources and Services Administration
IADL	instrumental activity of daily living
I/DD	intellectual and developmental disabilities
IPE	interprofessional education
LGBT	lesbian, gay, bisexual, and transgender
LTSS	long-term services and supports
MFP	Money Follows the Person
NFCSP	National Family Caregiver Support Program
NHATS	National Health and Aging Trends Study
NIH	National Institutes of Health
NSOC	National Survey of Caregivers
OAA	Older Americans Act
PHR	personal health record
PTSD	post-traumatic stress disorder
RCT	randomized controlled trial
REACH	Resources for Enhancing Alzheimer's Caregiver Health
SNF	skilled nursing facility
SSA	Social Security Act
SUA	state unit on aging
TDI	Temporary Disability Insurance
VA	U.S. Department of Veterans Affairs
VAMC	Veterans Affairs Medical Center
VHA	Veterans Health Administration

GLOSSARY

Care recipient: Adults aged 65 or older, who need help from others due to functional or cognitive limitations, or a serious health condition.

Care team: Older adults and their families or friends (when desired by the older adult) and all health care and social service professionals who interact with individuals in their care.

Caregiver assessment: A systematic process of gathering information about a caregiving situation to identify the specific problems, needs, strengths, and resources of the family caregiver, as well as the caregiver's ability to contribute to the needs of the care recipient. A family caregiver assessment asks questions of the family caregiver. It does not ask questions of the care recipient about the family caregiver.

Caregiver or family caregiver[1]**:** Family caregivers are relatives, partners, friends, or neighbors who assist an older adult (referred to in this report as a care recipient) who needs help due to physical, mental, cognitive, or functional limitations. The caregiver's involvement is driven primarily by a personal relationship rather than by financial remuneration. Family caregivers may live with, or apart from, the person receiving care. Care may be episodic, or of short or long duration.

Caregiving: Providing help to an older adult who needs assistance because of physical, mental, cognitive health, or functional limitations, including help with self-care; carrying out medical/nursing tasks (e.g., medication management, tube feedings, wound care); locating, arranging, and coordinating services and supports; hiring and supervising direct care workers (e.g., home care aides); serving as an "advocate" for the care recipient during medical appointments or hospitalizations; communicating with health and social service providers; and implementing care plans.

Eldercare: Care of older adults who need daily help because of health or functioning reasons. Eldercare is generally provided by family members, but can also be provided by paid help in the home, or in care settings such as assisted living or nursing homes.

End-of-life care: Refers generally to the care received by people who are nearing the end of life. This care may include a range of services to address

[1] The term "caregiver" sometimes means health and social service professionals (e.g., physicians, nurses, or social workers) as well as direct care workers (e.g., home care aides) because they are paid for their services and have training to provide care to the older adult.

a person's medical, social, emotional, and spiritual needs. Disease-specific interventions as well as palliative and hospice care for those with advanced serious conditions are considered forms of end-of-life care.

Family: Not only people related by blood or marriage, but also close friends, partners, companions, and others whom individuals would want as part of their care team.

Family leave: A period of time away from a job for specified family reasons such as to care for a spouse, child, or parent who has a serious health condition. Family leave can be paid or unpaid.

Family responsibilities discrimination (or caregiver discrimination): Employment discrimination against someone based on his or her family caregiving responsibilities and the assumption that caregivers are not dependable or less productive than their peers.

"Frail" and **"frailty":** A clinical syndrome characterized by the presence of at least three of the following: unintentional weight loss (10 lbs. in the past 12 months), self-reported exhaustion, weakness (grip strength), slow walking speed, and low physical activity.

"High-need" care recipients: Older adults who have probable dementia or need help with at least two self-care activities (i.e., bathing, dressing, eating, toileting, getting in and out of bed).

Long-term services and supports (LTSS): An array of paid and unpaid personal care, health care, and social services generally provided over a sustained period of time to people of all ages with chronic conditions and with functional limitations. Services can include personal care (e.g., bathing or dressing), help with medication management, paying bills, transportation, meal preparation, and health maintenance tasks. Services can be provided in a variety of settings such as nursing homes, residential care facilities, and individual homes.

Paid sick leave: Provides pay protection to sick or injured workers for a fixed number of paid sick days per year. Some employers also allow workers to use sick leave to care for an ill family member, or to accompany a family member to a medical appointment.

Palliative care: Care that provides relief from pain and other symptoms, supports quality of life, and is focused on people with serious advanced illness and their families. Palliative care may begin early in the course of treatment for a serious illness and may be delivered in a number of ways across the continuum of health care settings, including in the home, nursing homes, long-term acute care facilities, acute care hospitals, and outpatient clinics.

Patient-centered care: Health care that establishes a partnership among practitioners, patients, and their families (when appropriate) to ensure that decisions respect patients' wants, needs, and preferences and that patients have the education and support they need to make decisions and participate in their own care.

Person- and family-centered care: An approach to the planning and delivery of care across settings and time that is centered in collaborative partnerships among individuals, their defined family, and providers of care. It supports health and well-being by being consistent with, respectful of, and responsive to an individual's priorities, goals, needs, cultural traditions, family situation, and values. Core domains of person- and family-centered care include the support and involvement of family as defined by each individual.

Respite care: Services designed to allow family caregivers to have time away from their caregiving role. Respite can be provided at home, through adult day services in the community, or by short-term stays in a facility or retreat setting. Respite is planned or emergency services that result in some measurable improvement in the well-being of the caregiver, care recipient, and/or family system.

Appendix B

Committee and Staff Biographies

COMMITTEE MEMBER BIOGRAPHIES

Richard Schulz, Ph.D. (*Chair*), is Distinguished Service Professor of Psychiatry, director of the University Center for Social and Urban Research, director of Gerontology, and associate director of the Aging Institute of the University of Pittsburgh Medical Center Senior Services and the University of Pittsburgh. Dr. Schulz's work has focused on social-psychological aspects of aging, including the impact of disabling late-life disease on individuals and their families. He has been funded by the National Institutes of Health for more than three decades to conduct descriptive longitudinal and intervention research on diverse older populations representing illnesses such as cancer, spinal cord injury, stroke, Alzheimer's disease, heart disease, and arthritis. In the past decade, he has become interested in supportive interventions, including technology-based approaches designed to enhance individual functioning and quality of life of both individuals and their relatives. Dr. Schulz has been a leading contributor to the literature on the health effects of caregiving, Alzheimer's disease caregiving, and intervention studies for caregivers of persons with Alzheimer's disease. This body of work is reflected in more than 300 publications, which have appeared in major medical, psychology, and aging journals, including the *New England Journal of Medicine*, *Journal of the American Medical Association*, and *Archives of Internal Medicine*. He is also the author of numerous books, including the *Handbook of Alzheimer's Caregiver Intervention Research* and the *Quality of Life Technology Handbook*. Dr. Schulz is the recipient of several honors, including the Kleemeier Award for Research on Aging from the Gerontological Society of America, the M. Powell Lawton Distinguished Contribution Award for Applied Gerontology from the American Psychological Association, and the Developmental Health Award for Research on Health in Later Life from the American Psychological Association. He earned his Ph.D. in Social Psychology from Duke University.

María P. Aranda, Ph.D., M.S.W., M.P.A., joined the University of Southern California (USC) School of Social Work faculty in 1995 and holds a joint appointment with the USC Leonard Davis School of Gerontology. Dr. Aranda's research and teaching interests address the interplays among chronic illness, social resources, and psychological well-being in low-income minority populations. Dr. Aranda has served as Principal Investigator or Co-Investigator on several key studies funded by and/or in collaboration with the National Institute of Mental Health, National Cancer Institute, National Institute on Aging, Individual-Centered Outcomes Research Institute, Southern California, The John A. Hartford Foundation/The Gerontological Society of America, National Institute of Rehabilitation and Research, Alzheimer's Association/Health Resources and Services Administration, Los Angeles County Department of Mental Health, and Larson Endowment for Innovative Research. Overall, her research addresses the study of psychosocial care of adult and late-life psychiatric disorders, linguistic and cultural adaptations of behavioral health services, and evidence-based interventions. Dr. Aranda has 30 years of licensed clinical experience providing assessment and treatment services to middle-aged and older adults with co-morbid medical and psychiatric illness. She is a national trainer on evidence-based psychosocial treatments such as Problem Solving Treatment and Chronic Disease Self-Management. She has served on local and national boards and committees dedicated to the enhancement of practice, policy, research, and advocacy related to historically underrepresented minority populations. Dr. Aranda received her undergraduate degree in Social Work from the California State University, Los Angeles. She obtained her M.S.W., M.P.A., and Ph.D. from the University of Southern California.

Susan Beane, M.D., is the vice president and medical director of Healthfirst, Inc., a nonprofit, managed-care organization that provides health care coverage to individuals and families in the New York City metropolitan area through low- or no-cost government-sponsored health insurance programs, including Child Health Plus, Family Health Plus, Medicaid, and Medicare Advantage. Dr. Beane is a primary care physician and board-certified internist. She focuses on care management and clinical provider partnerships, especially programs designed to improve the delivery of vital, evidence-based health care to Healthfirst members. Prior to joining Healthfirst, Dr.

Beane served as chief medical officer for the Affinity Health Plan for 5 years. Before that, she was medical director at AmeriChoice and HIP USA. Dr. Beane is a graduate of Princeton University and Columbia University College of Physicians and Surgeons.

Sara J. Czaja, Ph.D., is a professor in the Departments of Psychiatry & Behavioral Sciences, and Industrial Engineering at the University of Miami and scientific director of the Center on Aging at the University of Miami. She has an extensive background in scientific investigation related to family caregiving, functional performance of older adults, innovative use of technology in intervention research, supervision of both laboratory and field research, and administration of large-scale research programs. She is also the director of the Center on Research and Education for Aging and Technology Enhancement (CREATE). CREATE is funded by the National Institute on Aging and involves collaboration with the Georgia Institute of Technology and Florida State University. The focus of CREATE is on making technology more accessible, useful, and usable for older adults. Dr. Czaja's research interests include aging and cognition, caregiving, human–computer interaction, training, and functional assessment. In addition, she is a Fellow of the American Psychological Association, the Human Factors and Ergonomics Society, and the Gerontological Society of America. She is the past chair of the Risk Prevention and Behavior Scientific Review Panel of the National Institutes of Health. She is also the current president of Division 20 (Adult Development and Aging) of the American Psychology Association. She is a member of the National Academies of Sciences, Engineering, and Medicine's Board on Human Systems Integration and has served on several National Research Council and Institute of Medicine committees.

Brian M. Duke, M.H.A., M.B.E., is system director, Senior Services with Main Line Health, leading a service line to meet the needs of older people throughout the care continuum and developing population health strategies and person- and family-centered approaches for care delivery. Mr. Duke came to Main Line Health following service as Secretary of the Pennsylvania Department of Aging. During his service he oversaw the delivery of services and benefits for older Pennsylvanians through a network of 52 area agencies on aging, and advocated for the interests of older people at all levels of government. He chaired the Pennsylvania Alzheimer's Disease Planning Committee and co-chaired the Pennsylvania Long-Term Care Commission. Prior to his service as Secretary, Mr. Duke was director of the Bucks County Area Agency on Aging, leading the delivery of social services that helped older people to age and live well in their homes and communities. Prior to that he served as executive director of the New Jersey

Foundation for Aging, a statewide public charity dedicated to improving the quality of life of older adults. Mr. Duke served as a consultant to the U.S. Administration on Aging and the AARP Foundation in the development of statewide caregiver coalitions in 12 states. He also co-chaired the Caring Community—a coalition of 100 organizations convened by WHYY, the public broadcasting station serving the greater Philadelphia region—producing award-winning programs and community outreach. Mr. Duke served as a consultant with the Family Caregiver: Outreach and Assistance in Our Communities project undertaken by the Penn State University Agricultural and Extension Education Programs to define strategies to engage and help family caregivers in rural regions. He is the author of the *Caregiver Coalitions Advocacy Guide: Uniting Voices, Building Community* with the National Alliance for Caregiving. Mr. Duke served as director of Geriatric Program Initiatives with the Institute on Aging of the University of Pennsylvania. Previously, he worked in the field of hospital administration for 20 years. He participates at the national, state, and local levels to foster effective strategies to support family caregivers, encourage aging well, and build community partnerships. He holds a B.S. in Business Administration from the University of Scranton, an M.H.A. (Health Administration) from The George Washington University, and an M.B.E. (Bioethics) from the University of Pennsylvania.

Judy Feder, Ph.D., is a professor of public policy and founding dean of the McCourt School of Public Policy at Georgetown University. Dr. Feder has a long and distinguished career in health policy. A widely published scholar, she served as staff director of the U.S. Bipartisan Commission on Comprehensive Health Care (Pepper Commission); as Principal Deputy Assistant Secretary for Planning and Evaluation at the U.S. Department of Health and Human Services in former President Bill Clinton's first term; and as a Senior Fellow at the Center for American Progress (2008-2011). She is currently an Institute Fellow at the Urban Institute. In 2012, Dr. Feder served on the Congressional Commission on Long-Term Care. She is a member of the National Academy of Medicine, the National Academy of Public Administration, and the National Academy of Social Insurance; a former chair and board member of AcademyHealth; a member of the Center for American Progress Action Fund Board, the Board of the National Academy of Social Insurance, and the Hamilton Project's Advisory Council; and a senior advisor to the Kaiser Commission on Medicaid and the Uninsured. Dr. Feder is a political scientist, with a B.A. from Brandeis University, and a master's degree and Ph.D. from Harvard University.

Lynn Friss Feinberg, M.S.W., is a senior strategic policy advisor at the AARP Public Policy Institute, providing research, policy analysis, and technical assistance on issues related to family caregiving and long-term services and supports. Ms. Feinberg came to AARP from the National Partnership for Women & Families, where she served as the first director of the Campaign for Better Care, an initiative to improve care in the United States for vulnerable older adults with multiple chronic conditions and their families. Previously, Ms. Feinberg was the deputy director of the National Center on Caregiving at the San Francisco-based Family Caregiver Alliance (FCA), where she was a leader in family-centered care and dementia issues, with special expertise in developing and replicating family caregiver support programs and translating research to promote policy change. During more than two decades at FCA, she directed the National Consensus Project for Caregiver Assessment, and led the first 50-state study on publicly funded caregiving programs in the nation, which was funded by the U.S. Administration on Aging from 2002 to 2004. In 2007-2008, Ms. Feinberg was selected as the John Heinz Senate Fellow in Aging, serving in the office of U.S. Senator Barbara Boxer (D-CA). She received the American Society on Aging's Leadership Award in 2006, and the Paul Nathanson Distinguished Advocate Award from Justice in Aging in 2015, for her career work on family care issues. Ms. Feinberg has published and lectured widely on family care policy and practice, and has served on numerous advisory boards and committees to address aging and caregiving issues. Currently, Ms. Feinberg is immediate past chair of the American Society on Aging, a fellow of the Gerontological Society of America, and an elected member of the National Academy for Social Insurance. Ms. Feinberg holds a master's degree in Social Welfare and Gerontology from the University of California, Berkeley.

Laura N. Gitlin, Ph.D., an applied research sociologist, is the director of the Center for Innovative Care in Aging and a professor with joint appointments in the Johns Hopkins School of Nursing and School of Medicine. Dr. Gitlin is nationally and internationally recognized for her research on developing, testing, and implementing novel nonpharmacologic interventions to improve the quality of life of persons with dementia and their family caregivers, enhance daily functioning in older adults with a disability, and address mental health disparities among minority groups. She is a well-funded researcher, having received continuous research and training grants from federal agencies and private foundations for nearly 30 years. A theme throughout her research is applying a social-ecological perspective and person-directed approach as well as collaborating with community organizations and health professionals to maximize the relevance and impact of intervention strategies. She is also involved in translating and implementing her team's proven interventions for delivery in different social service and practice settings globally and in the United States.

Lisa P. Gwyther, M.S.W., is the founder and director of the Duke Family Support Program (FSP). She has also served as president of the Gerontological Society of America. FSP provides critical education and support for individuals with Alzheimer's and other dementias, their families, and the health care and aging service networks that work with them. She is also co-leader of the Clinical Professional Unit for Social Work in the Duke Department of Psychiatry and Behavioral Sciences and she directs the Duke Employee Elder Care Consultation Service. In 1993, Ms. Gwyther served as the first John Heinz Public Policy Fellow in Health and Aging and worked on the health staff of then-Senate Majority Leader George J. Mitchell. Her current research interests include community translation of evidence-based dementia caregiver interventions, early-stage Alzheimer's programming, and nonpharmacological approaches to dementia-related behavioral symptoms. Ms. Gwyther received her bachelor's degree in Psychology as well as a master's degree in Social Work from Case Western Reserve University.

Rodger Herdman, M.D., is a retired physician with a distinguished career in both federal and state health policy. Dr. Herdman held positions as assistant professor and professor of pediatrics, respectively, at the University of Minnesota and the Albany Medical College between 1966 and 1979. In 1969, he was appointed director of the New York State Kidney Disease Institute in Albany. During 1969-1977, he served as deputy commissioner of the New York State Department of Health, responsible for research, departmental health care facilities, and the state's Medicaid program at various times. In 1977, he was named New York state's director of public health. From 1979 until joining the U.S. Congress's Office of Technology Assessment (OTA), he was a vice president of the Memorial Sloan-Kettering Cancer Center. In 1983, he was appointed assistant director of OTA for Health and Life Sciences and then acting director and director from 1993 to 1996. After the closure of OTA, he joined the Institute of Medicine (IOM) as a senior scholar and directed studies on graduate medical education, organ transplantation, silicone breast implants, and the U.S. Department of Veterans Affairs national formulary. On completing those studies, Dr. Herdman was appointed director of the IOM/National Research Council National Cancer Policy Board from 2000 through 2005. From 2005 to 2009, he initiated and directed the IOM National Cancer Policy Forum, which differed from the Board by including members from federal and private-sector agencies or organizations in addition to at-large academic/industry members. From 2007 to 2014, he served as director of the IOM Board on Health Care Services in addition to his other duties. Dr. Herdman graduated from Yale University, Magna Cum Laude, Phi Beta Kappa, and from Yale University School of Medicine. He interned in Pediatrics at the University of Minnesota, was a medical officer, U.S. Navy, and thereafter, completed a residency in Pediatrics and continued with a medical Fellowship in Immunology and Nephrology at Minnesota.

Ladson Hinton, M.D., is a geriatric psychiatrist, clinical and services researcher, and social scientist. Over the past two decades, Dr. Hinton has conducted interdisciplinary research to better understand the cultural and social dimensions of late-life depression, dementia-related illness, and caregiving experience among older adults and their families. He has applied this knowledge to develop innovative and culturally appropriate intervention approaches to overcome gaps and disparities in health care. Dr. Hinton has received national recognition for his expertise on the cultural aspects of geriatric mental health and family caregiving and has received multiple awards from the National Institutes of Health as a Principal Investigator. He is currently the Principal Investigator for a National Institute of Mental Health (NIMH) study titled "A Family-Based Primary Care Intervention to Enhance Older Men's Depression Care" and is co-directing a project (CARE-Partners) to develop and implement innovative new community- and family-centered models of care for depression in older adults through a grant from the California-based Archstone Foundation. Dr. Hinton is the director of the University of California (UC), Davis, Latino Aging Research Resource Center, one of seven national Resource Centers for Minority Aging Research funded by the National Institute on Aging (NIA), and he also directs the Education Core for the NIA-funded UC Davis Alzheimer's Disease Center. He chairs the Distinguished Scholars Advisory Board for the University of Southern California Roybal Institute on Aging and is an associate of the Harvard Asia Center, where he is engaged in a collaborative global health project to develop new models for eldercare in Asia. Dr. Hinton received his M.D. from Tulane University and completed his Psychiatric residency at UC San Francisco. He received postdoctoral training in the Robert Wood Johnson Clinical Scholars Program at UC San Francisco and in the NIMH-funded "Clinically-Relevant Medical Anthropology Program" at Harvard Medical School, where he conducted seminal work on dementia caregiving in ethnically diverse families. At UC Davis he was Co-Principal Investigator of the Sacramento Area Latino Study on Aging (SALSA), where his work focused on how Mexican-American families are impacted by and deal with dementia behavioral problems, work that later informed the development and testing of a culturally tailored educational intervention for Latino dementia caregivers. His community work includes co-founding the UC Davis Spanish Mini-Medical School, partnering with the Asian Community Center to enhance dementia care services, and serving on the Chapter Board of Directors of the Northern California Alzheimer's Association (2008-2012).

Peter Kemper, Ph.D., is an economist and expert on policy and delivery of long-term services and supports (LTSS). He has led a number of studies on the lifetime risk of needing LTSS, nursing home use, and expenditures for LTSS. His research on home care includes the evaluation of Channeling, a large randomized study that tested the effect of public financing of home care for older adults. Other research analyzes state options for the design of home care programs, case management in home care, the effect of state Medicaid home care spending on unmet need for personal care, and options for improving the jobs of direct care workers. Dr. Kemper has extensive experience designing complex evaluation and data collection projects. As Principal Investigator of the Community Tracking Study, he developed the overall study design and designed consumer, physician, and employer surveys. He also designed the evaluation of Better Jobs Better Care demonstration and directed surveys of home care aides, their supervisors, and clinical managers, and designed an employment information reporting system used to track job turnover. Dr. Kemper retired from Pennsylvania State University in 2011 to serve as Deputy Assistant Secretary for Disability, Aging, and Long-Term Care Policy in the Office of the Assistant Secretary for Planning and Evaluation at the U.S. Department of Health and Human Services. He had previously served as a commissioner on the Medicare Payment Advisory Commission and as a workgroup leader on the Clinton health reform effort. Before coming to Penn State, he was the vice president of the Center for Studying Health System Change, director of the Division of Long-Term Care Studies at the Agency for Health Care Policy and Research, and director of the Madison Office of Mathematica. He earned a bachelor's degree in Mathematics at Oberlin College and a doctorate in Economics at Yale University.

Linda O. Nichols, Ph.D., is the co-director of the Caregiver Center at the Memphis Veterans Affairs Medical Center and a professor of Preventive and Internal Medicine at the University of Tennessee Health Science Center. The Caregiver Center at the Memphis VA Medical Center provides training to U.S. Department of Veterans Affairs (VA) staff across the country to work with caregivers of individuals with dementia, spinal cord injuries or disorders, multiple sclerosis, and post-traumatic stress disorder, and with families of post-9/11 veterans. Dr. Nichols is a health services researcher and medical anthropologist focusing on dementia caregiving and the challenges faced by military families during and after deployment. Her research is funded by the VA, the U.S. Department of Defense, and the National Institute on Aging. In 2011, her research became the basis for the Caregiver Center's evidence-based national service programs for the Veterans Health Administration as part of the implementation of the VA's caregiver legislation. Dr. Nichols received her Ph.D. in Anthropology from Washington University in St. Louis.

Carol Rodat, M.A., is the New York policy director for the Paraprofessional Healthcare Institute (PHI), a national organization dedicated to strengthening the direct care workforce that provides services and supports to older adults and people with disabilities. She is responsible for advocacy, research, and analysis on behalf of New York's direct care workers and long-term services and supports consumers. Ms. Rodat has more than 30 years of policy experience, having worked in the field of child welfare for the Child Welfare League of America in Washington, DC, and as executive director of Hospital Trustees of New York State, where she initiated one of the first quality improvement projects in the state's hospitals. Before joining PHI, she was the president of the Home Care Association of New York State, a nonprofit organization active in state and federal home care policy. She has published several reports and studies on the importance of the long-term services and supports workforce and testified frequently on the role of the direct care worker. Recently, she participated in a multiyear learning collaborative designed to improve the attention to and services for family caregivers and is currently working on identifying the roles that families and home care aides can play in the integration of care.

Charles P. Sabatino, J.D., is the director of the American Bar Association's (ABA's) Commission on Law and Aging. Since 1984, he has been responsible for the ABA Commission's research, project development, consultation, and education in areas of health law, long-term services and supports, guardianship and capacity issues, surrogate decision making, legal services delivery for older adults, and professional ethics. He is also a part-time adjunct professor at Georgetown University Law Center, where he has taught Law and Aging since 1987. He is a Fellow and former president of the National Academy of Elder Law Attorneys and a board member of the Washington, DC-based Coalition to Transform Advanced Care, co-chairing its Public Policy Working Group. Mr. Sabatino received his B.A. from Cornell University and his J.D. from Georgetown University Law Center and is a member of the Virginia and Washington, DC bars.

Karen Schumacher, Ph.D., R.N., is a professor in the College of Nursing at the University of Nebraska Medical Center and an associate member of the Fred and Pamela Buffett Cancer Center. Dr. Schumacher's clinical background is in home health care nursing. She worked extensively with family caregivers of older adults as a clinical nurse specialist at Vanderbilt University Medical Center and as a home health care nurse at Community Health Services, Inc., in Nashville. Her research now focuses on family caregiving for individuals with cancer. Her studies examine the caregiving skills needed to provide care at home during and after cancer treatment, as well as the similarities and differences in rural and urban caregiving. A concurrent research focus is management of cancer pain by individuals and family caregivers. Her research has been funded by the National Institutes of Health and the American Cancer Society. Dr. Schumacher has extensive experience as a nurse educator, having served as a faculty member at Vanderbilt University, the University of California, San Francisco (UCSF), and the University of Pennsylvania. While at the University of Pennsylvania, she served for 1 year as the Beatrice Renfield Visiting Nurse Scholar at the Visiting Nurse Service of New York. Dr. Schumacher received her bachelor's degree in Nursing from Vanderbilt University, her master's degree in Community Health Nursing from the University of Colorado, and her Ph.D. from UCSF. She completed a postdoctoral fellowship at Oregon Health & Science University.

Alan Stevens, Ph.D., is the Vernon D. Holleman-Lewis M. Rampy Centennial Chair in Gerontology at Baylor Scott & White Health, the largest nonprofit health care system in Texas. He is also professor of Medicine and Public Health at the Texas A&M University System Health Science Center. Dr. Stevens serves as the director of the Center for Applied Health Research (CAHR), a joint endeavor of Baylor Scott & White Health, the Texas A&M College of Medicine, and the Central Texas Veterans Health Care System. CAHR conducts and facilitates collaborative projects in the areas of translational and outcomes research. Dr. Stevens also heads the Center's Program on Aging and Care, which develops and implements evidence-based clinical interventions for older adults and their caregivers, and he is the director of the National Institutes of Health-funded Community Research Center for Senior Health. Dr. Stevens is the appointed co-chair of the Hartford Change AGEnts Initiative, headquartered at the Gerontological Society of America. In 2012, Dr. Stevens was appointed for a 3-year term to the Board of Directors of the Texas Institute of Health Care Quality and Efficiency. Dr. Stevens completed his graduate training at the University of New Orleans, earning a master's degree and a Doctorate of Philosophy in Applied Developmental Psychology. Prior to joining Baylor Scott & White Health and Texas A&M in 2005, he was an associate professor of medicine at the University of Alabama at Birmingham.

Donna Wagner, Ph.D., dean of the College of Health and Social Services, New Mexico State University, has been examining family caregiving and workplace eldercare programs since the mid-1980s. She is a Fellow of both the Gerontological Society of America and the Association for Gerontology in Higher Education (AGHE), currently serving as president of AGHE.

Dr. Wagner's research has included studies on long-distance caregiving, employed caregivers and the development of workplace programs, gender differences among employed caregivers, the efficacy of workplace eldercare programs, and the financial effects of family caregiving. She has published in the areas of rural caregiving, older caregivers, policy options to support caregivers, use of workplace programs, and programs and services for older adults. Dr. Wagner earned her B.A. in Psychology, as well as an M.A. and a Ph.D. in Urban Affairs from Portland State University, where she was affiliated with the Institute on Aging.

Jennifer L. Wolff, Ph.D., is a gerontologist and health services researcher who studies delivery of chronic care and long-term services and supports for older adults with complex health needs and late-life family caregiving. She has studied how the composition and experience of family caregivers has changed over time, how family caregivers navigate the medical system to facilitate health care for the individuals to whom they provide assistance, and the role of the medical community in supporting family caregivers. Dr. Wolff holds a primary appointment as associate professor in the Department of Health Policy and Management at the Johns Hopkins Bloomberg School of Public Health and is jointly appointed in the Johns Hopkins University School of Medicine Division of Geriatric Medicine and Gerontology. Dr. Wolff is a graduate of the Johns Hopkins Bloomberg School of Public Health, where she earned a doctoral degree in Health Services Research.

STAFF BIOGRAPHIES

Jill Eden, M.B.A., M.P.H. (*Study Director*), has been a senior program officer and study director at the National Academies of Sciences, Engineering, and Medicine since 2001. Her recent studies include *Graduate Medical Education That Meets the Nation's Health Needs* (2014), *The Mental Health and Substance Use Workforce for Older Adults: In Whose Hands?* (2012), *Finding What Works in Health Care: Standards for Systematic Reviews* (2011), *Initial National Priorities for Comparative Effectiveness Research* (2009), and *Knowing What Works in Health Care: A Roadmap for the Nation* (2008). Before joining the Academies, Ms. Eden worked in a variety of health policy research settings, including Mathematica Policy Research (MPR) and the U.S. Congress Office of Technology Assessment (OTA) and in health care financing at the New York City Health and Hospitals Corporation and Kaiser Foundation Health Plan (Southern California). At MPR, Ms. Eden directed studies on health plan accreditation, the State Children's Health Insurance Program, health care access and satisfaction in the military health system, the health care experiences of people who use community health centers, and the technical quality of state-specific, population-based surveys of health insurance coverage. At OTA, Ms. Eden authored or co-authored reports on individual cost sharing, Oregon's 1990 proposal to significantly expand Medicaid in the state, adolescent health, and the impact of HIV and AIDS on individual health insurance. Earlier in her career, Ms. Eden contributed to new benefits and rate development in Kaiser's southern California region and completed a 1-year hospital administration residency at the hospitals and clinics of a United Auto Workers health maintenance organization in Detroit. She received master's degrees from Columbia University's Graduate School of Business and the School of Public Health, and a bachelor's degree in Psychology from Barnard College.

Gus Zimmerman, M.P.P., is a research associate for the Board on Health Care Services and the Board on Health Sciences Policy of the National Academies of Sciences, Engineering, and Medicine. Prior to his current position, Mr. Zimmerman worked as a research assistant at the Menges Group, a private health care consulting firm. He has also worked in the U.S. House of Representatives and the National Coalition for LGBT Health. Mr. Zimmerman holds a bachelor's degree in Political Science from American University and a master's degree in Public Policy from Georgetown University, with concentrations in Health and Technology Policy.

Katye Magee, M.P.A., is a senior program assistant for the Board on Health Care Services and the Board on Health Sciences Policy of the National Academies of Sciences, Engineering, and Medicine. Prior to her current position, Ms. Magee completed her bachelor's degree at Tulane University, where she studied Public Health and English. She recently completed her master's of Public Administration at The George Washington University, with concentrations in health and social policy.

Sharyl Nass, Ph.D., serves as director of the Board on Health Care Services and director of the National Cancer Policy Forum at the National Academies of Sciences, Engineering, and Medicine. The Board considers the entire health care system in order to ensure the best possible care for all individuals. Its activities pertain to the organization, financing, effectiveness, workforce, and delivery of health care. For more than 15 years, Dr. Nass has worked on a broad range of health and science policy topics that include the quality and safety of health care and clinical trials, oversight of health research, developing technologies for precision medicine, and strategies for large-scale biomedical science. She has a Ph.D. from Georgetown University and undertook postdoctoral training at the Johns Hopkins University School of Medicine. She also holds a B.S. and an M.S. from the University of Wisconsin–Madison. In addition, she studied at the Max

Planck Institute in Germany under a Fellowship from the Heinrich Hertz-Stiftung Foundation. She was the 2007 recipient of the Cecil Award for Excellence in Health Policy Research, the 2010 recipient of a Distinguished Service Award from the Academies, and the 2012 recipient of the Institute of Medicine staff team achievement award (as the team leader).

Appendix C

Public Workshop Agendas

COMMITTEE ON FAMILY CAREGIVING FOR OLDER ADULTS

Perspectives on Family Caregiving for Older Adults

January 16, 2015
Keck Center
500 Fifth Street, NW
Room 100
Washington, DC 20001

8:30 AM **Welcome and Introductory Remarks** – *Terry Fulmer, Co-Chair, Committee on Family Caregiving for Older Adults*

8:35 AM **Panel 1: What Do Family Caregivers Experience, Want, and Need?**
Moderator: Lynn Friss Feinberg – Senior Strategic Policy Advisor, AARP Public Policy Institute

Objective – To learn about the experiences of family caregivers, including the types of tasks they are expected to perform, how those tasks are different now than in the past, the challenges they face, and what action should be taken to address their needs.

- *What Caregivers Want and Need* – Kathy Kelly – Executive Director, National Center on Caregiving, Family Caregiver Alliance

- *Home Alone: Family Caregivers Providing Complex Chronic Care Report* – Carol Levine – Director, Families and Health Care Project United Hospital Fund

- *Insights from Direct Experience as a Family Caregiver* – Kathy Kenyon – Family Caregiver

Q & A/Discussion

9:35 AM **Panel 2: Family Caregiver Interactions with the Health Care System**
Moderator: Jennifer Wolff – Associate Professor, Department of Health Policy and Management, Johns Hopkins Bloomberg School of Public Health

Objective – To learn about the barriers that family caregivers encounter in navigating health care and long-term services and supports systems on behalf of older adults and to also learn about two ways in which caregivers can be integrated into care systems.

- *Navigating the Health Care System* – Susan Reinhard – Senior Vice President, AARP; Director, AARP Public Policy Institute

- *Facilitating Access to Health Care Information* – Tom Delbanco – Co-Director, OpenNotes

- *Lessons from the CMMI Health Care Innovation Project on Alzheimer's and Dementia Care* – Zaldy S. Tan – Medical Director, University of California, Los Angeles' Alzheimer's and Dementia Care Program; Associate Professor, David Geffen School of Medicine, UCLA

Q & A/Discussion

10:35 AM **Panel 3: Selected Legal Issues in Family Caregiving**
Moderator: Charlie Sabatino – Director, American Bar Association, Commission on Law and Aging

Objective – To learn about selected legal issues that affect family caregivers.

- *Family Responsibility Discrimination in the Workplace* – Cynthia Calvert – Founder and Principal, WORKFORCE 21C; Senior Counsel, WorkLife Law

- *Surrogate Decision Making* – Nina Kohn – Professor of Law, Syracuse University College of Law; Member of American Bar Association Surrogate Decision-Making Committee and Chair, ABA Elder Rights Committee

- *Elder Abuse* – Marie-Therese Connolly – Director, Life Long Justice; Senior Scholar, Woodrow Wilson International Center for Scholars

Q & A/Discussion

11:45 AM **Closing Remarks** – *Richard Schulz, Co-Chair, Committee on Family Caregiving for Older Adults*

12:00 PM **ADJOURN**

COMMITTEE ON FAMILY CAREGIVING FOR OLDER ADULTS

The Diverse World of Family Caregiving

April 17, 2015
The Arnold and Mabel Beckman Center of The National Academies
100 Academy Drive
Irvine, CA 92617

8:30 AM **Welcome and Introductory Remarks** – *Richard Schulz Co-Chair, Committee on Family Caregiving for Older Adults*

8:35 AM **Panel 1: Changing Faces in America: Implications for Older Adults and Their Families**
Moderator: Ladson Hinton – Geriatric Psychiatrist and Professor, Department of Psychiatry and Behavioral Sciences, University of California, Davis

Objective – To learn about trends in the makeup of the U.S. population and their implications for family caregiving, and how to respond to an increasingly diverse, aging population.

- *Demographic Trends, Changes in Family Economic Well-Being, and Family Structures*
    - Eileen Crimmins – AARP Professor of Gerontology, Davis School of Gerontology, University of Southern California

- *Disability Trends in the Older Adult Population and Their Family Caregivers*
    - Marie A. Bernard – Deputy Director, National Institute on Aging of the National Institutes of Health

- *Caregiving Policy in a Diverse and Multicultural State*
    - Mariko Yamada – Former State Assembly member for California's 4th Assembly District

- *Meeting the Needs of Family Caregivers with Culturally Competent Interventions*
    - Heather Young – Associate Vice Chancellor for Nursing, Betty Irene Moore School of Nursing, University of California, Davis

Q & A/Discussion

9:55 AM **Panel 2: Perspectives from Providers: How Social Service Agencies Address Issues of Cultural Diversity**
Moderator: María Aranda – Associate Professor, University of Southern California School of Social Work

Objective – To learn about providing long-term services and supports to diverse family caregivers of older adults and to discuss the need to tailor services, the existence of best practices, and what role policy can play.

- *Providing Caregiver Support Services to Diverse Populations in Los Angeles*
    - Laura Trejo – General Manager, Los Angeles Department of Aging

- *Providing Caregiver Support Services to Asian and Pacific Islander American Families*
    - Donna L. Yee – Chief Executive Officer, Asian Community Center

- *Providing Caregiver Support Services to African American Families*
    - Donna Benton – Director, Older Adults Pacific Clinic

Q & A/Discussion

10:55 AM **Panel 3: Beyond Race and Ethnicity: Additional Issues of Diverse Populations**
Moderator: Brian Duke – System Director, Senior Services, Main Line Health

Objective – To learn about providing long-term services and supports to best meet the needs of rural caregivers, male caregivers, and lesbian, gay, bisexual, and transgender (LGBT) caregivers.

- *Family Caregiving from a Man's Perspective*
    - Winston Greene – Family Caregiver

- *Providing Caregiver Support Services in Rural Areas*
    - Cliff Burt – Caregiver Specialist, Georgia Division of Aging Services

- *LGBT Family Caregiving Experiences and Supportive Service Needs*
    - Karen Fredriksen-Goldsen – Professor and Director, Hartford Center of Excellence, University of Washington School of Social Work

Q & A/Discussion

11:55 AM **Closing Remarks –** *Ladson Hinton*

12:00 PM ADJOURN

Appendix D

Number of Years and Percentage of Adult Life Spent Caring for an Older Adult

Commissioned Analysis by Vicki A. Freedman, Ph.D.

INTRODUCTION

Adults may be called on to provide care to an older adult one or more times during their lifetime. Young adults may participate in the care of their grandparents; adults in their 50s and 60s may need to care for an aging parent or parent-in-law; and older adults may provide care to spouses or siblings. The number of years that adults can be expected to spend on average in a caregiving role in the United States has not been previously quantified.

This memo provides estimates for the United States of the average number of years expected and percentage of remaining life to be spent providing care to an adult age 65 or older with an activity limitation. Findings are presented for informal (family or unpaid non-relative) adult caregivers to older adults with one or more activity limitations and for an alternative (narrower) definition of caregiving to older adults who meet criteria for severe limitations.

GENERAL APPROACH

The estimates presented here draw on a widely used life table methodology developed for generating active life expectancy estimates.[1] Instead of generating years and percentage of life spent without disability, we use the methodology to calculate years and percentage of life spent caregiving.

[1]Details of the method are available in Sullivan (1971) and the statistical underpinnings developed in Imai and Soneji (2007). Step-by-step calculations are available in Jagger et al. (2006).

The method involves three steps. First, the proportion of adults providing care is calculated for 10-year age groups. Numerators are drawn from the 2011 National Survey of Caregiving (NSOC) linked to the National Health and Aging Trends Study (NHATS) and denominators are from the 2011 Current Population Survey (CPS). Then, life tables provided by the National Center for Health Statistics are used to generate person-years lived and life expectancy for each age group. Finally, caregiving rates are combined with the life table estimates to apportion life expectancy into the average number of years and percentage of remaining life expected to be providing care. Additional methodological details are provided in the technical appendix.

CAREGIVING DEFINITIONS

We include care provided to adults ages 65 and older who live in community or residential care settings (other than nursing homes) and received assistance in the prior month with self-care or mobility activities (eating, bathing, dressing, or toileting; getting out of bed; getting around inside; getting outside) or household activities (doing laundry, shopping for groceries or personal items, making hot meals, handling bills and banking, and keeping track of medications), the latter for health or functioning reasons. For the alternative definition, we include only care to older adults who live in community or residential care settings (other than nursing homes) and either have probable dementia or received assistance in the past month with two or more self-care activities (eating, bathing, dressing, toileting, or getting in or out of bed).

For both definitions, caregivers are family members or unpaid nonrelatives ages 20 and older who provided assistance in the past month with mobility, self-care, or household tasks; transportation; money matters other than bills or banking; or medical activities (sitting in with the sample person at physician visits; helping with insurance decisions).[2]

LIMITATIONS

The analysis has several limitations. First, estimates are sensitive to the definition of caregiving. Although we have demonstrated sensitivity to narrower definitions, using a broader definition that does not require the older adult to have a limitation or that includes a broader (or undefined) set of care tasks would yield higher estimates. Second, estimates of lifetime caregiving do not provide insights into the distribution of years spent caring

[2]We also generated a second set of alternative (narrow) estimates by imposing a minimum duration of receipt of help of 3 months or longer. See technical appendix for additional details.

and include those who never provide care. Thus, the estimates should be interpreted as population averages. Third, calculations apply current age-specific mortality and caregiving rates to a hypothetical cohort; hence, they are not intended to be forecasts of future experience. The stability of future caregiving rates will depend on a number of factors, including changes in late-life disability and mortality rates, average family size and composition, competing demands from work and family, the availability of formal caregivers, and cultural norms (Stone, 2015).

KEY FINDINGS

Proportion of Adults Providing Care to Older Adults

In 2011, approximately 18 million adults ages 20 and older—nearly 8 percent of all those age 20 and older—provided care to older adults with one or more activity limitations. The percentage of adults providing care ranges from less than 2 percent among those ages 20 to 29 to 16 percent among those ages 70 to 79 (Table D-1).

During mid-life (ages 40-69), women are more likely than men to provide care whereas men are more likely than women to provide care above age 80. Consequently, the chances of providing care peaks at different ages for men (nearly 16% older than age 70) and women (more than 18% among those ages 60 to 69).

About 8.5 million caregivers (48% of caregivers) provided care to an older adult with severe limitations. Percentages providing care are substantially lower using this narrower definition: the percentage ranges from less than 1 percent among those ages 20 to 29 to more than 7 percent among those ages 60 to 69 (last panel of Table D-1).

Number of Years and Percentage of Remaining Lifetime Providing Care to Older Adults

A 20-year-old adult can expect to spend on average 5.1 years—or nearly 9 percent of his or her remaining lifetime—caring for an older adult with an activity limitation (Table D-2). Over their lifetimes, women spend more years caring than men—on average 6.1 years or nearly 10 percent of their adult life—whereas men spend on average 4.1 years or just more than 7 percent of their adult life ($p<.05$ for difference in years).

The percentage of remaining life to be spent providing care peaks at different ages for men and women. For men, once they reach age 70, nearly 16 percent of remaining lifetime—or 1 to 2 years—is spent caring for an older adult. For women, this figure peaks between ages 50 and 69, when about 15 percent of remaining lifetime—or about 4 to 5 years—is spent caring.

TABLE D-1 Proportion Giving Care to Older Adults, by 10-Year Age Groups, 2011

	To Older Adults with One or More Activity Limitations[a]						To Older Adults with Severe Limitations[b]	
	All		Men		Women		All	
Caregiver's Age Group	Proportion Caregiving	SE	Proportion Caregiving	SE	Proportion Caregiving	SE	Proportion Caregiving	SE
20-29	0.016	0.0029	0.015	0.0041	0.018	0.0040	0.008	0.0022
30-39	0.027	0.0039	0.021	0.0045	0.033	0.0056	0.013	0.0028
40-49	0.068	0.0068	0.049	0.0075	0.086	0.0099	0.036	0.0049
50-59	0.115	0.0097	0.081	0.0079	0.147	0.0156	0.056	0.0069
60-69	0.149	0.0126	0.111	0.0115	0.184	0.0184	0.073	0.0088
70-79	0.160	0.0152	0.159	0.0191	0.161	0.0181	0.060	0.0089
80+	0.115	0.0137	0.157	0.0243	0.088	0.0153	0.061	0.0109
Caregivers (in millions)	17.7		6.8		10.9		8.5	
% of population caregiving	7.9%		6.3%		9.5%		3.8%	
(n)	1,971		660		1,311		1,018	

NOTE: Caregivers are family members or unpaid non-relatives ages 20 and older who provided assistance in the past month with mobility, self-care, or household tasks; transportation; money matters other than bills or banking; or medical activities (sitting in with the sample person at physician visits; helping with insurance decisions).

[a]Adults ages 65 and older who live in community or residential care settings (other than nursing homes) and received assistance in the prior month with self-care or mobility activities (eating, bathing, dressing, or toileting; getting out of bed; getting around inside; getting outside) or household activities (doing laundry, shopping for groceries or personal items, making hot meals, handling bills and banking, and keeping track of medications), the latter for health or functioning reasons.

[b]Adults ages 65 and older who live in community or residential care settings (other than nursing homes) and either have probable dementia or received assistance in the past month with two or more self-care activities (eating, bathing, dressing, toileting, or getting out of bed).

SOURCES: Estimates calculated from the 2011 Current Population Survey and the 2011 National Study of Caregiving (NSOC) linked to the National Health and Aging Trends Study, unweighted n for NSOC.

TABLE D-2 Expected Number of Years and Percentage of Remaining Life Caring for an Older Adult, 2011

Caregiver's Age Group	To Older Adults with One or More Activity Limitation(s)[a]						To Older Adults with Severe Limitations[b]	
	All Caregivers		Men		Women		All Caregivers	
	Years (95% CI)	% of Remaining Life	Years (95% CI)	% of Remaining Life	Years (95% CI)	% of Remaining Life	Years (95% CI)	% of Remaining Life
20-29	5.1 (4.7, 5.5)	8.6	4.1 (3.7, 4.5)	7.2	6.1 (5.5, 6.7)	9.9	2.4 (2.1, 2.7)	4.1
30-39	5.0 (4.6, 5.4)	10.0	4.0 (3.6, 4.5)	8.4	6.0 (5.4, 6.5)	11.5	2.4 (2.1, 2.6)	4.7
40-49	4.8 (4.4, 5.2)	11.9	3.9 (3.5, 4.3)	10.1	5.7 (5.1, 6.3)	13.4	2.3 (2.0, 2.5)	5.6
50-59	4.2 (3.8, 4.6)	13.5	3.5 (3.1, 3.9)	11.9	4.9 (4.4, 5.5)	14.9	2.0 (1.7, 2.2)	6.2
60-69	3.3 (3.0, 3.7)	14.4	2.9 (2.5, 3.4)	13.8	3.7 (3.2, 4.1)	15.0	1.5 (1.3, 1.7)	6.5
70-79	2.2 (1.8, 2.5)	14.1	2.2 (1.8, 2.7)	15.8	2.1 (1.7, 2.5)	12.8	0.9 (0.7, 1.1)	6.0
80+	1.0 (0.8, 1.3)	11.5	1.3 (0.9, 1.7)	15.7	0.8 (0.6, 1.1)	8.8	0.5 (0.4, 0.7)	6.1

NOTE: Caregivers are family members or unpaid non-relatives ages 20 and older who provided assistance in the last month with mobility, self-care, or household tasks; transportation; money matters other than bills or banking; or medical activities (sitting in with the sample person at physician visits; helping with insurance decisions).

[a]Adults ages 65 and older who live in community or residential care settings (other than nursing homes) and received assistance in the prior month with self-care or mobility activities (eating, bathing, dressing, or toileting; getting out of bed; getting around inside; getting outside) or household activities (doing laundry, shopping for groceries or personal items, making hot meals, handling bills and banking, and keeping track of medications), the latter for health or functioning reasons.

[b]Adults ages 65 and older who live in community or residential care settings (other than nursing homes) and either have probable dementia or received assistance in the past month with two or more self-care activities (eating, bathing, dressing, toileting, or getting out of bed).

SOURCES: Estimates calculated from the 2011 Current Population Survey and the 2011 National Study of Caregiving (NSOC) linked to the National Health and Aging Trends Study, unweighted n for NSOC.

On average, 2.4 years—or nearly half of the years spent providing care to an older adult (2.4/5.1 years)—is spent providing care to an older adult with severe limitations, defined as receiving help with two or more activities of daily living or having probable dementia (second to last column of Table D-2).

TECHNICAL APPENDIX
Methodology for Calculating Average Number of Years and Percentage of Adult Life Spent Caregiving

DATA SOURCES AND CAREGIVER DEFINITIONS

Source of Caregiving Information. Age-specific estimates of the proportion caregiving are calculated from two sources.

Numerators are drawn from the National Study of Caregiving (NSOC), a follow-back to the 2011 National Health and Aging Trends Study (NHATS).[3] NHATS is a nationally representative study of Medicare enrollees ages 65 or older living across all settings. The Round 1 response rate was 71 percent. NSOC is a follow-back telephone interview with all caregivers of eligible 2011 NHATS participants (see below for definition). NHATS respondents provided contact information for 68 percent of eligible caregivers. Sixty percent of those with contact information completed a telephone interview. NSOC provides non-response adjusted weights that are intended to adjust for the three levels of non-response so that the sample represents the total family caregiver population as identified in NHATS. For details see Kasper et al. (2013b).

Denominators (number of individuals in the non-institutionalized population by 10-year age groups) are drawn from the 2011 Current Population Survey (CPS) (U.S. Census Bureau, 2011).

Definition of Caregiving. NHATS participants were eligible for NSOC if they lived in the community or residential care settings other than nursing homes and received assistance in the past month with self-care or mobility activities (bathing, dressing, eating, toileting, getting out of bed, getting around inside, and going outside) or household activities (doing laundry, shopping for groceries or personal items, making hot meals, handling bills and banking, and keeping track of medications), the latter for health or functioning reasons.

Once eligible NHATS participants were identified, caregivers were eligible for NSOC if they were family members or unpaid non-relatives who provided assistance in the past month (according to the NHATS respondent) with mobility, self-care, household tasks, or transportation, or in the past year with money matters other than bills or banking or medical

[3]NHATS and NSOC are sponsored by the National Institute on Aging (grant number NIA U01AG32947) and were conducted by the Johns Hopkins University.

activities (sitting in with the sample person at physician visits; helping with insurance decisions).

Of the 2,007 caregivers interviewed in NSOC, we excluded 11 respondents who did not provide care in the past month (according to NSOC) and 25 who were younger than age 20. Of the remaining 1,971 caregivers included in the analysis, 31 were missing age.[4]

Alternative (Narrower) Definition of Caregiving to Older Adults with Severe Limitations. We also generated estimates for a narrower definition of the caregiving population that includes only those who cared for an older adult with severe limitations. This group of care recipients is defined as living in the community or in residential care (other than nursing homes) and either (1) receiving help with two or more out of five activities (getting out of bed, eating, toileting, bathing, or dressing) or (2) being classified as having probable dementia.[5] We also generated a second set of alternative (narrow) estimates that imposed a minimum duration of receipt of help of 3 months.[6]

CALCULATIONS

Choice of Age Interval. Ten-year age groups were chosen over smaller (e.g., 5-year) groups in order to ensure ample precision of estimates of the proportion providing care in each age group. For the broader definition of care for men and women together, there was also ample precision to repeat calculations using 5-year age intervals (presented at the end of this appendix).[7]

---

[4]Age at the NSOC interview was calculated from month and year of birth from NHATS for spouse caregivers and from NSOC for other types of caregivers. For 36 cases where age was missing from NSOC, the information was filled in based on age in NHATS. An additional 31 cases were still missing age, and assumed to be missing age at random (i.e., we assumed knowing their ages would not change the age distribution).

[5] NHATS participants were considered to have probable dementia if: the participant or the proxy reported a doctor's diagnosis of dementia or Alzheimer's disease; the participant received a score of 2 or more on a dementia screening instrument administered to a proxy; or the participant scored >=1.5 SD below the mean on at least two out of three domains on tests of memory, orientation, and executive functioning. These criteria have high sensitivity and specificity relative to a clinical diagnostic assessment (see Kasper et al., 2013b).

[6]In the second set of calculations, duration of help was assumed to be 3 or more months if the NHATS respondent received assistance for 3 or more months with any self-care activities (if they reported receiving assistance with eating, toileting, bathing, or dressing) or with any mobility activities (if they only reported receiving help getting out of bed). This additional restriction is intended to approximate the 90-day requirement in the definition of disability in the Health Insurance Portability and Accountability Act (Drabek and Marton, 2015).

[7]For all estimates, Relative Standard Errors (i.e., ratio of a standard error of an estimate to the estimate) are less than .30, a commonly used guideline in health surveys (Klein et al., 2002).

Proportion Caregiving and Standard Errors. To obtain estimates of the proportion caregiving, ${}_nc_x$, we divided the weighted number of caregivers from NSOC in each 10-year age group by the non-institutionalized population in each age group from the CPS for 2011 (see Table D-3).

Standard errors of proportions were calculated by taking the square root of the variance, according to the following formula: $var({}_nP_x*W*N/{}_nT_x) = (N\^2) * [(W\^2)*var({}_nP_x) + ({}_nP_x\^2)*var(W) + (var({}_nP_x)*var(W))] / ({}_nT_x\^2)$, where ${}_nP_x$ is the proportion of caregivers in age group x to x+n, W is the average weight for the caregiving sample, N is the number of caregivers in the sample, and ${}_nT_x$ is the number of adults in the population in age group x to x+n.[8] Table D-4 shows the unweighted and weighted sample sizes and the mean and standard error of the weight used in the calculations of the standard errors.

These calculations take into account uncertainty from two components in the numerators of the care rates: the distribution of caregivers across age groups (${}_nP_x$) and the mean population weight (W). Standard errors for ${}_nP_x$ and W were estimated using svy commands in Stata that take into account the complex design of NSOC. Population counts (from the CPS) are assumed to be fixed. The latter assumption should have minimal influence on the confidence intervals because the CPS relies on large sample sizes and produces point estimates very similar to the population counts from the 2010 Census.

Life Table Calculations. Unabridged (single year of age) life tables, available for 2010 for the entire population and by gender, were converted to abridged (10-year age category) life tables according to procedures described in Arias (2014). Because the focus of the caregiving calculations is adult life, we began the life table calculations at age 20; that is, the initial population (i.e., "radix") of the life table was assumed to begin at age 20 with 100,000 people (see Table D-5).

Expected Years of Care and Percentage of Remaining Life Spent Caring. Life expectancy was apportioned into years spent caring using Sullivan's method. First, we divided person-years expected to be lived in each age group (${}_nL_x$ in Table D-5) according to the proportion in each age group who provide care (${}_nc_x$ in Table D-6). Then, we calculated total years caring from age x forward by summing the person-years caring for the current age group to age 80+. We then calculated the expected number of years caring from age x by dividing the total years caring from age x forward by

[8]For gender-specific estimates, we used the proportion of women (men) caregivers in age group i, the average weight for women (men), the number of women (men) caregivers, and the number of women (men) in the population in age group i.

TABLE D-3 Calculation of Age-Specific Proportions Caregiving and Standard Errors[a]

Age (years)	Age Distribution of Caregivers (P)[b]	SE (P)[b]	Weighted Number of Caregivers[b]	Population (000s)[c]	Proportion Caregiving $_nc_x$	SE $_nc_x$
Caregivers to Older Adults with One or More Activity Limitations						
All						
20-29	0.039	0.0065	694,673	42,907	0.016	0.0029
30-39	0.060	0.0077	1,066,180	39,457	0.027	0.0039
40-49	0.163	0.0127	2,886,054	42,576	0.068	0.0068
50-59	0.269	0.0154	4,761,929	41,519	0.115	0.0097
60-69	0.250	0.0141	4,422,162	29,590	0.149	0.0126
70-79	0.148	0.0105	2,615,696	16,342	0.160	0.0152
80+	0.069	0.0071	1,225,864	10,676	0.115	0.0137
Men						
20-29	0.047	0.0130	321,344	21,877	0.015	0.0041
30-39	0.060	0.0124	405,133	19,609	0.021	0.0045
40-49	0.153	0.0213	1,032,939	20,972	0.049	0.0075
50-59	0.241	0.0182	1,632,888	20,194	0.081	0.0079
60-69	0.231	0.0191	1,563,215	14,047	0.111	0.0115
70-79	0.172	0.0176	1,162,429	7,307	0.159	0.0191
80+	0.097	0.0137	654,311	4,174	0.157	0.0243
Women						
20-29	0.034	0.0072	372,848	21,029	0.018	0.0040
30-39	0.061	0.0091	661,076	19,848	0.033	0.0056
40-49	0.170	0.0149	1,853,752	21,604	0.086	0.0099

50-59	0.287	0.0217	3,130,715	21,325	0.147	0.0156
60-69	0.262	0.0174	2,860,092	15,544	0.184	0.0184
70-79	0.133	0.0112	1,451,872	9,035	0.161	0.0181
80+	0.052	0.0082	569,945	6,502	0.088	0.0153
Caregivers to Older Adults with Severe Limitations[d]						
20-29	0.042	0.0102	352,627	42,907	0.008	0.0022
30-39	0.060	0.0118	511,955	39,457	0.013	0.0028
40-49	0.179	0.0177	1,522,016	42,576	0.036	0.0049
50-59	0.273	0.0211	2,316,811	41,519	0.056	0.0069
60-69	0.254	0.0190	2,156,373	29,590	0.073	0.0088
70-79	0.115	0.0131	9,758,11	16,342	0.060	0.0089
80+	0.076	0.0117	6,462,06	10,676	0.061	0.0109
Caregivers to Older Adults with Severe Limitations for 3 or More Months[d]						
20-29	0.038	0.0103	297,507	42,907	0.007	0.0020
30-39	0.064	0.0135	497,619	39,457	0.013	0.0029
40-49	0.179	0.0179	1,386,147	42,576	0.033	0.0044
50-59	0.270	0.0222	2,095,630	41,519	0.050	0.0062
60-69	0.258	0.0184	2,000,285	29,590	0.068	0.0078
70-79	0.112	0.0131	870,636	16,342	0.053	0.0079
80+	0.078	0.0128	605,843	10,676	0.057	0.0106

[a] See text for formula for calculating Standard Errors.
[b] SOURCE: 2011 National Study of Caregiving linked to the National Health and Aging Trends Study.
[c] SOURCE: U.S. Census Bureau 2011 Current Population Survey.
[d] See text for definition of severe limitations.

TABLE D-4 Sample Sizes, Weighted Population, and Mean Weight for Caregiving Samples

	Sample Size	Weighted Population of Caregivers	Mean Weight (SE)
Caregivers to older adults with one or more activity limitations			
All	1,971	17,672,559	8,966 (561)
Men	660	6,772,259	10,261 (638)
Women	1,311	10,900,300	8,314 (622)
Caregivers to older adult with severe limitations I[a]	1,018	8,481,799	8,331 (793)
Caregivers to older adult with severe limitations II[a]	953	7,753,666	8,136 (732)

[a]See text for definition of severe limitations.
SOURCE: 2011 National Study of Caregiving linked to the National Health and Aging Trends Study.

the number surviving to age x (column l_x in Table D-5). The percentage of remaining life to be spent caring was calculated by dividing the expected number of years caring from age x (in Table D-6) by the expectation of life at age x (in Table D-5). Step-by-step calculations (for active life expectancy) are available in Jagger et al. (2006).

Confidence Intervals for Expected Number of Years Caring. Table D-7 presents calculations of the standard error of the expected number of years caring. These calculations adopt the usual assumption that mortality rates (from vital statistics), which generate the life table estimates, are fixed. Step 1 (column 1) was to take the square of the number of person-years lived in each age group (${}_nL_x$ from Table D-5) and multiply that figure by the variance (squared standard error) of the proportion caregiving in that age group (SE(${}_nc_x$) calculated in Table D-3). In column 2 we sum the figures in column 1 from age x forward. The variance of the expected number of years caring is then column 2 divided by the squared number of people surviving to age x (l_x from Table D-5), and the standard error is the square root of this calculation. Confidence intervals of 95 percent are calculated using the standard approach of plus or minus 1.96 times the standard error of the estimate. A test statistic for differences in number of years caring between men and women (3.87) was calculated by dividing the difference in years caring (6.1-4.1) by the sum of the square roots of the variances (.218+.299).

Alternative Estimates Using 5-Year Age Groups. To examine the sensitivity of calculations to age group width, Tables D-8 through D-11 provide calculations using 5-year age groups for (all) caregivers providing care to an older adult with activity limitations. Findings regarding percentage of life spent caregiving are consistent with calculations using 10-year and 5-year age groups. For example, at age 80 there is only a .2 percentage point difference between the estimates based on 10-year (11.3 percent) and 5-year (11.5 percent) age groups.

TABLE D-5 Abridged Life Table Calculations, Adults Ages 20 and Older, 2010

Age (years)	Probability of Dying Between Ages *x* to *x* + *n*	Number Surviving to Age *x*	Number Dying Between Ages *x* to *x* + *n*	Person-Years Lived Between Ages *x* to *x* + *n*	Total Number of Person-Years Lived Above Age *x*	Expectation of Life at Age *x*
	${}_nq_x$	l_x	${}_nd_x$	${}_nL_x$	T_x	e_x
			All			
20-29	0.00909	100,000	909	995,570	5,939,745	59.4
30-39	0.01237	99,091	1,226	985,124	4,944,175	49.9
40-49	0.02586	97,865	2,531	967,442	3,959,051	40.5
50-59	0.05859	95,334	5,586	927,774	2,991,609	31.4
60-69	0.12054	89,748	10,819	848,067	2,063,835	23.0
70-79	0.26747	78,930	21,111	692,193	1,215,768	15.4
80+	1.00000	57,819	57,819	523,575	523,575	9.1
			Men			
20-29	0.01303	100,000	1,303	993,590	5,702,801	57.0
30-39	0.01602	98,697	1,582	979,388	4,709,211	47.7
40-49	0.03189	97,116	3,097	957,437	3,729,823	38.4
50-59	0.07367	94,019	6,927	908,627	2,772,386	29.5
60-69	0.14668	87,092	12,775	812,035	1,863,759	21.4
70-79	0.31301	74,317	23,262	635,119	1,051,724	14.2
80+	1.00000	51,055	51,055	416,606	416,606	8.2

Women						
20-29	0.00502	100,000	502	997,625	6,166,526	61.7
30-39	0.00872	99,498	867	991,009	5,168,900	51.9
40-49	0.01992	98,631	1,964	977,617	4,177,891	42.4
50-59	0.04409	96,666	4,262	947,025	3,200,274	33.1
60-69	0.09625	92,405	8,894	883,977	2,253,249	24.4
70-79	0.22886	83,510	19,112	748,357	1,369,272	16.4
80+	1.00000	64,399	64,399	620,914	620,914	9.6

SOURCE: Based on National Center for Health Statistics (Arias, 2014).

TABLE D-6 Calculation of Expected Number of Years and Proportion of Remaining Life Spent Caregiving

	Proportion Caregiving	SE	Person-Years Caring	Total Years Caring from Age x Forward	Expected Number of Years Caring from Age x	95% CI		Percentage of Remaining Life Caring
Age (years)	${}_{n}c_{x}$	$SE_{n}c_{x}$	${}_{n}c_{x} * {}_{n}L_{x}$	T_{cx}	e_{cx}	$e_{cx} - 1.96$ SE	$e_{cx} + 1.96$ SE	$e_{cx}/e_{x}*100$
Caregivers to Older Adults with One or More Activity Limitations								
All								
20-29	0.016	0.0029	16,118	512,379	5.1	4.7	5.5	8.6
30-39	0.027	0.0039	26,619	496,260	5.0	4.6	5.4	10.0
40-49	0.068	0.0068	65,579	469,641	4.8	4.4	5.2	11.9
50-59	0.115	0.0097	106,409	404,062	4.2	3.8	4.6	13.5
60-69	0.149	0.0126	126,742	297,653	3.3	3.0	3.7	14.4
70-79	0.160	0.0152	110,792	170,911	2.2	1.8	2.5	14.1
80+	0.115	0.0137	60,119	60,119	1.0	0.8	1.3	11.5
Men								
20-29	0.015	0.0041	14,595	412,169	4.1	3.7	4.5	7.2
30-39	0.021	0.0045	20,235	397,574	4.0	3.6	4.5	8.4
40-49	0.049	0.0075	47,157	377,339	3.9	3.5	4.3	10.1
50-59	0.081	0.0079	73,472	330,183	3.5	3.1	3.9	11.9
60-69	0.111	0.0115	90,367	256,711	2.9	2.5	3.4	13.8
70-79	0.159	0.0191	101,037	166,344	2.2	1.8	2.7	15.8
80+	0.157	0.0243	65,307	65,307	1.3	0.9	1.7	15.7
Women								
20-29	0.018	0.0040	17,688	610,949	6.1	5.5	6.7	9.9
30-39	0.033	0.0056	33,007	593,261	6.0	5.4	6.5	11.5

40-49	0.086	0.0099	83,885	560,253	5.7	5.1	6.3	13.4
50-59	0.147	0.0156	139,032	476,368	4.9	4.4	5.5	14.9
60-69	0.184	0.0184	162,651	337,336	3.7	3.2	4.1	15.0
70-79	0.161	0.0181	120,257	174,684	2.1	1.7	2.5	12.8
80+	0.088	0.0153	54,427	54,427	0.8	0.6	1.1	8.8
Caregivers to Older Adults with Severe Limitations[a]								
20-29	0.008	0.0022	8,182	242,146	2.4	2.1	2.7	4.1
30-39	0.013	0.0028	12,782	233,964	2.4	2.1	2.6	4.7
40-49	0.036	0.0049	34,584	221,182	2.3	2.0	2.5	5.6
50-59	0.056	0.0069	51,771	186,597	2.0	1.7	2.2	6.2
60-69	0.073	0.0088	61,803	134,826	1.5	1.3	1.7	6.5
70-79	0.060	0.0089	41,332	73,024	0.9	0.7	1.1	6.0
80+	0.061	0.0109	31,691	31,691	0.5	0.4	0.7	6.1
Caregivers to Older Adults with Severe Limitations for 3 or More Months[a]								
20-29	0.007	0.0020	6,903	221,571	2.2	2.0	2.5	3.7
30-39	0.013	0.0029	12,424	214,668	2.2	1.9	2.4	4.3
40-49	0.033	0.0044	31,497	202,244	2.1	1.8	2.3	5.7
50-59	0.050	0.0062	46,828	170,747	1.8	1.6	2.0	5.7
60-69	0.068	0.0078	57,329	123,918	1.4	1.2	1.6	6.0
70-79	0.053	0.0079	36,877	66,589	0.8	0.7	1.0	5.5
80+	0.057	0.0106	29,712	29,712	0.5	0.3	0.7	5.7

[a] See text for definition of severe limitations.

SOURCE: Proportion caring ${}_nc_x$ and standard errors SE (${}_nc_x$) calculated in Table D-3. ${}_nL_x$ calculated in Table D-7. Standard errors of e_{cx} calculated in Table D-7.

TABLE D-7 Calculation of Standard Error of Caregiving Life Expectancy

Age (years)	${}_nL_x$^2 * SE(${}_nc_x$)^2 (column 1)	Sum Col. 1 from Age x Forward (column 2)	V=col. 2/ l_x^2 (column 3)	SE= sqrt (column 3)
Caregivers to Older Adults with One or More Activity Limitations				
All				
20-29	8,245,389	422,867,873	0.0423	0.2056
30-39	14,497,857	414,622,484	0.0422	0.2055
40-49	42,859,716	400,124,627	0.0418	0.2044
50-59	81,257,655	357,264,911	0.0393	0.1983
60-69	113,761,156	276,007,256	0.0343	0.1851
70-79	110,473,754	162,246,101	0.0260	0.1614
80+	51,772,346	51,772,346	0.0155	0.1244
Men				
20-29	16,878,542	477,271,264	0.0477	0.2185
30-39	19,250,239	460,392,722	0.0473	0.2174
40-49	52,148,957	441,142,483	0.0468	0.2163
50-59	51,880,478	388,993,526	0.0440	0.2098
60-69	87,830,250	337,113,048	0.0444	0.2108
70-79	147,189,970	249,282,798	0.0451	0.2125
80+	102,092,828	102,092,828	0.0392	0.1979
Women				
20-29	15,681,031	896,191,523	0.0896	0.2994
30-39	30,630,022	880,510,492	0.0889	0.2982
40-49	93,628,007	849,880,470	0.0874	0.2956
50-59	218,740,540	756,252,464	0.0809	0.2845
60-69	264,412,916	537,511,924	0.0630	0.2509
70-79	183,393,283	273,099,007	0.0392	0.1979
80+	89,705,725	89,705,725	0.0216	0.1471
Caregivers to Older Adults with Severe Limitations[a]				
20-29	4,663,542	202,510,852	0.0203	0.1423
30-39	7,780,073	197,847,310	0.0201	0.1419
40-49	22,544,727	190,067,237	0.0198	0.1409
50-59	40,499,527	167,522,510	0.0184	0.1358
60-69	56,232,746	127,022,983	0.0158	0.1256
70-79	37,938,610	70,790,237	0.0114	0.1066
80+	32,851,627	32,851,627	0.0098	0.0991

TABLE D-7 Continued

Age (years)	${}_nL_x$^2 * SE(${}_nc_x$)^2 (column 1)	Sum Col. 1 from Age x Forward (column 2)	V=col. 2/ l_x^2 (column 3)	SE= sqrt (column 3)
Caregivers to Older Adults with Severe Limitations for 3 or More Months[a]				
20-29	3,863,784	166,956,322	0.0167	0.1292
30-39	8,135,709	163,092,538	0.0166	0.1289
40-49	18,001,446	154,956,829	0.0162	0.1272
50-59	32,703,580	136,955,383	0.0151	0.1228
60-69	43,504,373	104,251,803	0.0129	0.1138
70-79	29,781,218	60,747,430	0.0098	0.0987
80+	30,966,212	30,966,212	0.0093	0.0962

[a] See text for definition of severe limitations.

SOURCE: ${}_nL_x$ and l_x calculated in Table D-5; SE(${}_nc_x$) calculated in Table D-3.

TABLE D-8 Calculation of Age-Specific Caregiving Rates and Standard Errors: 5-Year Age Groups[a]

Age (years)	Age Distribution of Caregivers (*P*)[b]	SE (*P*)[b]	Weighted Number of Caregivers[b]	Population (000s)[c]	Proportion Caregiving $_nc_x$	SE $_nc_x$
			All Caregivers to Older Adults with One or More Activity Limitations			
20-24	0.022	0.0045	389,830	21,525	0.018	0.0038
25-29	0.017	0.0050	304,841	21,382	0.014	0.0043
30-34	0.022	0.0046	380,769	20,202	0.019	0.0042
35-39	0.039	0.0066	685,411	19,255	0.036	0.0065
40-44	0.055	0.0077	972,874	20,587	0.047	0.0072
45-49	0.108	0.0092	1,913,182	21,989	0.087	0.0092
50-54	0.135	0.0123	2,392,492	21,965	0.109	0.0120
55-59	0.134	0.0091	2,369,438	19,554	0.121	0.0112
60-64	0.141	0.0109	2,493,034	17,430	0.143	0.0142
65-69	0.109	0.0085	1,929,126	12,160	0.159	0.0159
70-74	0.081	0.0081	1,423,617	9,254	0.154	0.0182
75-79	0.067	0.0072	1,192,079	7,088	0.168	0.0208
80-84	0.041	0.0058	716,348	5,719	0.125	0.0196
85+	0.029	0.0042	509,516	4,957	0.103	0.0163

[a] See text for formula for calculating Standard Errors.
[b] SOURCE: 2011 National Study of Caregiving linked to the National Health and Aging Trends Study.
[c] SOURCE: 2011 Current Population Survey.

TABLE D-9 Abridged Life Table Calculations, Adults Ages 20 and Older, 2010: 5-Year Age Groups

Age (years)	Probability of Dying Between Ages *x* to *x* + *n*	Number Surviving to Age *x*	Number Dying Between Ages *x* to *x* + *n*	Person-Years Lived Between Ages *x* to *x* + *n*	Total Number of Person-Years Lived Above Age *x*	Expectation of Life at Age *x*
	${}_nq_x$	l_x	${}_nd_x$	${}_nL_x$	T_x	e_x
			All			
20-24	0.00432	100,000	432	498,921	5,939,745	59.4
25-29	0.00479	99,568	477	496,649	5,440,824	54.6
30-34	0.00550	99,091	545	494,095	4,944,175	49.9
35-39	0.00691	98,547	681	491,030	4,450,081	45.2
40-44	0.00998	97,865	977	486,885	3,959,051	40.5
45-49	0.01604	96,889	1,555	480,557	3,472,166	35.8
50-54	0.02434	95,334	2,321	470,869	2,991,609	31.4
55-59	0.03511	93,013	3,265	456,904	2,520,739	27.1
60-64	0.04985	89,748	4,474	437,557	2,063,835	23.0
65-69	0.07441	85,275	6,345	410,510	1,626,278	19.1
70-74	0.11232	78,930	8,865	372,485	1,215,768	15.4
75-79	0.17478	70,065	12,246	319,708	843,283	12.0
80-84	0.27438	57,819	15,864	249,432	523,575	9.1
85+	1.00000	41,954	41,954	274,143	274,143	6.5

SOURCE: Based on National Center for Health Statistics (Arias, 2014).

TABLE D-10 Calculation of Expected Number of Years and Percentage of Remaining Life Spent Caregiving: 5-Year Age Groups

	Proportion Caregiving	SE	Person-Years Caring	Total Years Caring from Age x Forward	Expected Number of Years Caring from Age x	95% CI		Percentage of Remaining Life Caring
Age (years)	${}_nc_x$	$SE_{n}c_x$	${}_nc_x * {}_nL_x$	T_{cx}	e_{cx}	$e_{cx} - 1.96$ SE	$e_{cx} + 1.96$ SE	e_{cx}/e_x*100
All Caregivers to Older Adults with One or More Activity Limitations								
20-24	0.018	0.0038	9,036	512,585	5.1	4.8	5.5	8.6
25-29	0.014	0.0043	7,081	503,549	5.1	4.7	5.4	9.3
30-34	0.019	0.0042	9,313	496,468	5.0	4.7	5.4	10.0
35-39	0.036	0.0065	17,479	487,156	4.9	4.6	5.3	10.9
40-44	0.047	0.0072	23,009	469,677	4.8	4.4	5.1	11.9
45-49	0.087	0.0092	41,812	446,668	4.6	4.3	5.0	12.9
50-54	0.109	0.0120	51,288	404,857	4.2	3.9	4.6	13.5
55-59	0.121	0.0112	55,365	353,568	3.8	3.5	4.1	14.0
60-64	0.143	0.0142	62,584	298,203	3.3	3.0	3.6	14.4
65-69	0.159	0.0159	65,125	235,619	2.8	2.5	3.1	14.5
70-74	0.154	0.0182	57,302	170,493	2.2	1.9	2.4	14.0
75-79	0.168	0.0208	53,769	113,191	1.6	1.4	1.9	13.4
80-84	0.125	0.0196	31,243	59,422	1.0	0.8	1.3	11.3
85+	0.103	0.0163	28,178	28,178	0.7	0.5	0.9	10.3

SOURCE: Caregiving rates ${}_nc_x$ and standard errors SE (${}_nc_x$) calculated in Table D-8. ${}_nL_x$ calculated in Table D-9. Standard errors of e_{cx} calculated in Table D-11.

TABLE D-11 Calculation of Standard Error of Caregiving Life Expectancy: 5-Year Age Groups

Age (years)	${}_nL_x$^2 * SE(${}_nc_x$)^2 (column 1)	Sum Column 1 From Age x Forward (column 2)	V = column 2/ l_x^2 (column 3)	SE = sqrt (column 3)
All Caregivers to Older Adults with One or More Activity Limitations				
20-24	3,676,837	327,861,567	0.0328	0.1811
25-29	4,476,599	324,184,730	0.0327	0.1808
30-34	4,272,712	319,708,131	0.0326	0.1804
35-39	10,118,905	315,435,419	0.0325	0.1802
40-44	12,378,426	305,316,514	0.0319	0.1785
45-49	19,448,278	292,938,088	0.0312	0.1767
50-54	32,138,131	273,489,811	0.0301	0.1735
55-59	26,296,162	241,351,680	0.0279	0.1670
60-64	38,806,361	215,055,518	0.0267	0.1634
65-69	42,639,829	176,249,158	0.0242	0.1557
70-74	45,808,760	133,609,329	0.0214	0.1464
75-79	44,136,656	87,800,569	0.0179	0.1337
80-84	23,803,772	43,663,914	0.0131	0.1143
85+	19,860,141	19,860,141	0.0113	0.1062

SOURCES: ${}_nL_x$ and l_x calculated in Table D-9; SE(${}_nc_x$) calculated in Table D-8.

REFERENCES

Arias, E. 2014. United States life tables, 2010. *National vital statistics reports* 63(7). Hyattsville, MD: National Center for Health Statistics. http://www.cdc.gov/nchs/data/nvsr/nvsr63/nvsr63_07.pdf (accessed October 10, 2015).

Drabek, J., and W. Marton. 2015. *Measuring the need for long-term services and supports research brief.* http://aspe.hhs.gov/sites/default/files/pdf/110376/MeasLTSSrb.pdf (accessed October 10, 2015).

Imai, K., and S. Soneji. 2007. On the estimation of disability-free life expectancy: Sullivan's Method and its extension. *Journal of the American Statistical Association* 102(80): 1199-1211.

Jagger, C., B. Cox, S. Le Roy, and EHEMU (European Health Expectancy Monitoring Unit). 2006. *Health expectancy calculation by the Sullivan Method*, 3rd ed. EHEMU Technical Report, September 2006. http://www.eurohex.eu/pdf/Sullivan_guide_final_jun2007.pdf.

Kasper, J. D., V. A. Freedman, and B. C. Spillman. 2013a. *Classification of persons by dementia status in the National Health and Aging Trends Study.* Technical Paper No. 5. http://www.nhats.org (accessed October 10, 2015).

Kasper, J. D., V. A. Freedman, and B. C. Spillman. 2013b. *National Study of Caregiving user guide.* Baltimore, MD: Johns Hopkins University School of Public Health. http://www.nhats.org (accessed October 10, 2015).

Klein, R. J., S. E. Proctor, M. A. Boudreault, and K. M. Turczyn. 2002. *Healthy People 2010 criteria for data suppression*, no. 24. http://www.cdc.gov/nchs/data/statnt/statnt24.pdf (accessed October 10, 2015).

National Health and Aging Trends Study. Produced and distributed by www.nhats.org with funding from the National Institute on Aging (grant number NIA U01AG32947).

National Study of Caregiving. Produced and distributed by www.nhats.org with funding from the U.S. Department of Health and Human Services' Office of the Assistant Secretary for Planning and Evaluation in cooperation with the National Institute on Aging (grant number NIA U01AG32947).

Stone, R. 2015. Factors affecting the future of family caregiving in the United States, edited by J. Gaugler and R. L. Kane. In *Family caregiving in the new normal.* Waltham, MA: Elsevier.

Sullivan, D. F. 1971. A single index of mortality and morbidity. *HSMHA Health Reports* 86:347-354.

U.S. Census Bureau. 2011. Current Population Survey, *Annual Social and Economic Supplement. Table 1.* http://www.census.gov/population/age/data/2011comp.html (accessed October 10, 2015).

Appendix E

Methodology: NHATS and NSOC Surveys

This report presents data on older adults and their family caregivers drawn from the public use files of the 2011 National Health and Aging Trends Study (NHATS) and the National Study of Caregiving (NSOC). They are two linked national studies led by the Johns Hopkins University Bloomberg School of Public Health, with data collection by Westat, and support from the National Institute on Aging for NHATS and the Assistant Secretary for Planning and Evaluation of the U.S. Department of Health and Human Services for NSOC (NHATS, 2015). Extensive technical documentation of the surveys' designs is available at: https://www.nhats.org/scripts/TechnicalPapers.htm and http://www.nhats.org.

NHATS is nationally representative of Medicare beneficiaries aged 65 years and older. Respondents (or their proxies) living in the community and in residential care settings, other than nursing homes, participated in a 2-hour in-person interview that included self-reports and validated performance-based measures of disability (Kasper et al., 2013a). For those living in nursing homes, an interview was conducted with a member of the facility staff to learn about the respondent's service environment. Study participants were asked whether and how they performed daily activities in the month before the interview. Among older adults who received assistance, a detailed helper roster was created listing the relationship and specific activities for each person providing assistance. Nursing home residents were not included in generating the helper roster.

NSOC respondents (i.e., family caregivers of the NHATS respondents) were family members or other unpaid helpers who provided assistance with mobility, self-care, household activities, transportation, or medically oriented tasks. A telephone interview was conducted with up to five family caregivers (i.e., "helpers") for each older adult. For older adults with more than five eligible helpers, the five helpers were selected at random.

Of 7,609 NHATS participants living in the community or in a residential care facility, 2,423 were included in the NSOC sampling frame, and 4,935 helpers met NSOC eligibility criteria. An NSOC non-response can arise from the NHATS participant (who may refuse to provide contact information for helpers) or his or her caregivers (who may refuse to participate) (Kasper et al., 2013a). The NHATS participants did not provide contact information for 1,573 eligible family caregivers, and 1,355 of the remaining 3,362 eligible family caregivers could not be located or refused to respond, yielding 68.1 percent and 59.7 percent of first-stage and second-stage response rates, respectively. In total, 2,007 family caregivers of 1,369 older adults responded in 2011 to the NSOC.

Observations from NHATS and NSOC are weighted to produce nationally representative estimates and to account for the surveys' complex sampling designs. Weights adjust for differential probabilities of selection at both the NHATS sample person and caregiver levels. The analyses presented in this report were conducted with statistical software (Stata v.12) using the survey sampling weights provided to NSOC users.

CLASSIFYING NHATS PARTICIPANTS BY DEMENTIA STATUS

Several analyses presented in this report distinguish among three groups of NHATS participants—those with probable dementia, possible dementia, or no dementia. NHATS assigns these categories based on the following:

- A report by the sample person or proxy respondent that a doctor told the sample person that he/she had dementia or Alzheimer's disease.
- A score indicating "probable dementia" on the AD8 Dementia Screening Interview (which was administered to proxy respondents to the NHATS interview). The AD8 is a brief informant interview used to detect dementia (Galvin et al., 2005, 2006).
- Cognitive tests that evaluate the sample person's memory (immediate and delayed 10-word recall), orientation (date, month, year, and day of the week; naming the President and Vice President), and executive function (clock drawing test).

A report by either the NHATS participant or a proxy respondent that a doctor told the sample person that he/she had dementia or Alzheimer's disease was used to classify persons as having probable dementia (Kasper et al., 2013b). Proxy respondents not reporting a diagnosis who gave answers to the AD8 who met criteria for likely dementia (a score of 2 or higher) also were classified as having probable dementia. For all others—self-respondents not reporting a diagnosis and a small number (n = 79) with proxy respondents who had no diagnosis reported and did not meet AD8 criteria, but had test information—score cut-points applied to cognitive tests assessing three domains (memory, orientation, executive functioning) were used. Impairment was defined as scores at or below 1.5 standard deviations (SDs) from the mean for self-respondents. Impairment in at least two cognitive domains was required for probable dementia; a cut-point of <1.5 SDs below the mean in one domain was used for cognitive impairment, indicating possible dementia.

REFERENCES

Galvin, J., C. Roe, K. Powlishta, M. Coats, S. Muich, E. Grant, J. Miller, M. Storandt, and J. Morris. 2005. The AD8: A brief informant interview to detect dementia. *Neurology* 65(4):559-564.

Galvin, J. E., C. M. Roe, C. Xiong, and J. C. Morris. 2006. Validity and reliability of the AD8 informant interview in dementia. *Neurology* 67(11):1942-1948.

Kasper, J. D., V. A. Freedman, and B. C. Spillman. 2013a. *National Study of Caregiving (NSOC) user guide.* Baltimore, MD: Johns Hopkins University School of Public Health.

Kasper, J. D., V. A. Freedman, and B. C. Spillman. 2013b. *Classification of persons by dementia status in the National Health and Aging Trends Study.* https://www.nhats.org/scripts/documents/NHATS_Dementia_Technical_Paper_5_Jul2013.pdf (accessed May 20, 2015).

NHATS (National Health and Aging Trends Study). 2015. *NHATS FAQ.* http://www.nhats.org/scripts/participant/NHATSFAQ.htm (accessed August 23, 2016).

Appendix F

Caregiving: The Odyssey of Becoming More Human

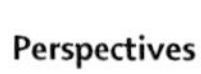

The art of medicine

Caregiving: the odyssey of becoming more human

"Let the more loving one be me."

W H Auden, *The More Loving One*

I lead her across the living room, holding her hand behind my back, so that I can navigate the two of us between chairs, sofas, end tables, over Persian rugs, through the passageway and into the kitchen. I help her find and carefully place herself in a chair, one of four at the oval-shaped oak table. She turns the wrong way, forcing the chair outward; I push her legs around and in, under the table's edge. The sun streams through the bank of windows. The brightness of the light and its warmth, on a freezing winter's day, make her smile. She turns toward me. The uneven pupils in Joan Kleinman's green-brown eyes look above and beyond my head, searching for my face. Gently I turn her head towards me. I grin as she raises her eyebrows in recognition, shakes her long brown hair and the soft warmth of her sudden happiness lights up her still strikingly beautiful face. "Wonderful!" she whispers. "I'm a Palo Alto, a California girl. I like it warm."

I place a fork in her right hand and guide it to the poached egg in the deep bowl. I have already cut up the toast, so that I can help her spear pieces of bread and soak up the yolk. She can't find the tea cup in front of her, so I move her hand next to its handle. The Darjeeling tea glows hot and golden red in the Chinese tea cup. "Wonderful!" she again whispers.

Later, while I am trying to decide what she should wear, Joan frowns, fussing with her feet. "These nails are too long. And where are my shoes? I need to find my shoes?" She stands before about 18 pairs on a rack, shoes her unseeing brain can't recognise. "Don't get agitated," I interject with foreboding. "Do you want a Zyprexa?"

"No! No pills. Why do I need pills. I'm healthy."

"Joan, you have Alzheimer's disease. You're not healthy. You have a brain disease. A serious problem." I can barely conceal the frustration in my voice.

"Why did God do this to me? I've always been good. I never did anything to cause this. Should I kill myself?" She says it in such a way as to signal to me, as she has before, that this is a statement of pain and a cry for help, not an earnest question to discuss or to make plans. In fact it means the opposite: because, as in the past, she quickly changes tone. "If you love then you can do it! We can live and love."

"We can do it" I repeat, each time a little bit more weakly, enduring the unendurable. And so, another morning begins, another day of caregiving and care-receiving between a 67-year-old man and a 69-year-old woman who have lived together passionately and collaboratively for 43 years, absorbed in an intense relationship—intellectual, aesthetic, sexual, emotional, moral. What has made it possible to get even this far are our two adult children, their spouses, my 95-year-old mother, my brother, and our four grandchildren who sometimes take the hand of their often uncomprehending grandmother, because she is standing alone, lost, and lead her back into the protective, enabling circle of our family.

For 5 years we have lived through the progressive neurodegenerative disorder that has unspooled the neural networks of Joan's brain. It originated in the occipital lobes at the far back of the brain. The pathology of undoing has inexorably worked its way forward to the parietal and temporal lobes on the sides of the brain, and finally to the frontal lobes that mount up behind the forehead, through the layers of neurons and nodes of connecting neural nets that structure and retain memories, focus attention, balance emotion with common sense, underwrite judgment, and make possible the ordinariness of reading, writing, telling stories, understanding jokes, recognising people, orienting oneself in space and in time, but also within emotional and moral coordinates, and, of course, doing things in the world.

This trail of unravelled brain structure and mounting dysfunction is, in physical terms, only one of inches; yet its silent, implacable wrecking creates entirely new conditions for living a life and being with others. Joan has an atypical form of Alzheimer's disease. She is, as I write, functionally blind. She cannot find her way in our home, where she has lived since 1982. She often misinterprets those objects she does see, treating a chair as if it were a table or the floor lamp a person. Left unaccompanied, she walks into doors and has banged her legs so hard into low tables she didn't see that she has caused deep contusions. Once, at our son's house, she opened a door and fell down a flight of unseen stairs, breaking her pelvis; at the onset of the disease, she ran into the street, where a pick-up truck ran over her right foot.

Joan can't, on her own, find her way out of the bedroom. Yet, once safely in my hands or those of our trusted home health aide, she can walk effectively. A China scholar who translates and interprets ancient texts, she can no longer read. A wife and mother whose fierce commitment to the family was its moral backbone, she now struggles to be part of family functions and can sometimes seem impassive and cut off from us. Formerly the primary caregiver for her husband and children, she is now the care-receiver. She may no longer be who she was even 5 years ago, but her subjectivity has not so much disappeared—there is much of her personality that is still present—as altered. And that alteration has affected what had been for four decades an all-consuming relationship—our identity and orientation. I still cannot accept to treat her as if she can no longer share the sensibility and narrative we have created over four decades, and yet, more and more frequently, she can't.

She is happy much of the time. It is me, the caregiver, who, more often, is sad and despairing.

She is a source of great concern to each of us, her family members, about how to best manage her condition. We grieve what we have lost and fear what we know lies ahead. We have each of us gone through feelings of loss, anger, and frustration. We have been marked by a special kind of pain. But we have also experienced a deepening sense of responsibility, gratitude for all that we had lived through together, love, solidarity, and a shared sensibility that we have resisted what is beyond our control and are, individually and collectively, more for it. This is not meant as a self-satisfying summing up—there is no final summary yet and the proper genre is tragedy, as millions who are engaged in these everyday practices know.

I am writing principally about people like me who give care to loved ones who suffer the infirmities of advanced age, serious disabilities, terminal illnesses, and the devastating consequences of such health catastrophes as stroke or dementia. Faced with these crises, family and close friends become responsible for assistance with all the practical, mundane activities of daily living: dressing, feeding, bathing, toileting, ambulating, communicating, and interfacing with the health-care system. Caregivers protect the vulnerable and dependent. To use the experience-distorting technical language: they offer cognitive, behavioural, and emotional support. And because caregiving is so tiring, and emotionally draining, effective caregiving requires that caregivers themselves receive practical and emotional support.

But, to use the close experiential language of actually doing it, caregiving is also a defining moral practice. It is a practice of empathic imagination, responsibility, witnessing, and solidarity with those in great need. It is a moral practice that makes caregivers, and at times even the care-receivers, more present and thereby fully human. If the ancient Chinese perception is right that we are not born fully human, but only become so as we cultivate ourselves and our relations with others—and that we must do so in a threatening world where things often go terribly wrong and where what we are able to control is very limited—then caregiving is one of those relationships and practices of self-cultivation that make us, even as we experience our limits and failures, more human. It completes (not absolutely, but as a kind of burnishing of what we really are—warts and all) our humanity. And if that Chinese perspective is also right (as I believe it is), when it claims that by building our humanity, we humanise the world, then our own ethical cultivation at the very least fosters that of others and holds the potential, through those relationships, of deepening meaning, beauty, and goodness in our experience of the world.

I am not a naive moralist. I've had far too much experience of the demands, tensions, and downright failures of caregiving to fall into sentimentality and utopianism. Caregiving is not easy. It consumes time, energy, and financial resources.

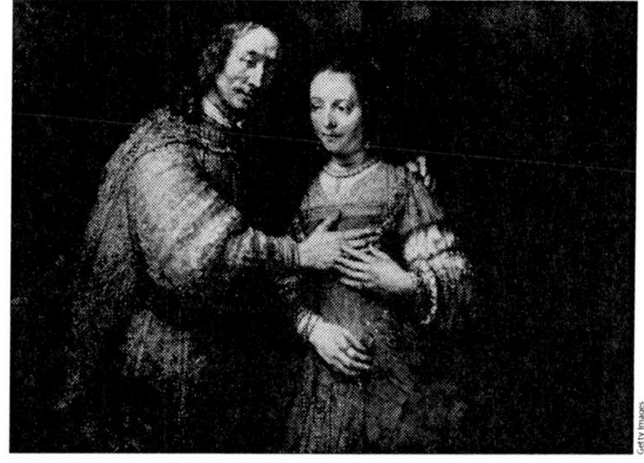

Getty Images

Rembrandt Harmensz van Rijn, *The Jewish Bride* (1667)

It sucks out strength and determination. It turns simple ideas of efficacy and hope into big question marks. It can amplify anguish and desperation. It can divide the self. It can bring out family conflicts. It can separate out those who care from those who can't or won't handle it. It is very difficult. It is also far more complex, uncertain, and unbounded than professional medical and nursing models suggest. I know about the moral core of caregiving not nearly so much from my professional life as a psychiatrist and medical anthropologist, nor principally from the research literature and my own studies, but primarily because of my new life of practice as the primary caregiver for Joan Kleinman.

I learned to be a caregiver by doing it, because I had to do it; it was there to do. I think this is how most people learn to be caregivers, for people who are elderly, disabled, or chronically or terminally ill. But of course this is also how parents, especially mothers, learn to care for children. My point is not so dissimilar to what William James claimed was how we learn to feel emotions: we move, we respond, we act. Our muscles (voluntary and involuntary) move. And so out of practices comes affect. And out of practices comes caregiving. We are caregivers because we practise caregiving. It is all the little concrete things I described in caring for my wife that taken together and over time constitute my caregiving, that make me a caregiver. So much depends on those concrete things: the doing, the feeling, the shadings, the symphonic complexity, the inadequacy, the living at every moment and over what can be such a long journey of the incompleteness yet the presence of a caregiver.

Arthur Kleinman
Harvard Medical School, Cambridge, MA 02138, USA
kleinman@wjh.harvard.edu

Further reading

Abel EK. Hearts of Wisdom: American Women Caring for Kin 1850–1940. Cambridge, MA: Harvard University Press, 2000.

Alterra A. The Caregiver: A Life with Alzheimer's. Foreword by Arthur Kleinman. Ithica and London: ILR Press/Cornell University Press, 2007.

Kleinman A. What Really Matters: Living a Moral Life Amidst Uncertainty and Danger. New York: Oxford University Press, 2006.

Reiff D. Swimming in a Sea of Death: A Son's Memoir. New York: Simon and Schuster, 2008.

Tronto JC. Moral Boundaries: A Political Argument for an Ethic of Care. New York and London: Routledge, Chapman and Hall, 1993.

Appendix G

Caregiving Stories

The caregiving experience is highly individual and dependent on personal and family circumstances. These vignettes and personal stories describe the experiences of real individuals caring for an older adult.

WHEN AN OLDER ADULT HAS DEMENTIA

One Daughter's Experience[1]

Before Mom moved in . . .

"We are busy with Social Security, Medicare, lawyer, bank, apartment prep. From what I've heard, Mom is doing pretty well. Her down times seem to come and go, but the delusions don't seem to be quite as dark. When speaking to her on the phone she seems genuinely happy about moving to New York and living with us."

After Mom moved in . . .

"It's been stressful for quite a while. I cared for dad, my 2 uncles, and my husband. My husband is helping me so much now by being a great

[1] As the committee began its work, Ruthie R. offered to share her emails to her cousin (a committee member) documenting her ongoing journey of caring for her mother after she had been diagnosed with dementia. The following are excerpts covering a more than 4-year period between April 2009 and January 2015.

shopper and chef. Mom has gained about 11 pounds since coming here. Much of what I'm feeling is the slow release of years of stress. Writing down my thoughts is new to me."

After a hip fracture . . .

"I am so angry that my head might explode. At about 5:30, I was handed a bunch of papers by the head of the rehab department at the hospital where my mom has started physical therapy. We all thought this was a great idea. But apparently her Medigap policy denied this coverage. I have requested a 'fast track' appeal. She has already started the rehab work 2x a day. I hope they keep going with the treatment while this nightmare unfolds. I hate this."

While she was still at the rehab center . . .

"Mom did well in physical therapy, on her second day. She walked up and down the hall with a walker, according to her roommate, a former home health aide herself. I have one question. She keeps getting up out of bed, even though her bed and wheelchair are alarmed. The alarms don't phase her. It doesn't seem to stick when she is told to stay in bed, or not to stand up. . . . The staff come in to help, but a momentary delay could produce another fall (god forbid) . . . thank goodness for her roommate who is incredibly patient. Are there other devices/methods? Suggestions? I'm wondering what can be done at home too . . ."

After she returned home . . .

"Generally, things are good. There's an element of unknown that we deal with all the time. Schedules mean nothing unless there's an appointment, etc. I know I'm supposed to have a 'regular' schedule of things to do, but her energy changes from day to day—moment to moment. I'm rolling with it, and trying not to overthink and let her direct whenever possible."

After 1 year at home . . .

"I've lost my career. I've got permanent WIWAS (Will I ever Work Again Syndrome). It really has me down today. Sure, I think about working. I have help a few hours a day, I should be able to do something. But thinking about being among (young) people, wondering if I still have the skills, worrying why anyone would want to hire me, I break out in hives. I'm a pretty good caregiver, bobbing and weaving my way through bureaucracies, tracking down answers to questions with dogged determination, tackling confusing paperwork, keeping it all straight, trying to get what I can for my mom, with appointments, keeping her happy, well-fed, and somewhat on track, I haven't been polishing my skills, resume or portfolio. I should feel good about caregiving and the work of getting to this point with her. Just 2 years ago we were in a desperate place."

After 4 years . . .

"Things are at a slightly different stage. Mom has slowed down, with a little more confusion at times, more sleepiness, less balance, more use of the walker especially outside. She is still very sweet and has a smile and a nice word for everyone. Thank goodness for the St. Charles Senior Center, where they talk about how remarkable Sylvia is, and how they all love her. Rarely is she agitated, but it happens."

A Husband and Father with the Challenging Behavioral Symptoms of Dementia[2]

"Gabriela and Saúl have five daughters, all of whom lived in the same city as their parents. While all of the daughters participated in caring for their parents, they assumed different tasks: one daughter handled her father's medical appointments and other professional care; one oversaw finances and bill paying; and the other three took care of groceries, meals, household repairs, entertainment, and social outings. Every week, one daughter, Yolanda, spent one of her days off from work with her mother, taking stock and planning for the forthcoming week.

Sometime after his physician diagnosed him with Alzheimer's disease, Saúl began to exhibit aggressive behavior. He was put on psychotropic medications that helped some but tended to make him tired. Two of Saúl's behaviors were especially distressing to Gabriela. One was his lack of hygiene and resistance to bathing or wearing clean clothes. He insisted on wearing dirty pajamas to adult daycare. The second difficult behavior was his obsession with paper. Wherever Saúl went, he collected old newspapers, free brochures, and pamphlets, grabbing handfuls that he stored at home on shelves and in filing cabinets and dresser drawers. Gabriela could no longer put away clothes or other items. On garbage pick-up days, Saúl scrambled through bins to retrieve any papers that she had thrown away. Gabriela tried continually to bathe him or help him into a clean shirt.

---

[2] Apesoa-Varano, C., J. C. Barker, and L. Hinton. 2012. Mexican-American families and dementia: An exploration of "work" in response to dementia-related aggressive behavior. In *Aging, health, and longevity in the Mexican-Origin population*, edited by J. L. Angel, F. Torres-Gil, and K. Markides. New York: Springer. Pp. 277-291.

On these occasions, Saúl would yell 'strong words' at her or get angry. Gabriela surreptitiously threw things away, placing them in big plastic bags in the garage for her daughters to remove when they visited. Saúl's hoarding behavior triggered his first incident of violence. One day while he was at adult daycare, an office attendant tried to stop him from taking office records and documents. Saúl grabbed her by the throat and tried to strangle her. On another occasion, Gabriela was struggling with Saúl over a broom that she had been using when he grabbed it in a threatening manner and yelled at her. Very frightened, she locked herself in her room and called her daughters.

Gabriela was continually worried and stressed. Yolanda often gently reminded Gabriela that they had learned that aggressive behavior was an aspect of Alzheimer's disease and that it would get worse. She urged her mother to be patient and to not take Saúl's behavior personally. Yolanda would patiently explain to her mother that 'He knows that he doesn't want something to happen but he no longer has the ability to articulate that he doesn't want something taken away from him, so he resorts to showing it by getting angry.' While agreeing, Gabriela would nevertheless say, 'it's that I just can't get it into my head that he's not the same man. I just can't!' Gabriela delegated the management of Saúl's behavior at daycare or outside the house to her daughters. 'I am getting old,' she said, 'so don't let me know what goes on there at [the daycare center] because it could give me a heart attack.' Gabriela feared not only for her own safety but also that the daycare center would no longer accept Saúl. She also worried that her difficulties managing Saúl's behavior would make her appear unfit to care for him and lead to his institutionalization."

A WIFE HELPS MANAGE HER HUSBAND'S CANCER TREATMENT[3]

"Marjorie was a caregiver for her husband Ralph during his treatment for cancer. Marjorie and Ralph are a couple in their late 60s who live in a rural area 60 miles from any cancer specialist and hundreds of miles from a cancer center. Marjorie's caregiving experience was characterized by intense involvement during periods of active treatment punctuated by interludes when Ralph was feeling well and life returned to some semblance of normal. The intensive periods of caregiving involved assisting with self-care, providing emotional support, performing medical and nursing tasks, frequently driving long distances, identifying and coordinating home

[3] Schumacher, K., M. Z. Cohen, B. S. Fletcher, and W. M. Lydiatt. 2010. *Family caregiving in the car and away from home*. Paper presented at Council for the Advancement of Nursing Science State of the Science Congress on Nursing Research, Washington, DC.

care services and other community resources, navigating local and distant healthcare systems, working out financial arrangements for cancer treatment, and applying for Medicaid. Marjorie served as the eyes and ears of health professionals when acute changes in Ralph's condition occurred at home. She monitored Ralph's condition, communicated her observations to doctors and nurses by phone, and took Ralph to an emergency room when necessary. Even during the interludes of more normal life, Marjorie remained vigilant about Ralph's health and well-being.

When Ralph was initially diagnosed with cancer, he was treated with surgery followed by radiation and chemotherapy. He was found to have diabetes during his hospitalization for surgery. He was discharged from the hospital late in the day, so the first time Marjorie tested his blood sugar and administered insulin without a nurse present in the car; it was dark during the 6-hour drive home. At home, Marjorie monitored the surgical incision and when she noticed drainage, she reported it to Ralph's physicians. She coordinated the treatment plan for the draining incision with physicians near home and the oncologic surgeon in the cancer center 6 hours away, and carried out their instructions at home. After the incision healed, Ralph received his radiation and chemotherapy treatments closer to home. However, the closest radiation treatment facility was still too far away to drive daily, so Ralph and Marjorie stayed in a motel 5 days a week, returning home on the weekends. Marjorie did the driving, played a key role in managing the radiation and chemotherapy side effects, tried to make sure Ralph got good nutrition in their temporary living quarters (taking into account that he had diabetes as well as cancer), and tried to think of ways to keep their spirits up while away from their family and friends. Constant vigilance was required, as Ralph suffered from severe nausea and vomiting and had an episode of delirium as a side effect from one of his medications.

Following the radiation and chemotherapy treatments, Ralph and Marjorie enjoyed an interlude of nearly normal activities at home for a while. However, the cancer recurred a year later. After considering all the alternatives, Ralph chose to have additional surgery, followed by more radiation and chemotherapy. The specialized treatment and follow-up meant traveling to the distant cancer center. Once again, Marjorie and Ralph lived in a motel room. More caregiving was required this time, including managing tube feedings, oxygen equipment, oral suctioning, and a regimen of 10 new medications, in addition to constant vigilance, symptom and side effect management, and emotional support. Marjorie provided a level of family caregiving that makes modern cancer treatment possible for rural-dwelling individuals."

TWO STORIES OF JOB DISCRIMINATION[4]

"One caller to WorkLife Law's employee hotline took intermittent Family and Medical Leave Act leave to care for his wife. After he informed his employer that his wife would be going on long-term disability, his new supervisor told him that he must be in the office from 8 a.m. to 5 p.m. and that he could no longer flex his hours, telecommute, or work from home—despite the fact that the employer permitted and even encouraged all similarly situated employees to do so. The caller had been telecommuting, working from home, and flexing his hours for well over a decade with no detriment to his performance."

"The largest individual jury verdict in an FRD [Family Responsibilities Discrimination] case to date ($11.65 million) involved a hospital maintenance worker, Chris Schultz, who was fired in 2002 while caring for his father with Alzheimer's disease and mother with congestive heart problems and severe diabetes. To help manage his parents' care, he asked to take intermittent leave, to which he was entitled under the federal Family and Medical Leave Act (FMLA). While he was on leave to care for his parents, his supervisor suddenly instituted a new quota system that was impossible for Schultz to meet. As a result, Schultz was fired for poor performance after 26 years as a dedicated employee with a record of excellent evaluations—the year before he began taking leave, his picture hung in the lobby as the hospital's outstanding worker of 1999."

---

[4] Williams, J. C., R. Devaux, P. Petrac, and L. Feinberg. 2012. *Protecting family caregivers from employment discrimination*. Washington, DC: AARP Public Policy Institute. http://www.aarp.org/home-family/caregiving/info-08-2012/insight-protecting-family-caregivers-from-employment-discrimination-AARP-ppi-health.html (accessed August 23, 2016).

Appendix H

HIPAA and Caregivers' Access to Information

The Health Insurance Portability and Accountability Act of 1996 (HIPAA) mandated the creation of privacy standards for personally identifiable health information. The set of privacy regulations promulgated under HIPAA, known as the Privacy Rule (45 CFR Part 164), defines the types of uses and disclosures of an individual's health information that are permitted by health care providers and health plans. In other words, it determines who can look at and receive an individual's health information, including family members and friends of the person. The regulations include limits on who can get one's information, mechanisms for correcting information in an individual's record, and a requirement to disclose who has seen it. The regulations are enforced by the U.S. Department of Health and Human Services (HHS) Office of Civil Rights. Health care providers and plans covered under the rule are referred to as "covered entities." The discussion below addresses only adults, not minors, in accordance with the committee's charge and focus on adults age 65 and older.

The Privacy Rule, along with two related HHS rules addressing security and breach notification, seek to protect the privacy and security of persons seeking or receiving health care. The HIPAA penalties primarily target failures to preserve privacy and security, not failures to disclose information. There are only two mandatory disclosures under the Privacy Rule: disclosure to the individual (and certain representatives authorized by the individual) and disclosure to the Secretary of HHS for purposes of investigating compliance.[1] All other disclosures under the Act are permissive and guided by a principle of minimum necessary disclosure.[2] Health care providers exercise considerable discretion, and providers tend to be very cautious about disclosure. The Privacy Rule makes no mention of caregivers in its provisions. Instead, it provides someone serving as caregiver with three possible avenues of access to a care recipient's protected health information.

PERSONAL REPRESENTATIVES

A caregiver who is the individual's "personal representative" has the authority, under applicable law, to act on behalf of an individual in making decisions related to health care and has the same rights of access.[3] The rule defers to state law to determine who has authority to act on behalf of the individual with respect to health care decisions. There are three primary ways that state law confers authority on another to make health care decisions on behalf of an individual:

1. **Through health care advance directives,** specifically health care powers of attorney. Anyone appointed health care agent or proxy under such a document should have all the rights to access and control of information that the individual has. However, this authority commences only when the advance directive appointing the agent becomes effective. In some states, the appointment of a health care agent can be immediately effective, but in most states the appointment becomes effective only at the point the person loses capacity to make health care decisions. Because many people may need and want their health care proxy to have access to their health infor-

[1] 45 CFR § 164.502. "Covered entities: Required disclosures. A covered entity is required to disclose protected health information: (i) To an individual, when requested under, and required by § 164.524 or § 164.528; and (ii) When required by the Secretary under subpart C of part 160 of this subchapter to investigate or determine the covered entity's compliance with this subchapter."

[2] 45 CFR § 164.502. "When using or disclosing protected health information or when requesting protected health information from another covered entity or business associate, a covered entity or business associate must make reasonable efforts to limit protected health information to the minimum necessary to accomplish the intended purpose of the use, disclosure, or request."

[3] 45 CFR § 164.502(g). A covered entity must "treat a personal representative as the individual for purposes of this subchapter. . . . If under applicable law a person has authority to act on behalf of an individual who is an adult or an emancipated minor in making decisions related to health care, a covered entity must treat such person as a personal representative under this subchapter, with respect to protected health information relevant to such personal representation." An exception to this rule is provided in cases of suspected abuse, neglect, or endangerment by the personal representative.

mation prior to the point of their losing capacity to make health care decisions, their expectations and the expectations of their appointed proxy may be frustrated.

2. **Through default surrogate decision-making laws (or case law).** Most, but not all, states specify a hierarchy of next of kin who have authority to make health care decisions when no one has been formally appointed. Default surrogates also have all the rights to access and control of information that the individual has. However, it may not always be clear who the default surrogate is, especially where information about the family is limited or there is more than one possible surrogate at the same level of the hierarchy (e.g., multiple adult children). Moreover, some states have no specified hierarchy (e.g., California, Colorado, Hawaii) and depend on identifying the surrogate by consensus. As with health care powers of attorney, the authority of a default surrogate commences only when the individual has lost capacity to make health care decisions.
3. **Through guardianship law.** Judicial proceedings to appoint a guardian are usually a measure of last resort for individuals who have lost capacity to manage their affairs. Courts normally prefer to appoint a close family member as guardian. But, the guardian has only as much or as little authority as the guardianship order specifies.[4]

Failure of the provider or health plan to disclose information to one's known and presently authorized personal representative is a violation of the HIPAA Privacy Rule, unless the covered entity has a reasonable belief that either: (1) the individual has been or may be subjected to domestic violence, abuse, or neglect by such person; or (2) treating such person as the personal representative could endanger the individual; and the covered entity, in the exercise of professional judgment, decides that it is not in the best interest of the individual to treat the person as the individual's personal representative.[5]

HIPAA AUTHORIZATIONS AND DIRECTED RIGHT TO ACCESS

The second avenue of access is for anyone to whom the individual has given a valid HIPAA authorization or a directed right to access. A HIPAA authorization is a document normally provided by one's health care provider, signed by the individual, that identifies the scope of information that

[4] For deceased individuals, a person appointed executor or administrator of the individual's estate also bears the status of personal representative.

[5] 45 CFR § 164.502.

may be disclosed, to whom, and for what purposes, and it meets other specifications under the Privacy Rule. A family caregiver bearing a HIPAA authorization does not stand in the shoes of the individual, as does a personal representative, for the Privacy Rule is permissive and the principle of minimum necessary disclosure applies. Thus, a caregiver relying on a HIPAA authorization may still encounter barriers to access.

A directed right to access is an authorization by the individual to another person to give the person a right of access to one's personal health information. If given to another, the right of access is mandatory. Health care providers must disclose unless an exception applies. Exceptions are limited to personal notes of mental health care professionals, maintained separately from medical records, and information in connection with a civil, criminal, or administrative action/proceeding. The right to access must be in writing, but its required elements are very simple. It must be signed by the individual, and clearly identify the designated person and where to the send the personal health information (Samuels, 2016).

FAMILY AND FRIENDS

The third avenue of access is for other family and friends who are not formally appointed personal representatives or designated persons under a written authorization, but who are involved in the person's health care or payment for health care in some way. Under this part of the rule, one's health care provider may share relevant information about the individual if

1. the individual (who is the subject of the confidential information) gives the provider permission to share the information (a person can also prohibit sharing with specified individuals);
2. the individual is present and does not object to sharing the information with the other person; or
3. the individual is not present, and the provider determines, based on professional judgment, that it is in the individual's best interest to share information with the other person.

How much information is shared is also a matter of professional judgment, based on the circumstances, but is to be limited to just the information that the person involved needs to know about the person's care or payment. When someone other than a friend or family member is involved, the health care provider must be reasonably sure that the person asked that individual to be involved in his or her care or payment for care.[6]

[6] 45 CFR § 164.510.

The HHS Office for Civil Rights provides the following examples of the third circumstance:

- An emergency room doctor may discuss a person's treatment in front of the person's friend if the person asks that her friend come into the treatment room.
- A doctor's office may discuss a person's bill with the individual's adult daughter who is with her father at his medical appointment and has questions about the charges.
- A doctor may discuss the medications a person needs to take with the person's health aide who has accompanied the person to a medical appointment.
- A doctor may give information about a person's mobility limitations to the person's sister who is driving the individual home from the hospital.
- A nurse may discuss a person's health status with the person's brother if she informs him that she is going to do so and the person does not object, but a nurse may not discuss a person's condition with the person's brother after the person has stated she does not want her family to know about her condition.

When a language interpreter is needed, information can generally be disclosed to the interpreter according to regulatory guidance (HHS, 2008a,b).

Under the Family and Friends Rule, health care providers exercise substantial discretion in determining what, if any, health information can be shared. This discretion can impede caregivers' access to needed information. Variability in disclosure can depend on the health care provider's professional knowledge, familiarity with the family, personal attitudes, perceptions, and biases.

Caregiver problems in gaining access to needed health information appear to be fairly common based on anecdotes, but reliable data on the frequency and nature of problems are non-existent. The HHS Office for Civil Rights reported that its enforcement database tracks only breaches of privacy and security, not failures to disclose information.[7] Because most failures to disclose information are permissive exercises of discretion, they are not violations of the Privacy Rule.

The Veterans Health Administration (VHA) also complies with HIPAA regulations, as well as other federal laws, and has guidelines for veterans' facilities that are parallel to those of the HHS Office for Civil Rights (VHA,

[7] Committee Briefing, M. Gordon-Nguyen, and C. Heide, HHS Office of Civil Rights, April 28, 2015.

2006). However, in a Privacy Fact Sheet, VHA does address caregivers and how to identify them, although one purpose of the guidance is to identify caregivers who may be eligible to participate in support and educational groups or other VA family support services (VHA Information Access and Privacy Office, 2009).

In summary, caregivers have no special status under the HIPAA Privacy Rule, although their role as caregiver is relevant to providers' exercise of professional judgment over disclosure. Fulfilling the role of caregiver sometimes requires ready access to much if not all of the person's health information. The HHS Office for Civil Rights could facilitate caregivers' access to information if it were to provide administrative guidance to covered entities about the importance of the role of family caregivers and their need for complete and timely access to protected health information. This would encourage providers to exercise their professional judgment in permitting access to information for caregivers, consistent with the best interests of the care recipient. Such guidance under the Privacy Rule would help to establish caregivers as recognized members of the care team.

Training offered in both the public and private sectors on the requirements of the HIPAA Privacy Rule could likewise address the essential role in care delivery and support played by family caregivers, and include guidance on identifying caregivers and sharing information with caregivers more inclusively, consistent with the best interests of the care recipient.

In providing explicit recognition of caregivers, the HHS Office for Civil Rights could note that caregivers are already recognized in other federal laws for various purposes, for example:

- for assistance and support services for caregivers from the U.S. Department of Veterans Affairs [38 USC § 1720G];
- under Social Services Block Grants to States [42 USC § 1397j];
- under the National Family Caregiver Support Program pursuant to the Older Americans Act [42 USC § 3030s-1]; and
- under the Public Health Service's Lifespan Respite Program for caregivers [42 USC § 300ii].

REFERENCES

HHS (U.S. Department of Health and Human Services). 2008a. *Health information privacy FAQs number 530.* http://www.hhs.gov/hipaa/for-professionals/faq/530/when-does-hipaa-allow-a-health-care-provider-to-dicuss-information-with-family/index.html (accessed June 23, 2016).

HHS. 2008b. *Health information privacy FAQs number 536.* http://www.hhs.gov/hipaa/for-professionals/faq/536/may-a-health-care-provider-share-information-with-an-interpreter/index.html (accessed June 23, 2016).

Samuels, J. 2016. *Understanding individuals' right under HIPAA to access their health information.* http://www.hhs.gov/blog/2016/01/07/understanding-individuals-right-under-hipaa-access-their.html (accessed June 23, 2016).

VHA (Veterans Health Administration). 2006. *Handbook 1605.1, Privacy and release of information.* Washington, DC: U.S. Department of Veterans Affairs.

VHA Information Access and Privacy Office. 2009. *Privacy fact sheet: Sharing information with caregivers.* Vol. 09, No. 7. Washington, DC: U.S. Department of Veterans Affairs.